The Exotic Animal Respiratory System

Guest Editors

SUSAN E. OROSZ, PhD, DVM, Dipl. ABVP–Avian,
Dipl. ECZM–Avian
CATHY A. JOHNSON-DELANEY, DVM, Dipl.
ABVP–Avian and Exotic Companion Mammal

VETERINARY CLINICS OF NORTH AMERICA: EXOTIC ANIMAL PRACTICE

www.vetexotic.theclinics.com

Consulting Editor
AGNES E. RUPLEY, DVM, Dipl. ABVP–Avian

May 2011 • Volume 14 • Number 2

SAUNDERS an imprint of ELSEVIER, Inc.

W.B. SAUNDERS COMPANY

A Division of Elsevier Inc.

1600 John F. Kennedy Boulevard ● Suite 1800 ● Philadelphia, Pennsylvania 19103-2899

http://www.vetexotic.theclinics.com

**VETERINARY CLINICS OF NORTH AMERICA: EXOTIC ANIMAL PRACTICE Volume 14, Number 2
May 2011 ISSN 1094-9194, ISBN-13: 978-1-4557-0521-4**

Editor: John Vassallo; j.vassallo@elsevier.com

Veterinary Clinics of North America: Exotic Animal Practice (ISSN 1094-9194) is published in January, May, and September by Elsevier, Inc., 360 Park Avenue South, New York, NY 10010-1710. Subscription prices are $212.00 per year for US individuals, $345.00 per year for US institutions, $108.00 per year for US students and residents, $253.00 per year for Canadian individuals, $407.00 per year for Canadian institutions, $285.00 per year for international individuals, $407.00 per year for international institutions and $139.00 per year for Canadian and foreign students/residents. To receive student/resident rate, orders must be accompanied by name of affiliated institution, date of term, and the *signature* of program/residency coordinator on institution letterhead. Orders will be billed at individual rate until proof of status is received. Foreign air speed delivery is included in all *Clinics* subscription prices. All prices are subject to change without notice. **POSTMASTER:** Send address changes to *Veterinary Clinics of North America: Exotic Animal Practice*, Elsevier Health Sciences Division, Subscription Customer Service, 3251 Riverport Lane, Maryland Heights, MO 63043. **Customer Service: Telephone: 1-800-654-2452** (U.S. and Canada); **1-314-447-8871** (outside U.S. and Canada). **Fax: 1-314-447-8029. E-mail: journalscustomerservice-usa@elsevier.com** (for print support); **journalsonlinesupport-usa@elsevier.com** (for online support).

Reprints. For copies of 100 or more of articles in this publication, please contact the Commercial Reprints Department, Elsevier Inc., 360 Park Avenue South, New York, New York 10010-1710. Tel.: (212)-633-3813; Fax: (212)-633-1935; E-mail: reprints@elsevier.com.

Veterinary Clinics of North America: Exotic Animal Practice is covered in *MEDLINE/PubMed (Index Medicus)*.

Printed and bound by CPI Group (UK) Ltd, Croydon, CR0 4YY
Transferred to Digital Print 2011

Contributors

CONSULTING EDITOR

AGNES E. RUPLEY, DVM
Diplomate, American Board of Veterinary Practitioners-Avian Practice; Director and
Chief Veterinarian, All Pets Medical & Laser Surgical Center, College Station, Texas

GUEST EDITORS

SUSAN E. OROSZ, PhD, DVM
Diplomate, American Board of Veterinary Practitioners-Avian Practice; Diplomate,
European College of Zoological Medicine-Avian; Owner, Bird and Exotic Pet Wellness
Center, Toledo, Ohio

CATHY A. JOHNSON-DELANEY, DVM
Diplomate, American Board of Veterinary Practitioners-Avian Practice; Diplomate,
American Board of Veterinary Practitioners-Exotic Companion Mammal Practice;
Eastside Avian and Exotic Animal Medical Center, Kirkland, Washington

AUTHORS

TRACY BENNETT, DVM
Diplomate, American Board of Veterinary Practitioners-Avian Practice; Bird and Exotic
Clinic of Seattle, Seattle, Washington

VITTORIO CAPELLO, DVM
Diplomate, European College of Zoological Medicine-Small Mammal; Diplomate,
American Board of Veterinary Practitioners-Exotic Companion Mammal Practice; Clinica
Veterinaria S. Siro; Clinica Veterinaria Gran Sasso, Milan, Italy

DAN H. JOHNSON, DVM
Diplomate, American Board of Veterinary Practitioners-Exotic Companion Mammal
Practice; Owner, Avian and Exotic Animal Care, Raleigh, North Carolina

CATHY A. JOHNSON-DELANEY, DVM
Diplomate, American Board of Veterinary Practitioners-Avian Practice; Diplomate,
American Board of Veterinary Practitioners-Exotic Companion Mammal Practice;
Eastside Avian and Exotic Animal Medical Center, Kirkland, Washington

MELISSA A. KLING, DVM
Director, Laboratory Animal Resources, Mercer University Medical School, Division
of Basic Medicine; Executive Director, Association of Exotic Mammal Veterinarians,
Macon, Georgia

ANGELA M. LENNOX, DVM
Diplomate, American Board of Veterinary Practitioners-Avian Practice; Avian and Exotic
Animal Clinic, Indianapolis, Indiana

MARLA LICHTENBERGER, DVM
Diplomate, American College of Veterinary Emergency and Critical Care; Owner, Milwaukee Emergency Medicine Center for Animals, Greenfield, Wisconsin

SUSAN E. OROSZ, PhD, DVM
Diplomate, American Board of Veterinary Practitioners-Avian Practice; Diplomate, European College of Zoological Medicine-Avian; Owner, Bird and Exotic Pet Wellness Center, Toledo, Ohio

HELEN E. ROBERTS, DVM
Aquatic Veterinary Services of WNY, 5 Corners Animal Hospital, Orchard Park, New York

JUERGEN SCHUMACHER, Dr. Med.Vet
Diplomate, American College of Zoological Medicine; Diplomate, European College of Zoological Medicine Herpetology; Professor and Director, Avian and Zoologic Medicine Service, Department of Small Animal Clinical Sciences, College of Veterinary Medicine, The University of Tennessee, Knoxville, Tennessee

STEPHEN A. SMITH, DVM, PhD
Professor of Aquatic Medicine/Fish Health, Department of Biomedical Sciences and Pathobiology, Virginia-Maryland Regional College of Veterinary Medicine, Virginia Tech, Blacksburg, Virginia

ENRIQUE YARTO-JARAMILLO, DVM, MSc
Private Practice, Centro Veterinario; Professor of Wild Animal and Exotic Pet Medicine, Department of Ethology, Wildlife and Laboratory Animals, School of Veterinary Medicine, National Autonomus University of Mexico, Mexico, DF, Mexico

Contents

Preface: The Exotic Animal Respiratory System ix

Susan E. Orosz and Cathy A. Johnson-Delaney

Disorders of the Respiratory System in Pet and Ornamental Fish 179

Helen E. Roberts and Stephen A. Smith

The respiratory organ of fish is the gill. In addition to respiration, the gills also perform functions of acid-base regulation, osmoregulation, and excretion of nitrogenous compounds. Because of their intimate association with the environment, the gills are often the primary target organ of pollutants, poor water quality, infectious disease agents, and noninfectious problems, making examination of the gills essential to the complete examination of sick individual fish and fish populations. The degree of response of the gill tissue depends on type, severity, and degree of injury and functional changes will precede morphologic changes. Antemortem tests and water quality testing can, and should, be performed on clinically affected fish whenever possible.

Respiratory Medicine of Reptiles 207

Juergen Schumacher

Noninfectious and infectious causes have been implicated in the development of respiratory tract disease in reptiles. Treatment modalities in reptiles have to account for species differences in response to therapeutic agents as well as interpretation of diagnostic findings. Data on effective drugs and dosages for the treatment of respiratory diseases are often lacking in reptiles. Recently, advances have been made on the application of advanced imaging modalities, especially computed tomography for the diagnosis and treatment monitoring of reptiles. This article describes common infectious and noninfectious causes of respiratory disease in reptiles, including diagnostic and therapeutic regimen.

The Chelonian Respiratory System 225

Tracy Bennett

This article reviews anatomy, physiology, diagnostic techniques, and specific disease syndromes of the chelonian respiratory system. Respiratory disease is common in chelonians and is a cause of significant morbidity and mortality in these animals. Mycoplasma, herpesvirus, and iridovirus are reviewed in depth.

Avian Respiratory Distress: Etiology, Diagnosis, and Treatment 241

Susan E. Orosz and Marla Lichtenberger

Respiratory distress is usually a life-threatening emergency in any species and this is particularly important in avian species because of their unique anatomy and physiology. In the emergency room, observation of breathing patterns, respiratory sounds, and a brief physical examination are the most important tools for the diagnosis and treatment of respiratory distress in avian patients. These tools will help the clinician localize the lesion. This discussion focuses on the 5 anatomic divisions of the respiratory system and provides clinically important anatomic and physiologic principles and diagnosis and treatment protocols for the common diseases occurring in each part.

Rabbit Respiratory System: Clinical Anatomy, Physiology and Disease   257

Cathy A. Johnson-Delaney and Susan E. Orosz

Rabbits are obligate nose breathers due to their epiglottis positioned rostrally to the soft palate. Any obstruction within the nasal cavity will produce a respiratory wheeze with increased respiratory effort. Respiratory diseases are a major cause of morbidity and mortality in rabbits. This article focuses on these diseases and their causative pathogens.

Hedgehogs and Sugar Gliders: Respiratory Anatomy, Physiology, and Disease   267

Dan H. Johnson

This article discusses the respiratory anatomy, physiology, and disease of African pygmy hedgehogs (*Atelerix albiventris*) and sugar gliders (*Petaurus breviceps*), two species commonly seen in exotic animal practice. Where appropriate, information from closely related species is mentioned because cross-susceptibility is likely and because these additional species may also be encountered in practice. Other body systems and processes are discussed insofar as they relate to, or affect, respiratory function. Although some topics, such as special senses, hibernation, or vocalization, may seem out of place, in each case the information relates back to respiration in some important way.

A Review of Respiratory System Anatomy, Physiology, and Disease in the Mouse, Rat, Hamster, and Gerbil   287

Melissa A. Kling

The purpose of this article is to provide for practitioners a comprehensive overview of respiratory diseases, both infectious and noninfectious, in the mouse, rat, hamster, and gerbil. The information presented will also be useful for veterinarians pursuing board certification. Anatomy and physiology are briefly addressed, as those two facets alone could encompass an entire article for these species.

Respiratory System Anatomy, Physiology, and Disease: Guinea Pigs and Chinchillas   339

Enrique Yarto-Jaramillo

Respiratory diseases are common in guinea pigs and chinchillas. There are multifactorial causes of respiratory involvement in these species of rodents, from infectious (bacterial, viral, and fungal) to neoplastic causes. Toxicoses and diseases affecting other systems may also induce respiratory signs. Knowledge of biology, including husbandry, nutritional requirements, and behavior, are important clues for the clinician to determine the role these issues may play in the development, progression, and prognosis of respiratory clinical cases in rodents. Current approaches in the diagnosis and therapy for respiratory disease in small mammals warrant more research concerning response-to-treatment reports.

Ferret Respiratory System: Clinical Anatomy, Physiology, and Disease   357

Cathy A. Johnson-Delaney and Susan E. Orosz

The upper and lower respiratory tracts of ferrets have several similarities to humans, and therefore have been used as a research model for respiratory function. This article describes the clinical anatomy and physiology, and common respiratory diseases of the ferret.

Diagnostic Imaging of the Respiratory System in Exotic Companion Mammals   369

Vittorio Capello and Angela M. Lennox

The level of care for smaller companion mammals has increased significantly during the past few years. Today, exotic companion mammals are acknowledged as a specific area of zoologic medicine. Owner demands for a higher level of care is increasing dramatically. Because most of these patients are small (less than 2 kg), this represents a great challenge, in particular for the field of diagnostic imaging. This article reviews the 5 main diagnostic imaging modalities currently available for investigation of the respiratory system of exotic companion mammals: radiography, ultrasonography, endoscopy, computed tomography, and magnetic resonance.

Index   391

FORTHCOMING ISSUES

September 2011
Zoonoses, Public Health and the Exotic Animal Practitioner
Marcy J. Souza, DVM, MPH, DABVP-Avian, *Guest Editor*

January 2012
Mycobacteriosis
Miguel D. Saggese, DVM, PhD, *Guest Editor*

May 2012
Pediatrics
Kristine Kuchinski, DVM, PhD, *Guest Editor*

RECENT ISSUES

January 2011
Analgesia and Pain Management
Joanne Paul-Murphy, DVM, Dipl. ACZM, *Guest Editor*

September 2010
Advances and Updates in Internal Medicine
Kemba Marshall, DVM, DABVP–Avian, *Guest Editor*

May 2010
Endoscopy and Endosurgery
Stephen J. Divers, BVetMed, DZooMed, DACZM, DipECZM(herp), FRCVS, *Guest Editor*

RELATED INTEREST

Veterinary Clinics of North America: Small Animal Practice (Volume 40, Issue 6, November 2010)
Current Topics in Canine and Feline Infectious Diseases
Stephen C. Barr, BVSc, MVS, PhD, *Guest Editor*

THE CLINICS ARE NOW AVAILABLE ONLINE!

Access your subscription at:
www.theclinics.com

Preface

The Exotic Animal Respiratory System

Our goal with this issue was to provide the veterinary readership timely information concerning the respiratory system of a diverse group of exotic animals. It has been 11 years since *Veterinary Clinics of North America: Exotic Animal Practice* has addressed respiratory medicine of exotics. Any clinician knows that respiratory diseases are behind many common presenting problems.

The anatomy and physiology of the respiratory tree have been included in many of the articles to provide the underpinning of knowledge to better diagnose and treat respiratory diseases in exotics. We have included anatomical drawings and figures as well. The information presented should provide a basis of understanding for the new-to-the-field clinician and additional new information to those that have been practicing in the field for a while. We also want to encourage those that are new to refer to those with experience as all animals, including exotics, deserve quality care. We are entering a new era where we have a number of board certifications in various disciplines in exotics. We have drawn on some of those diplomates as authors and others that have long-term experience in their respective areas. We hope that this issue devoted to the respiratory system of exotic animals in health and those patients with disease will provide veterinarians timely and important information to enhance their diagnostic and therapeutic success.

Susan E. Orosz, PhD, DVM, Dipl. ABVP–Avian, Dipl. ECZM–Avian
Bird and Exotic Pet Wellness Center
5166 Monroe Street, Suite 305
Toledo, OH 43623, USA

Cathy A. Johnson-Delaney, DVM, Dipl. ABVP–Avian and Exotic Companion Mammal
Eastside Avian and Exotic Animal Medical Center
12930 NE 125th Way
Kirkland, WA 98034, USA

E-mail addresses:
drsusanorosz@aol.com (S.E. Orosz)
cajddvm@hotmail.com (C.A. Johnson-Delaney)

Vet Clin Exot Anim 14 (2011) ix
doi:10.1016/j.cvex.2011.03.011
1094-9194/11/$ – see front matter © 2011 Elsevier Inc. All rights reserved.

Disorders of the Respiratory System in Pet and Ornamental Fish

Helen E. Roberts, DVM[a],*, Stephen A. Smith, DVM, PhD[b]

KEYWORDS

- Pet fish • Ornamental fish • Branchitis • Gill
- Wet mount cytology • Hypoxia • Respiratory disorders
- Pathology

Living in an aquatic environment where oxygen is in less supply and harder to extract than in a terrestrial one, fish have developed a respiratory system that is much more efficient than terrestrial vertebrates. The gills of fish are a unique organ system and serve several functions including respiration, osmoregulation, excretion of nitrogenous wastes, and acid-base regulation.[1] The gills are the primary site of oxygen exchange in fish and are in intimate contact with the aquatic environment. In most cases, the separation between the water and the tissues of the fish is only a few cell layers thick. Gills are a common target for assault by infectious and noninfectious disease processes.[2] Nonlethal diagnostic biopsy of the gills can identify pathologic changes, provide samples for bacterial culture/identification/sensitivity testing, aid in fungal element identification, provide samples for viral testing, and provide parasitic organisms for identification.[3–6] This diagnostic test is so important that it should be included as part of every diagnostic workup performed on a fish.

ANATOMY AND PHYSIOLOGY

The respiratory system of most fish species includes the gill arches, 2 opercula, and the buccal cavity, all located in the cranial portion of the body. Most teleosts (including pet and ornamental fish) have 4 respiratory gill arches and 1 dorsally located, nonrespiratory pseudobranch.[1,2,7–9] The arches are supported by a bony skeleton and are protected by a specialized, moveable flap called an operculum. Each respiratory

[a] Aquatic Veterinary Services of WNY, 5 Corners Animal Hospital, 2799 Southwestern Boulevard, Suite 100, Orchard Park, NY 14127, USA
[b] Department of Biomedical Sciences and Pathobiology, Virginia-Maryland Regional College of Veterinary Medicine, Phase II, Duck Pond Drive, Virginia Tech, Blacksburg, VA 24061-0442, USA
* Corresponding author.
E-mail address: nyfishdoc@aol.com

Vet Clin Exot Anim 14 (2011) 179–206
doi:10.1016/j.cvex.2011.03.004
vetexotic.theclinics.com

arch has 2 rows of gill filaments (or primary lamellae) that project from the arch, like the "teeth of a comb,"[10] with numerous rows of secondary lamellae extending perpendicular from these primary lamellae (**Fig. 1**).[1–3] The secondary lamellae consist of epithelial cells (usually 1 or 2 layers) surrounding a central vascular space, supported by contractile pillar cells.[2,3,10] It is at the secondary lamellae where gas exchange occurs. Comparatively large gills (with a corresponding increased lamellar surface area) can be found in some very active fish (eg, tuna) and fish with a relative tolerance for hypoxia.[11,12] The lamellar epithelium is thin and its external surface is covered with microridges that serve to further increase the surface area for respiration.[2,10,13] A protective biofilm consisting of mucus and other cellular and chemical components covers this epithelium. This layer and the underlying lamellar epithelium are very sensitive to stress and environmental changes.[2]

Blood flow to the gills comes directly from the heart via the ventral aorta. The lamellar blood channels are so small in diameter that erythrocytes move through the capillaries one red blood cell at a time. Because nearly the entire cardiac output enters the gills, traumatic injury to the gills can negatively affect the health of the fish and can be potentially fatal.[1,9,11,14] This is an important consideration when attempting nonlethal gill sampling for diagnostic purposes. A complex system theorized to involve interactions between many hormones and the autonomic nervous system serves to control lamellar perfusion in the gills.[1,10] A counter-current system between the blood flow and water flow creates an efficient transfer of oxygen by passive diffusion from a relatively higher oxygen concentration in the water to a lower concentration in the bloodstream. Video demonstrations of blood flow through the gills can be found on the Internet as a supplement to an article by Evans and colleagues.[15] A small amount of blood is also delivered to a central venous sinus via alternate pathways for delivering nutrients to the gill tissue.[1,2] Abductor and adductor muscles allow the fish to spread the gill filaments and change the flow of water over the gills in times of higher oxygen demand.[2,14,16]

The highly vascular and semipermeable nature of the gills may be exploited as a drug delivery method. In one study, topical gill application of a spawning hormone was used in small tropical fish where injections were not feasible.[17] Another example is the spray delivery of a highly concentrated anesthetic solution to the gills for sedation or anesthesia. This method is used most often in public aquariums for large elasmobranchs, but can be used in a variety of species where immersion in the anesthetic solution is impractical or cost prohibitive.[18]

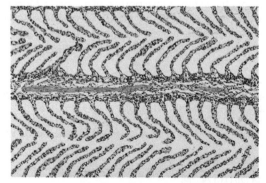

Fig. 1. Histologic view of a normal gill section with secondary lamellae seen extending perpendicularly from primary lamellae (H&E, original magnification ×400).

Air-breathing fish, or labyrinth fish, and some catfish have developed very vascular accessory organs that serve to extract oxygen from the air at the surface of the water.[2,3,19] This ability can help with oxygen extraction from the air when the aquatic environment becomes hypoxic or can aid gas exchange in species that bury themselves in mud during dry seasons.[16,18,20] Air-breathing fish can be obligate air breathers (must have access above the water surface) or facultative air breathers (only breath air when the dissolved oxygen level of the water is very low).[21] Examples of pet fish in this group include bettas (*Betta splendens*) (**Fig. 2**), paradise fish (*Macropodus opercularis*), and gouramis (multiple species). Prolonged and unpredictable induction of anesthesia may occur in these species when using an anesthetic in an aqueous solution.[18]

Respiration in fish is continuous and unidirectional (compared with the bidirectional mechanism in mammals): water flows into the buccal cavity, flows past the gill tissue, and exits via the opercular opening.[2,3,9,14] This type of respiratory cycling is called a dual-phase pump.[9] During the first phase, the mouth is open and the opercula are closed, water enters the expanding buccal and opercular cavities.[3,9] In the second phase, the mouth closes, the opercula open, and the buccal cavity contracts forcing the water to flow over the gills and exit via the opercular opening.[3,9] Some fish species such as tuna use ram gill ventilation (open mouth swimming) as a primary means of respiration instead of the dual-phase pump, whereas other species resort to this method only when swimming rapidly or when in a strong current.[2,9,22] Ram ventilation can reduce the energy expenditure required for respiration.[1,22] Fish can also cough, temporarily reversing the flow of water over the gills.[3,23] Coughing can be triggered by mechanical and chemical stimulation of the gills.[10] An increased coughing rate has been associated with irritant pollution,[10] gill parasitism, bacterial gill disease,[24] and excess mucus[3] and could be a more sensitive indicator than an increased opercular rate of general stress in fish.[23]

RESPONSE OF GILLS TO INJURY AND CLINICAL SIGNS OF GILL DISEASE

Gills are delicate, highly vascularized organs that are always in direct contact with the external environment. Because of this, gills are highly susceptible to invasion by various infectious agents; damage from environmental toxins, irritants, and pollutants; and the adverse effects of stress. Common causes of stress in pet and ornamental

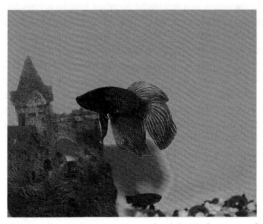

Fig. 2. *Betta splendens* has an accessory organ, the labyrinth organ, for breathing atmospheric air.

fish include capture and handling, overcrowding, poor water quality, overfeeding, inadequate husbandry and maintenance, and interspecies and intraspecies incompatibility. In response to stress, fish undergo a similar stress-induced hormone response as other pet species that includes the release of catecholamines and glucocorticoids.[25–27] Catecholamine-mediated reactions to stress include increased blood flow to the gills in an effort to improve oxygen uptake,[25,27] increased heart and respiratory rates, and altered permeability of the gills.[27] Some of these changes can occur rapidly. It is important to note that functional changes will occur before detectable morphologic changes. For example, hyperventilation induced by hypoxia can occur within seconds.[1] The acute changes induced by hypoxic conditions are an attempt to maintain adequate oxygenation of the fish despite a lowered oxygen concentration in the environment.[28,29] A reflex bradycardia is often observed with hypoxia and may occur in an attempt to reduce blood flow to the gills and favorably increase gas exchange.[29]

Oxygen depletion can be a common occurrence in aquatic environments and is a major cause of stress and hypoxia in fish. In pet and ornamental fish, some situations that cause hypoxia include transport and shipping, as well as plant/algae overgrowth in ponds or aquaria.[26] Clinically, hypoxic conditions can occur as an adverse effect of therapeutic treatments, such as formalin, or after a massive algae die-off following the use of an algaecide. Mechanical failure of aeration equipment, pumps, or filtration equipment can also contribute to hypoxic conditions.[30]

Lesions that can occur in the gills in response to injury include color change because of congestion or thinning of blood, diffuse or focal necrosis, telangiectasia (dilation of the terminal blood vessels), edema, hemorrhage, lamellar thickening and fusion, epithelial hypertrophy and hyperplasia, and increased mucus secretion.[2,8,13,26] Increased mucus production may initially be beneficial, as the mucus may bind some toxins found in the water or prevent some pathogens from attaching to the gill.[8] Most of these can be seen grossly or during wet mount cytologic examination. To complicate matters, many gill lesions seen on histopathological examination can also be a result of artifacts from processing and improper fixation of specimens or poor euthanasia technique.[2,13]

One interesting response to environmental hypoxia has been reported in the Crucian carp (Carassius carassius), the goldfish (Carassius auratus), the mangrove killifish (Kryptolebias marmoratus), and the giant Amazonian fish (Arapaima gigas).[31] In these species, secondary lamellae are normally located inside a cellular mass, effectively reducing the respiratory surface area.[26,31] During times of environmental hypoxia, the interlamellar cell mass recedes, exposing the lamellae, and thus increasing the efficiency of oxygen uptake via the increased functional area.

Most clinical signs of injury to the gills are a reflection of hypoxic environmental conditions or a relative hypoxia and can be readily observed without direct manipulation of the fish. **Table 1** lists common, nonspecific clinical signs that can be associated with diseases and injury to the gills. It is important to remember that the gills perform more than just a respiratory function, so diseases that affect the gills can also cause clinical signs related to the disruption of osmoregulation, acid-base imbalances, and nitrogenous waste accumulation in the body.

DIAGNOSTIC EVALUATION OF RESPIRATORY DISEASE

All evaluations of clinically ill fish start with a good history and physical examination. Historical questions should be broad in nature and investigate life support systems (eg, filters, water and air pumps) and maintenance, husbandry and management

Table 1
Clinical signs associated with diseases of the gills[a]

Clinical Sign	Description	Comments
Abnormal dark coloration	Darker than normal for particular species, reproductive status, and color phase	General stress Systemic disease Poor water quality
Coughing	Rapid opercular flaring that moves water in a reversed directional flow over the gills	Occasional coughing is normal, increased rate can be indicative of disease Exposure to gill irritants Gill parasitism Stress
Flared opercula	Opercula open, exposing the gill tissue	Severe hypoxia, usually agonal Goiter, pharyngeal foreign body
Flashing	Rubbing the body on bottom of tank or pond exposing the ventral aspect (a "flash" of pale color of the ventrum)	Parasitism Poor water quality
Gasping	Exaggerated and repeated opening and closing of the mouth	Hypoxia Relative hypoxia (anemia, nitrite poisoning) Poor water quality Many gill disorders
Gathering at water inflow sites/facing into water current	Congregation at areas of moving water-waterfalls, water inflow pipes, water fountains, and so forth	May be an attempt to find increased oxygen concentration or increased water flow over the gills
Gilling	Increased opercular rate	Nonspecific sign of stress Hypoxic or conditions that create a relative hypoxia
Jumping	Jumping out of the water Desiccated fish may be found on the floor or edge of the pond	Startled fish Poor water quality (low oxygen, low pH) Parasitism toxic or caustic substances
Mucus production increased	The increased mucus layer can impart a hazy or dull appearance to the gills	May see trailing strands of mucus exiting the operculum
Piping	Open mouthed gulping at the air: water interface	See also "Gasping" Do not confuse with normal bubble nest building seen in fish such as bettas

[a] These signs are not pathognomonic for gill disease and can be present in many diseases of fish.

practices, number of fish and variety of species, recent changes or treatments, presence of new fish, and the duration and course of disease.[3,4,32,33] Life support system failures including the misuse of ozone can contribute to or be a direct cause of respiratory disease in fish.[3]

Examination should first include observation of the live fish without any direct handling of the affected fish. Clinical signs as listed in **Table 1** may be observed. Physical examination of the fish follows observation. Rinsed, powder-free nitrile, vinyl, or latex gloves should be worn to reduce any damage to the fish's skin and to reduce the risk of zoonotic disease transmission (**Fig. 3**).[34] If the examination takes more

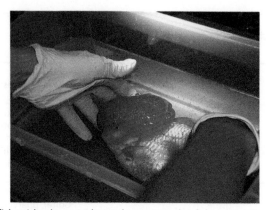

Fig. 3. Handling fish with gloves reduces damage to the fish's slime coat and protects the practitioner from zoonotic disease transmission.

than a few minutes, the fish should periodically be placed in water or should be irrigated with water to prevent desiccation of the external surfaces and gill tissue. Fish will usually resist manipulation of the opercula and gills for examination purposes so sedation or anesthesia is recommended unless the patient is considered a high-risk candidate for anesthesia. The opercula and surrounding tissue should be carefully examined for any lesions. Abnormal examination findings that may be seen on gross examination of the gills include focal, patchy, or diffuse necrosis; focal or diffuse color changes; increased mucus production; missing sections of gill filaments; the presence of multicellular parasites or nodular lesions; and focal or diffuse swelling of the gill (**Figs. 4** and **5**).

Water quality testing should also be performed for the complete evaluation of sick fish. There are many environmental abnormalities that can lead to respiratory distress. General testing parameters should include dissolved oxygen (DO), ammonia, nitrite, nitrate, and pH. Salinity measurements should be added for general testing of marine systems. Further testing can include tests for the presence of heavy metals (including copper) and chlorine/chloramine.

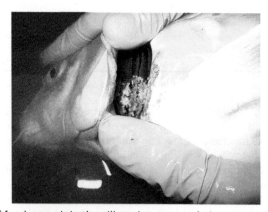

Fig. 4. An area of focal necrosis in the gills owing to a predation attempt on a koi (*Cyprinus carpio*).

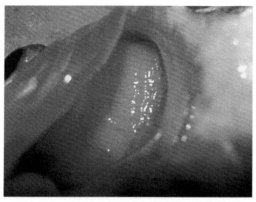

Fig. 5. The extreme pallor of these gills from a goldfish (*Carassius auratus*) is suggestive of anemia.

Diagnostic testing, including wet mount cytologic preps of the gills, are also considered part of the minimum database in the evaluation of sick fish. The gill biopsy is essential for any case of respiratory disease and should be evaluated in all but the most seriously morbid cases. A gill biopsy allows for evaluation of gill morphology and for the presence of parasites. Only a very small piece of gill tissue needs to be sampled during a nonlethal examination. Hemorrhage is not usually a concern unless a large amount of tissue is removed or the patient is a mature or gravid fish.[3–6]

Gill biopsy for the wet mount examination procedure is completed as follows[3–6] (**Figs. 6** and **7**):

1. Place a drop of water from the aquarium or pond on a clean slide.
2. Using gloved hands, gently lift the operculum of the sedated or anesthetized fish to reveal the gills. Gill rakers should be examined carefully during the physical examination, as many larger parasites will lodge in these areas.
3. With fine scissors such as iris tenotomy or suture removal scissors, snip a tiny section from the distal end of a few primary lamellae.
4. Place the gill tissue in the water drop on the prepared slide and place a coverslip over the tissue.
5. Examine the unstained slide immediately for evidence of parasites, fungi, or bacteria.

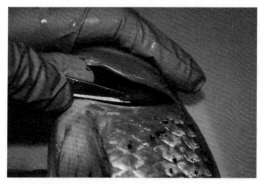

Fig. 6. A small section of gill tissue is removed for a wet mount preparation.

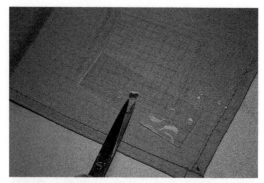

Fig. 7. A tiny piece of gill tissue is placed in the water drop for a wet mount examination.

6. The sample can also be examined for gill architecture. Gill pathology such as hyperplasia, hypertrophy, necrosis, lamellar fusion, excess mucus and telangiectasia may be observed.
7. In extremely large fish, one may need to scrape only the surface of the gills.

Another nonlethal technique for evaluation of the gills is with the use of rigid endoscopy. The scope is placed under the operculum and the practitioner can visualize the gills in situ as water flows over them.[35] With the magnification of the endoscope, the erythrocytes can be observed moving through the secondary lamellae and it may also be possible to see some external gill parasites.[35]

Hematological parameters associated with prolonged or severe hypoxia (and subsequent respiratory disease) include polycythemia, polychromasia, and anemia.[36,37] Serum biochemical changes that may be observed during hypoxia include increases in ammonia, potassium, calcium, magnesium, and phosphate.[37] An increased hematocrit has been reported in obligate air-breathing fish.[38] Hypoglycemia and a reduction in serum lipid values have also been reported with hypoxia.[37] An elevation of blood urea nitrogen (BUN) has been associated with copper-induced gill damage irrespective of any renal damage.[38,39] It is important to note that interpretation of hematological parameters and serum or plasma chemistry values can be difficult because not many profiles have been established for the multitude of species kept as pet and ornamental fish. In addition, interpretation of hematological and chemistry information is further complicated by alterations that may occur in the values owing to handling, stress, environmental temperatures, sex, breeding status, diet, use of anesthesia, and overall water quality.[5,36,37]

If a necropsy is performed, large sections of a gill arch can be removed and placed in formalin or other fixative for histopathology or other media for purposes of viral testing or bacterial culture and identification.

COMMON DISEASES OF THE GILLS
Infectious Diseases

Parasitic diseases
Parasitic diseases are the most common infectious diseases diagnosed in fish. The most common method of introduction is failure to quarantine and treat new additions to a pond or aquaria. Most of the parasites listed in the following paragraphs do not specifically target the gills but can be found in numerous locations on the body. An advantage to colonizing the gill epithelium is the protection offered to the easily damaged tissues by the opercula. Clinical signs suggestive of parasitic infestations

of the gills include flashing, increased mucus production, ulcerations and scale loss, and other general signs of dyspnea (see **Table 1**). A more complete description of parasitic diseases in fish can be found in a previous edition of the *Veterinary Clinics of North America, Exotic Animal Practice* series.[40]

Ichthyophthirius multifiliis, a holotrichous ciliated protozoan, is the most common parasite of fish and infects a large number of freshwater fish in a wide range of aquatic environments. "Ich," also known as "Ick" or "white spot disease," has a direct, complex life cycle that is temperature dependent. *Cryptocaryon irritans* is the marine version of this parasite. The disease derives its common name from the typical 1.0 mm white nodules (0.5 mm nodules for *Cryptocaryon*) seen distributed over the skin and gills of the fish (**Fig. 8**). Both parasites cause nearly identical pathology and clinical signs. At water temperatures typical of what can be found in tropical fish aquaria (25°C/77°F), the parasite can complete its life cycle in 3 to 6 days.[40] The life stage found on a fish, the trophont, is embedded in the epithelial tissues of the gill and is protected from external treatments.[40] Only the free-swimming life stage, the theront, is susceptible to treatment. Clinical signs are typical of external parasitism and include flashing, excess mucus production, cutaneous lesions, frayed fins and tail, dyspnea, lethargy, osmoregulatory insufficiency, and death.[24,40–42] Diagnosis is made by examination of a wet mount cytology preparation of the skin and gills. The parasite is easily identified by the characteristic slow, rolling motion and unique shape of its nucleus. The nucleus of *Ichthyophthirius* has a horseshoe shape, whereas the nucleus of *Cryptocaryon* is lobulated with 4 beadlike segments (**Fig. 9**).[40]

Trichodinid parasites are commonly diagnosed ciliated protozoans of both marine and freshwater fish species that primarily parasitize the skin and gills. These parasites are often seen in conditions that promote high levels of organic debris in the water, overcrowding, and poor husbandry practices.[40,43] Clinical signs are those typical of external parasitism and diagnosis is made by examination of a gill biopsy wet mount preparation. The circular, ciliated parasite with a characteristic internal circular denticular ring moves rapidly in the wet mount preparation, in a rotating whirling pattern, and has been described as a "scrubbing bubble" or flying saucer (**Fig. 10**).[40,43]

Chilodonella sp (*Brooklynella* sp is the marine counterpart) is another ciliated protozoan parasite that can be found on the gills of fish. Observation of the flattened parasite with several distinct bands of cilia in a wet mount cytologic preparation is diagnostic. Gill pathology seen with this parasitic infestation includes hyperplasia and fusion of the lamellae.[40]

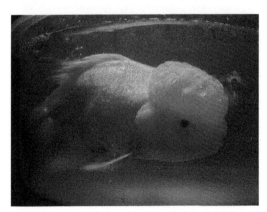

Fig. 8. A goldfish (*Carassius auratus*) infected with *Ichthyophthirius multifiliis.*

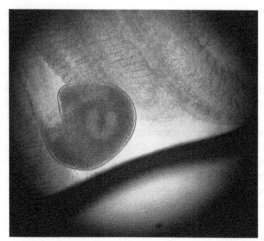

Fig. 9. A wet mount prep showing *Ichthyophthirius* in the gill tissue, magnification ×40.

Sessile or sedentary ciliates of clinical importance in causing respiratory disease in fish include *Epistylis* and *Capriniana*.[4,24,40] These ciliates are usually found on fish held in ponds where large amounts of organic debris are present.[40] *Epistylis* appears as a gelatinous to white cottony mass on the operculum and other locations. Wet mount cytology will help differentiate this ciliate from *Saprolegnia* (a fungal cause of gill disease) and *Flavobacterium columnare* (a bacterial cause of gill disease).[24,44] *Capriniana piscium* has a predilection for gill tissue and causes severe respiratory distress in affected fish by mechanically blocking gill tissue.[24,40]

Ichthyobodo sp (previously known as *Costia*) can cause severe respiratory distress and heavy mucus production when it colonizes gill tissue. The flagellated protozoan is approximately equal in size to a red blood cell and demonstrates a flickering-type motion in wet mounts. The parasite may be seen concurrently with other diseases causing debilitation in the fish, including koi herpesvirus (KHV) infections and bacterial sepsis. Two other parasitic flagellated *Cryptobia* species, *C branchialis* and *C agitans*, have been reported to specifically colonize gill tissue.[24,40]

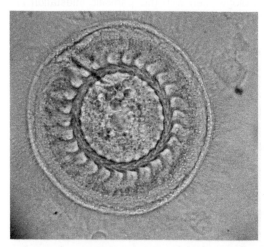

Fig. 10. *Trichodina* sp as seen in a wet mount prep, original magnification ×40.

Another group of protozoan parasites that causes respiratory disease includes the parasitic dinoflagellates, *Amyloodinium ocellatum* (marine) and *Piscinoodinium* sp (freshwater). Both have life cycles similar to *Ichthyophthirius* and only the free-swimming life stage is susceptible to treatment. Disease caused by these organisms is referred to as "velvet" or "rust" because of the characteristic gross appearance of the affected fish. Infestation of the gills can cause severe pathology, including edema, hyperplasia, inflammation, hemorrhage, and necrosis of the gill filaments.[4,24,40]

Monogenean flatworms, are a frequent finding in the gills of freshwater and marine pet and ornamental fish species. The most common genera infecting freshwater pet fish are *Dactylogyrus*, the oviparous "gill fluke" (**Fig. 11**), and *Gyrodactylus*, the viviparous "skin fluke." Neither parasite is location specific and can be found both on the skin and gills of affected fish. The author has seen heavy *Dactylogyrus* infestations most often on imported fancy goldfish and *Gyrodactylus* in other species, such as koi and discus (*Symphysodon* sp). The capsalid marine flukes, *Benedenia* sp and *Neobenedenia* sp, can be found colonizing the skin and gills of affected fish. Clinical signs of monogenean infestations are nonspecific and can range from mild flashing and coughing to heavy mucus production, lethargy, secondary bacteremia, cutaneous lesions, and death.[4,24,40–43] Diagnosis is most often made by examination of a gill biopsy wet mount preparation. Marine capsalids may also be seen after a freshwater dip, a common procedure used in quarantine protocols of newly acquired marine fish. The pale-colored parasites dislodge from their attachments on the fish and can be seen in the fish's water when viewed against a dark background.[40]

Other parasites that have been reported to cause gill problems include the parasitic intracellular microsporidians that can cause respiratory disease in fish, including *Pleistophora* sp, *Glugea* sp, and *Heterosporis* sp. Diagnosis is made with histopathology and wet mount examination of the lesions. The myxosporean, *Myxobolus intrachondrealis*, has been identified in the gill cartilage of the common carp, *Cyprinus carpio*.[45] Other *Myxobolus* sp may be identified as a cause of disease of the gills and associated structures.

Larval digenetic trematodes such as *Neascus* sp and *Clinostomum* sp may also infest the gill tissue. Mild infestations cause minimal pathology but a heavy infestation

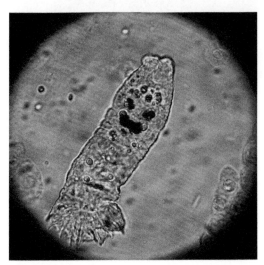

Fig. 11. *Dactylogyrus* sp ("gill fluke") as seen in a wet mount prep, original magnification ×40. Note the characteristic black eyespots and posterior holdfast organ of this species.

can lead to tissue damage and secondary infections.[40,41] Crustacean parasites that may be seen on the gills include *Lernaea* sp (ie, anchor worm), *Argulus* sp (ie, fish louse), the copepod *Ergasilus* sp in freshwater systems, and the isopod *Gnathia* sp in marine systems.[3,40,41] Leeches may also occasionally be found attached to the opercula and gill tissue of pond-reared fish (**Fig. 12**).[3]

Bacterial diseases

Bacterial diseases in fish are fairly common and outbreaks are usually a secondary complication of immunosuppression after stressful events. Pathogenic bacteria that are isolated from gill lesions are frequently organisms that are ubiquitous in the environment.[40,46] Probably the most common bacterial disease of freshwater fish is *Aeromonas hydrophilia*, a Gram-negative bacterium that causes a disease syndrome commonly known as "motile *Aeromonas* septicemia," "red sore disease," "hemorrhagic septicemia," or "ulcer disease."[47] This pathogen initially affects the gills and skin of the fish, then progressively becomes a septicemia infecting many internal organs. The clinical manifestations in the gill may include pale-colored gills to focal or widespread hemorrhagic and necrotic areas of the gills.

Another bacterial disease of the gills, commonly termed "bacterial gill disease," is caused by *Flavobacterium branchiophilia* (a species previously placed in the genus *Cytophagus*, then *Flexibacter*).[47] This Gram-negative bacteria predominantly affects the external surface of the gill causing the number of epithelia and mucus cells to increase. The space between the lamellae becomes filled in with proliferative cellular tissue, which reduces the surface area of the gill and consequently reduces the ability of the gill to allow diffusion of gasses across the tissue. Necrosis of the gill tissue will

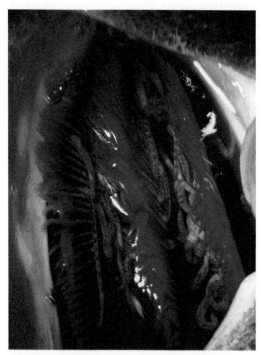

Fig. 12. Leeches (species unknown) found on the gills of a wolf eel (*Anarrhichthys ocellatus*). (*Courtesy of* Dr T. Miller-Morgan.)

sometimes occur in severe cases. Basically, fish find it hard to breath and often face the water current to maximize water flow through the oral and branchial cavities. Numerous scenarios can lead to this bacteria becoming established in a population of fish, such as overcrowding, elevated metabolic waste products, accumulation of organic material in the water column, and increased water temperatures. Another bacteria in this group, *Flavobacterium columnare*, can also affect the gill, causing a disease known as "columnaris" or "cotton-wool" disease. This bacterium colonizes the surface of the gill where it often imparts a distinctive yellowish color to the gill. In wet mount preparations, the bacteria are commonly observed in characteristic hay-stacklike clusters of filamentous, flexing organisms. This pathogen causes necrosis of the cells at the distal end of the gill filament and progresses to involve the entire filament. Like *F branchiophilia*, predisposing factors include crowding, poor water quality, and increased water temperatures.

Chronic mycobacteriosis may also manifest as an infection of the gills.[48] This can be seen grossly as small white nodules among the gill filaments, in wet mounts as discrete granulomas within the gill tissue, or in histopathology as granulomas with acid-fast bacteria (**Fig. 13**). This bacterial group (*M marinum, M fortuitum*, and so forth) is an important zoonotic pathogen in fish, and pet fish clients should be made aware of the potential human health hazard.[34,48]

Viral diseases

Viral diseases of fish typically produce nonspecific local and general clinical signs and lesions. The most common method of introduction into a naïve population is by failing to isolate and quarantine new animals at viral permissive water temperatures. Most viruses have a specific water temperature range required for spreading the infection to new fish. There are no specific treatments indicated for viral disease outbreaks, although increasing the water temperature outside the specific viral range has been associated with abatement of clinical signs in cases of goldfish herpesvirus and KHV.[49,50] Surviving fish should not be considered "cured" because they can become latent carriers and spread the disease by shedding the virus, infecting naïve fish. Viral diseases of importance that are known to cause lesions in the gills include goldfish herpesvirus (Cyprinid Herpes Virus 2 [CyHV-2], herpes viral hematopoietic necrosis [HVHN]), KHV (Cyprinid Herpes Virus 3 [CyHV-3], carp interstitial nephritis), *Megalocytivirus,* and Spring Viremia of Carp (SVCV). Viral hemorrhagic septicemia (VHS) has been isolated from many species of marine and freshwater fish. Although generally

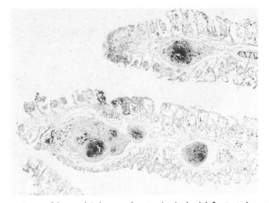

Fig. 13. Histologic section of branchial mycobacteriosis (acid-fast stain, original magnification ×400) showing several granulomas.

not a differential for disease outbreaks in ornamental fish populations, the virus has anecdotally been reported in koi but has not been confirmed.[49]

Goldfish herpesvirus disease outbreaks can occur in all varieties of goldfish and have been detected in the United Kingdom, the United States, Taiwan, Japan, and Australia.[50] Outbreaks generally occur in water temperatures higher than 15°C and can cause acute mortalities, from 50% to 100%.[49,51] Goodwin and colleagues[50] reported that high mortalities were most often associated with shipping stress and acute temperature drops. In addition to the common clinical signs of lethargy and anorexia, affected fish often have multifocal pale, patchy gill lesions. Necropsy reveals splenomegaly with white nodules in the splenic tissue, ascites, and swollen kidneys.[49–51] A quantitative polymerase chain reaction (PCR) test developed by the University of Arkansas is available for confirmation of the disease.[49,52]

KHV has been associated with massive fish mortalities in naïve populations. The virus shows a global distribution and has been found in wild common carp populations in addition to koi, the ornamental variety of *Cyprinus carpio*. Most infections occur in water temperatures between 16°C and 28°C following exposure to an infected fish.[49,53] Failure to quarantine new additions at viral permissive water temperatures is the most common historical finding. Concomitant infection with parasites and secondary bacterial and fungal infections are common. Clinical signs include respiratory distress (piping, gasping, elevated opercular rate), cutaneous ulcerations and hemorrhages, loss of scales, enophthalmos, lethargy, and anorexia. Typical gill lesions include widespread patchy necrosis, areas of hemorrhage, swelling, and excessive mucus (**Fig. 14**).[49,54] The virus survives in water, mud, and feces of infected fish for prolonged periods.[49,55] Draining and drying ponds for several weeks in addition to cleaning and disinfecting tanks and equipment has been recommended. Diagnosis can be made by history, observation of the clinical signs, and the use of PCR testing, virus neutralization tests, or virus isolation.[49,54] A commercial enzyme-linked immunosorbent assay (ELISA) test that detects antibodies to KHV is available to aid in the identification of clinical carriers but false negatives can occur if the fish is tested early in the course of the disease.[49] This test may be combined with quarantine at permissive temperatures to screen for uninfected or KHV carrier fish. An effective vaccine is currently being investigated by several researchers. Goldfish housed with KHV-infected koi have tested positive via PCR for KHV, making them and other species potential vectors in spreading the disease.[49,56,57]

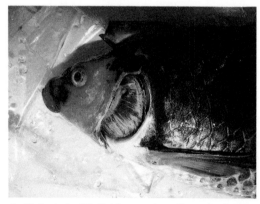

Fig. 14. Gills from a koi infected with Koi herpesvirus. Note the focal areas of necrosis and hemorrhage.

Megalocytivirus is a genus of iridoviruses that has been shown to cause systemic disease in many species of marine and freshwater fish, including several ornamental species commonly kept as pets. Clinical signs are nonspecific and may include lethargy, anemia, hemorrhage of the gills, and high mortalities.[49,55] Large, basophilic cytomegalic cells can be observed on microscopic examination of the gill and other organs.[58]

There is no specific treatment for viral diseases. Improving husbandry practices and water quality, treating secondary or concurrent diseases, and reducing stress may result in a favorable outcome in some infections. Prevention is best and can be achieved through screening suppliers of fish, antemortem testing of fish for exposure when such tests exist, quarantine of all new introductions, and practicing good biosecurity techniques.

Fungal diseases

Fungal pathogens of the gill are generally considered to be opportunistic infections and are usually associated with adverse environmental conditions, poor aeration, or physical trauma. However, fish exposed to intensive culture situations, poor nutrition, temperature shock, external parasites, spawning activity, or other activities causing immunosuppression are generally more susceptible to fungal infections. Most fungal pathogens of pet and ornamental fish belong to the Class Oomycetes in either the genera *Saprolegnia* or *Aphanomyces*.[59,60] The fungal mass is composed of branched, nonseptate fungal hyphae and accumulated debris from the water that becomes trapped in the fungal hyphae. The characteristic gross pathology observed with this type of infection is a white to gray cottonlike mycelial mass on the surface of the gill. This is often associated with an underlying focal, superficial erosion of the gill epithelium. Sometimes these fungal pathogens, especially *Aphanomyces* sp, may become more aggressive and invade the deeper tissues of the gill. When this happens, there is usually no grossly visible external cottony growth on the surface of the gill, as the hyphae penetrate into the dermis, underlying muscle, and viscera of the fish.

In addition, 2 species of the genera *Branchiomyces (B sanguinis, B demingrans)* are considered primary pathogens of gill epithelial tissue. These fungal infections, commonly called "gill rot" or "branchiomycosis," are usually associated with poor water quality conditions or poor feeding practices (**Fig. 15**). Infections of the gill may present as hemorrhagic swellings and progress to necrosis of large areas of the gill owing to infarction of local blood vessels. Infections of the gill may also invade other tissues of the branchial cavity such as the pseudobranch and thymus.

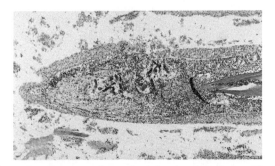

Fig. 15. Histologic section (hematoxylin-eosin stained, original magnification ×400) of gill tissue infected with *Branchiomyces* sp showing general swelling and loss of normal filament architecture. The hyphal elements (dark pink structures) of the fungus can be seen in the center of the affected tissue.

Noninfectious Diseases

Environmental problems

Many different environmental issues can negatively affect gill morphology and function. Water quality problems such as ammonia, nitrite and nitrate toxicity, supersaturation of gases, and turbidity can significantly reduce the ability of gasses, ions, and minerals to diffuse across the gill surface. The water quality toxicities and turbidity chemically and physically irritate the gill tissues and cause them to become hyperplastic. As the epithelial tissues of the gill become thickened, diffusion across the gills becomes more difficult, affecting oxygen uptake and carbon dioxide and ammonia excretion. Thus, the fish not only becomes hypoxic, but also hyperammonemic and acidotic with resulting homeostatic imbalances. The 3 major water quality toxicities (ie, ammonia, nitrite, and nitrate) are difficult to distinguish either grossly or histologically (**Fig. 16**), but all can be acutely or chronically stressful to fish depending on the concentration and time of exposure and all can be lethal. Wet mounts of gill biopsies may have an increased amount of mucus, a thickened appearance to the gill lamellae, and clubbing and fusion of gill filaments. Additionally, nitrite toxicity, which can sometimes cause methemoglobinemia (ie, brown blood disease), may cause the gills to become a dark red to chocolate-brown color once the methemoglobinemia reaches concentrations of 40% or higher.[61]

Supersaturation of gases in the water column is another problem that can affect the function of the gills. This problem, commonly called "gas bubble disease" manifests as bubbles in the capillaries of the gills and fins, air bubbles in the eye, and raised bubbles in the skin. The elevated gas concentrations above atmospheric levels can be caused by insufficient aeration of water obtained from deep wells or springs; leaks in pumps, valves, or water lines; or sudden water temperature changes. Various gases may be involved, although elevated nitrogen concentrations seem to be the most common, and may be both chronically stressful and acutely lethal to fish. Wet mounts of gill biopsies will reveal air bubbles within the lumen of the capillaries, which prevents normal flow of blood though the vessels (**Fig. 17**).

Water pH parameters outside an optimal range (species dependent) can cause changes in the gills and increase the toxicity of some pollutants in the water.[8,61,62] A low pH causes increased mucus production and changes typical of a stress-induced response in the gills. Acidic water also favors higher toxicity of heavy metal pollutants.[8,61] High water pH can cause hypertrophy of the goblet and epithelial cells in the gills leading to excessive mucus production and swelling.[8,61]

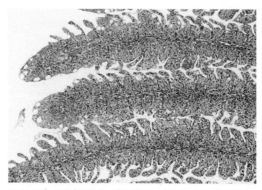

Fig. 16. Histologic section from the gill of a fish with water quality (ammonia or nitrite) toxicity. Note the thickened appearance, lamellar fusion, and hyperplasia (H&E, original magnification ×40).

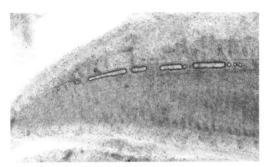

Fig. 17. Gas bubble disease. Note the air bubbles found in the capillary lumen of a secondary lamella caused by supersaturation of gases in the water column (original magnification ×100).

The gills are a major site for damage caused by pollutants in the water. Contaminants and/or toxins that can cause gill damage and subsequent signs of respiratory distress include chlorine; heavy metals, including copper, iron, zinc, mercury, and aluminum; formalin; potassium permanganate; and detergents. Heavy metals contamination of the environment results in structural damage of the gill epithelium.[8] Chlorine is found in many municipal water supplies where it has been added for its disinfectant properties.[63,64] Chlorine is toxic to fish and can result in severe pathologic changes in the gill tissue. Lesions commonly seen include epithelial lifting, hypertrophy, hyperplasia, lamellar fusion, excess mucus production, and necrosis.[3,63,65] The most common finding is failure to use a dechlorinator when adding water, setting up a new system, or performing a water change in aquaria and ponds. Diagnosis is made on historical findings, physical examination findings, and water testing for chlorine.

Copper is a heavy metal that can be introduced into systems as a therapeutic agent, algaecide, decoration, or it may exist as a component of the plumbing system. Copper toxicity results in edema of the gills, in addition to immunosuppression and liver and kidney damage. Measurement of toxic levels of the free copper ion in the water with field test kits can support a diagnosis. Copper is more toxic when used in systems with low alkalinity and low pH.[62,64] Zinc toxicity may also occur when fish are housed in galvanized tubs or in display ponds where the public can toss coins into the water. Zinc and copper toxic effects are additive.[62,64] Other heavy metals that cause gill pathology include aluminum (when present in acidic water it can cause gill necrosis) and iron and manganese (where high levels of each can favor iron and manganese oxide precipitates depositing on the gills, causing lamellar fusion and necrosis).[62,64] A sample of water can be submitted to an environmental lab for heavy metal testing for definitive diagnosis, although this testing can run several hundred dollars.

Potassium permanganate, a common water treatment used to treat pond fish, can also cause precipitation of manganese oxides when used in systems with a high water pH. Another water treatment and therapeutic agent, formalin, can cause gill irritation and reduce dissolved oxygen content in ponds. Formalin is more toxic in aquaria and ponds with soft, acidic water and at high temperatures.[64] Species vary in their sensitivity to formalin.

Nutritional diseases
Suboptimal nutrition can also affect the gill. A pathologic condition (ie, nutritional gill disease) caused by a deficiency of pantothenic acid in older feed has been reported

to affect the gills of catfish and trout.[66,67] Gross lesions included hyperplasia of the proximal portions of the gill filaments causing the gill filaments to become swollen and bulbous. The resulting clubbing and fusion of the gill filaments interferes with gaseous exchange and the fish become lethargic and anorexic. Dry feeds that have been stored for extended periods of time or exposed to high temperatures are usually the cause of the problem. Fortunately, the condition appears to be reversible with the use of fresh feed, although recovery may be a gradual process. Although this specific problem has not been reported in pet fish, it is assumed that the same type of pathology would occur if pet or ornamental fish were fed a diet deficient in pantothenic acid.

In addition to being nutritionally deficient in some cases, fish food can also become contaminated with various toxic agents including mycotoxins, pesticides, and herbicides, leading to toxicities in fish. For example, aflatoxin, a mycotoxin produced by *Aspergillus* sp, has been shown to cause necrotic changes in the gills.[68]

Neoplastic diseases

Neoplasia of the gills and the surrounding tissue is a relatively rare occurrence.[3,69] The consequence to respiration depends on the location and size of the lesion, degree of invasiveness, and/or mechanical interference of respiration. Papillomas, squamous cell carcinomas, chondromas, branchioblastomas, and pseudobranchial adenomas have all been reported to occur in multiple fish species.[3,69,70] Thyroid hyperplasia can cause compression of the gills and distension of the opercula.[4] **Fig. 18** shows a koi, *Cyprinus carpio*, with a neoplastic mass in the gill cavity.

Miscellaneous diseases and conditions

There are several other situations that can involve the gills and affect respiration and disease susceptibility. Missing or deformed opercula can be a result of a genetic defect, traumatic injury, and deficiencies of Vitamins A and C (**Fig. 19**).[3,71,72] In one article, osseous metaplasia caused swelling of the gills in a goldfish, *C auratus*.[73] Many species of ornamental fish root in the pond or aquaria substrate. Occasionally, a piece of substrate can become lodged in the oral cavity or pharyngeal region causing signs of respiratory distress owing to interference of the normal gill and opercula function (**Fig. 20**).[3]

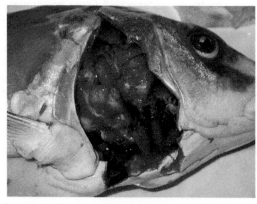

Fig. 18. A neoplastic mass in the branchial cavity of a koi (*Cyprinus carpio*). (*Courtesy of* Dr T. Miller-Morgan.)

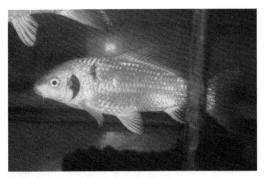

Fig. 19. Opercular defect in a koi (*Cyprinus carpio*).

TREATMENT OF RESPIRATORY DISORDERS IN FISH

Treatment of respiratory disorders requires an accurate diagnosis and understanding of the role any environmental disorders may have. Inaccurate diagnoses can delay appropriate treatment and risk increasing morbidity in the population. Many treatments used to treat ornamental and pet fish are not approved by the US Food and Drug Administration, thus the client should be informed of any known adverse effects, and consent to treat should be obtained before instituting therapy. Water or immersion-type treatments should be closely monitored for any adverse reactions in the fish or the biofiltration system. Some treatments also have the potential to cause gill irritation or toxicity. In the treatment of parasitic diseases, it is recommended not to bypass the filtration system because of the possible hidden presence of life stages "hiding" in the filtration system. Supplemental aeration is recommended whenever possible to maximize respiratory efficiency. When fish have been removed to a newly set-up hospital or isolation tank for treatment, there is a possibility of water quality abnormalities developing from a nonactivated filter that can lead to a worsening of the clinical signs. Routine water quality monitoring is needed in these systems.

Medications commonly used in the treatment of diseases of the gills can be found in **Table 2**.

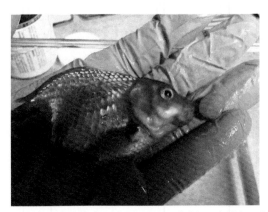

Fig. 20. Piece of gravel removed from the pharynx of this goldfish exhibiting respiratory distress.

Table 2
Formulary for the treatment of selected respiratory diseases in fish[a]

Condition(s)	Treatment[a]	Dosage(s)	Comments
Bacterial diseases			
	Amikacin[40,72]	5 mg/kg IM q 12 h	Has not been studied pharmacokinetically in pet fish, used frequently by hobbyists
	Aztreonam[40,72]	100 mg/kg IM, ICe q 48 h	Used by koi hobbyists
	Ceftazidime[73]	20–30 mg/kg IM q 72 h	Not studied pharmacokinetically in pet fish Used commonly by fish veterinarians
	Enrofloxacin[35,73–75]	5–10 mg/kg IM, ICe q 48–72 h 5 mg/kg PO every 24–48 h 2.5 mg/L × 5 h every 24–48 h	Only studied pharmacokinetically in koi and pacu, but used commonly by fish veterinarians in many species Resistance becoming an issue in bacterial infections in koi
	Florfenicol[76–78]	Red Pacu: 20–30 mg/kg IM q 24 h Koi: 25 mg/kg q 24–48 h; shorter half-life in three-spot gourami may necessitate more frequent dosing 50 mg/kg PO q 24 h in koi; shorter half-life in gourami may necessitate q 12-h dosing Minimal absorption as bath treatment in koi[77]	Studied pharmacokinetically in red pacu, koi, and three-spot gourami Available in food as a veterinary feed directive (VFD) (Aquaflor) with specific legal constraints. Cannot be prescribed for extralabel use
	Hydrogen peroxide 35% (35% Perox-Aid)[78,79]		FDA approved for use for bacterial gill disease and columnaris disease in specific species
	Oxytetracycline[35,80–82]	7 mg/kg IM q 24 h 1.12 g/lb food/d for 10 d 750–3780 mg/10 gallons for 6–12 h, repeat daily for 10 d (dose will depend on hardness of water) 50%–75% water changes between treatments[35]	Studied pharmacokinetically in red pacu Increased Ca and Mg inactivate, not useful in marine systems as bath treatment Available as a medicated food, Terramycin 200 for fish Water can become yellow with use of oxytetracycline Bacterial resistance common

	Sulfadimethoxine/ ormethoprim[40,72,82]	50 mg/kg/d for 5 d	Not useful as bath treatment Not studied pharmacokinetically in pet fish Medicated feed available (Romet B, Romet-30)
Fungal diseases			
	Formalin[73,78,83,84]	(See section on parasites for dosing information)	
	Hydrogen peroxide 35%[78,79]	Egg treatment: 500–1000 mg/L dip for 15 min	A trial bioassay is recommended before widespread use
	[a]Malachite green[44,58,73,84-86]	1–2 mg/L 30–60-min bath treatment 0.1 mg/L prolonged immersion 0.5 mg/L 60-min bath 0.3 mg/L 24-h bath 100 mg/L topical application	Carcinogenic, teratogenic, respiratory poison, and stains objects Can be toxic to gill tissue Reported toxicity in eggs near hatching, small marine fish, young fry, some tetra, catfish, scaleless fish, loach species, and plants Toxicity enhanced with warmer water temperatures and low pH Can be toxic when combined with formalin Use zinc-free solution Remove from water with activated carbon Rinse after topical application
	Sodium chloride[58]	10–50 g/L for 1–2 min bath	Kills the infectious zoospore, not the fungal hyphae on the fish
Parasitic diseases			
Freshwater external protozoan parasites	Sodium chloride solution ("saltwater," hypersalinity treatment)[40,87]	3–6 g/L prolonged immersion 10–30 g/L dip (5–10 min or until fish is stressed)	Can also reduce osmoregulatory stress Dip is often used in quarantine protocols
Freshwater external protozoan and crustacean ectoparasites Fungal diseases (saprolegniasis)	Formalin (37% formaldehyde)[73,78,83,84]	0.125–0.25 mL/L Bath q 24 h × 2–3 days for up to 60 min 0.015–0.025 mL/L (15–25 ppm) prolonged immersion, every 2–3 d	Carcinogenic, human health concerns *Depletes oxygen*, additional aeration required Some fish very sensitive Not for use in stressed fish

(continued on next page)

Table 2
(continued)

Condition(s)	Treatment[a]	Dosage(s)	Comments
	Formalin (cont.)		Toxicity enhanced with low water pH and low alkalinity Do not use if white precipitate forms Contraindicated >27°C (80°F) Toxic to invertebrates
External protozoan, dinoflagellate, monogenean, and crustacean pathogens of marine and freshwater fish	Hydrogen peroxide 35%	50–100 mg/L for 30–60 min for 3 consecutive days	Investigational claims can be evaluated at: http://www.fws.gov/fisheries/aadap/summaryHistory11-669.htm (AADAP = Aquatic Animal Drug Approval Program)
Marine protozoan ectoparasites and some monogenean infestations	Freshwater (hyposalinity)[87]	Dip (duration in minutes)	Not effective against all protozoans A common quarantine procedure
Marine protozoan ectoparasites and dinoflagellates	Copper[40,84]	0.2 mg/L free copper ion prolonged immersion 100 mg/L bath	Not recommended for freshwater systems Bound to inorganic compounds Toxic to invertebrates Elasmobranchs may react adversely Copper levels should be monitored Solubility affected by pH and alkalinity Immunosuppressive and toxic to gill tissue

External infections ectoparasites (protozoan, monogeneans)	Potassium permanganate[40]	2 mg/L prolonged immersion 5–20 mg/L 1-h bath	Inactivated by organic compounds in water Caustic Toxic in high pH water Stains Can be toxic in some fish species Can cause blindness in humans (powder) Watch for signs of stress in patients with use Safer products are available
Monogenean	Closantel 5 mg/mL and mebendazole 75 mg/mL (Supaverm, Janssen Animal Health)[40,59]	1 mL/400 L bath treatment	Caution-Koi ONLY! Fatal to goldfish. Not studied pharmacokinetically in fish Not FDA approved, not commercially available in the United States Used by hobbyists
Monogenean	Praziquantel[35,40,73]	2–10 mg/L bath or prolonged immersion once weekly for 3–6 treatments	Treatment frequency and duration is determined by species of monogenean and water temperature
Dinoflagellates	Chloroquine[40]	10 mg/L prolonged immersion	Affects only the infectious dinospore stage Toxic to bacteria and invertebrates
General treatments			
	Sodium chloride	1 g/L prolonged immersion	Reduction of stress, nitrite toxicity
	Water changes		Indicated for environmental toxins (ammonia, copper, nitrite)

Abbreviations: FDA, Food and Drug Administration; ICe, intracoelomic; IM, intramuscularly; PO, by mouth; q, every.
[a] Some compounds should not be recommended for use by a veterinarian but are included here for completeness and because of their frequent use by laymen.

SUMMARY

The respiratory organ of fish is the gill. In addition to respiration, the gills also perform functions of acid-base regulation, osmoregulation, and excretion of nitrogenous compounds. Because of their intimate association with the environment, the gills are often the primary target organ of pollutants, poor water quality, infectious disease agents, and noninfectious problems, making examination of the gills essential to the complete examination of sick individual fish and fish populations. The degree of response of the gill tissue depends on type, severity, and degree of injury and functional changes will precede morphologic changes. Antemortem tests and water quality testing can and should be performed on clinically affected fish whenever possible.

REFERENCES

1. Evans DH, Piermarini PM, Choe KP. The multi-functional fish gill: dominant site of gas exchange, osmoregulation, acid-base regulation, and excretion of nitrogenous waste. Physiol Rev 2005;85:97–177.
2. Speare DJ, Ferguson HW. Gills and pseudobranchs. In: Ferguson HW, editor. Systemic pathology of fish: a text and atlas of normal tissues in teleosts and their responses in disease. 2nd edition. London: Scotian Press; 2006. p. 25–62.
3. Childs S, Whitaker BR. Respiratory disease. In: Wildgoose WH, editor. BSAVA manual of ornamental fish. 2nd edition. Gloucester (UK): British Small Animal Veterinary Association; 2001. p. 135–46.
4. Reavill D, Roberts H. Diagnostic cytology of fish. Vet Clin North Am Exotic Anim Pract 2007;10:207–34.
5. Roberts HE, Weber ES III, Smith SA. Nonlethal diagnostic techniques. In: Roberts HE, editor. Fundamentals of ornamental fish health. Ames (IA): Wiley-Blackwell; 2009. p. 172–84.
6. Smith SA. Nonlethal clinical techniques used in the diagnosis of diseases of fish. J Am Vet Med Assoc 2002;220:1203–6.
7. Stoskopf M. Anatomy. In: Stoskopf M, editor. Fish medicine. Philadelphia: WB Saunders; 1993. p. 2–30.
8. Evans DH. The fish gill: site of action and model for toxic effects of environmental pollutants. Environ Health Perspect 1987;71:47–58.
9. Strange RJ. Anatomy and physiology. In: Roberts HE, editor. Fundamentals of ornamental fish health. Ames (IA): Wiley-Blackwell; 2009. p. 5–24.
10. Ellis AE, Roberts RJ. The anatomy and physiology of teleosts. In: Roberts RJ, editor. Fish pathology. 3rd edition. London: WB Saunders; 2001. p. 12–54.
11. Nilsson GE. Commentary: gill remodeling in fish—a new fashion or an ancient secret? J Exp Biol 2007;210:2404–9.
12. Bernal D, Dickson KA, Shadwick RE, et al. Review: analysis of the evolutionary convergence for high performance swimming in lamnid sharks and tunas. Comp Biochem Physiol 2001;129:695–726.
13. Law M. When the gas won't pass: pathology of the gills. Presentation of the Eastern Fish Health Continuing Education Session. Shepherdstown (WV), May 28, 2010.
14. Taylor EW, Leite CA, McKenzie DJ, et al. Control of respiration in fish, amphibians, and reptiles. Braz J Med Biol Res 2010;43:409–24.
15. Evans DH, Piermarini PM, Choe KP. The multi-functional fish gill: dominant site of gas exchange, osmoregulation, acid-base regulation, and excretion of nitrogenous waste. Physiol Rev 2005;85:97–177. Supplemental movies. Available at: http://physrev.physiology.org/content/vol85/issue1/images/data/97/DC1/Filflow.mp4;

http://physrev.physiology.org/content/vol85/issue1/images/data/97/DC1/ETeffect. mp4. Accessed September 22, 2010.

16. Stoskopf M. Clinical physiology. In: Stoskopf M, editor. Fish medicine. Philadelphia: WB Saunders; 1993. p. 48–57.
17. Hill JE, Baldwin JD, Graves JS, et al. Preliminary observations of topical gill application of reproductive hormones for induced spawning of a tropical ornamental fish. N Am J Aquacult 2005;67:7–9.
18. Ross LG, Ross B. Anaesthesia of fish: I. Inhalation anaesthesia. In: Ross LG, Ross B, editors. Anaesthetic and sedative techniques for aquatic animals. 3rd edition. Oxford: Blackwell Publishing; 2008. p. 69–126.
19. Stoskopf M. Taxonomy and natural history of freshwater tropical fishes. In: Stoskopf M, editor. Fish medicine. Philadelphia: WB Saunders; 1993. p. 534–9.
20. Beleau M. Taxonomy and natural history of catfishes. In: Stoskopf M, editor. Fish medicine. Philadelphia: WB Saunders; 1993. p. 494–5.
21. Randle AM, Chapman LJ. Habitat use by the African anabantid fish *Ctenopoma muriei*: implications for costs of air breathing. Ecol Freshw Fish 2004;13:37–45.
22. Roberts JL. Active branchial and ram ventilation in fishes. Biol Bull 1975;148: 85–105.
23. Ross LG, Ross B. Defining stress in aquatic animals. In: Ross LG, Ross B, editors. Anaesthetic and sedative techniques for aquatic animals. 3rd edition. Oxford: Blackwell Publishing; 2008. p. 7–21.
24. Noga EJ. Problems 10-42. In: Noga EJ, editor. Fish disease: diagnosis and treatment. St Louis (MO): Mosby; 1996. p. 75–138.
25. Greenwell MG, Sherrill J, Clayton LA. Osmoregulation in fish. Mechanisms and clinical implications. Vet Clin North Am Exot Anim Pract 2003;6:169–89.
26. Harper C, Wolf JC. Morphologic effects of the stress response in fish. ILAR J 2009;50(4):387–96.
27. Pasnik D, Evans JJ, Klesius PH. Stress in fish. In: Roberts HE, editor. Fundamentals of ornamental fish health. Ames (IA): Wiley-Blackwell; 2009. p. 33–8.
28. Sandblom E, Axelsson M. Review. The venous circulation: a piscine perspective. Comp Biochem Physiol 2007;148(A):785–801.
29. Stecyk JAW, Farrell AP. Cardiorespiratory responses of the common carp (*Cyprinus carpio*) to severe hypoxia at three acclimation temperatures. J Exp Biol 2002; 205:759–68.
30. Cecil T. Environmental disorders. In: Wildgoose WH, editor. BSAVA manual of ornamental fish. 2nd edition. Gloucester (UK): British Small Animal Veterinary Association; 2001. p. 205–12.
31. Mitrovic D, Dymowska A, Nilsson G, et al. Physiological consequences of gill remodeling in goldfish (*Carassius auratus*) during exposure to long-term hypoxia. Am J Physiol Regul Integr Comp Physiol 2009;297:R224–34.
32. Butcher RL. General approach. In: Wildgoose WH, editor. BSAVA manual of ornamental fish. 2nd edition. Gloucester (UK): British Small Animal Veterinary Association; 2001. p. 63–7.
33. Roberts HE. History. In: Roberts HE, editor. Fundamentals of ornamental fish health. Ames (IA): Wiley-Blackwell; 2009. p. 158–60.
34. Lowry T, Smith S. Aquatic zoonoses associated with food, bait, ornamental, and tropical fish. J Am Vet Med Assoc 2007;231(6):876–80.
35. Sherrill J, Weber ES, Marty GD, et al. Fish cardiovascular physiology and disease. Vet Clin North Am Exot Anim Pract 2009;12:11–38.
36. Clauss TM, Dove AD, Arnold JE. Hematological disorders of fish. Vet Clin North Am Exot Anim Pract 2008;11:445–62.

37. Groff JM, Zinkl JG. Hematology and clinical chemistry of cyprinid fish: common carp and goldfish. Vet Clin North Am Exot Anim Pract 1999;2:741–76.

38. Stoskopf M. Clinical pathology of carp, goldfish, and koi. In: Stoskopf M, editor. Fish medicine. Philadelphia: WB Saunders; 1993. p. 450–3.

39. Nelson K, Jones J, Jacobson S, et al. Elevated blood urea nitrogen (BUN) levels in goldfish as an indicator of gill dysfunction. J Aqua Anim Health 1999; 11:52–60.

40. Roberts HE, Palmeiro BP. Bacterial and parasitic diseases of pet fish. Vet Clin North Am Exot Anim Pract 2009;12:609–38.

41. Smith SA, Roberts HE. Parasites of fish. In: Roberts HE, editor. Fundamentals of ornamental fish health. Ames (IA): Wiley-Blackwell; 2009. p. 102–12.

42. Longshaw M, Feist S. Parasitic diseases. In: Wildgoose WH, editor. BSAVA manual of ornamental fish health. 2nd edition. Gloucester (UK): BSAVA; 2001. p. 167–83.

43. Weber ES III, Govett P. Parasitology and necropsy of fish. Compend Contin Educ Vet 2009;31:E1–7.

44. Roberts HE. Fungal diseases in fish. In: Roberts HE, editor. Fundamentals of ornamental fish health. Ames (IA): Wiley-Blackwell; 2009. p. 137–43.

45. Molnar K. *Myxobolus intrachondrealis* sp. n. (Myxosporea: Myxobolidae), a parasite of the gill cartilage of the common carp, *Cyprinus carpio*. Folia Parasitol 2000; 47:167–71.

46. Noga EJ. Problems 44-54. In: Noga EJ, editor. Fish disease: diagnosis and treatment. St Louis (MO): Mosby; 1996. p. 75–138.

47. Woo PT, Bruno DW. Viral, bacterial and fungal infections. In: Fish diseases and disorders, vol. 3. 2nd edition. Oxfordshire (UK): CABI, Inc; 2010. p. 1000.

48. Smith SA. Mycobacterial infections in pet fish. Semin Avian Exot Pet 1997;6:40–5.

49. Palmeiro B, Weber ES. Viral pathogens of fish. In: Roberts HE, editor. Fundamentals of ornamental fish health. Ames (IA): Wiley-Blackwell; 2009. p. 113–24.

50. Goodwin AE, Sadler J, Merry GE, et al. Herpesviral haematopoietic necrosis virus (CyHV-2) infection: case studies from commercial goldfish farms. J Fish Dis 2009; 32:271–8.

51. Jeffery KR, Bateman K, Feist SW, et al. Isolation of a cyprinid herpesvirus 2 from goldfish, *Carassius auratus* (L.), in the UK. J Fish Dis 2007;30:649–56.

52. Goodwin AE, Merry GE, Sadler J. Detection of the herpesviral haematopoietic necrosis disease agent (*Cyprinid herpesvirus 2*) in moribund and healthy goldfish: validation of a quantitative PCR diagnostic method. Dis Aquat Org 2006; 69:137–43.

53. St-Hilaire S, Beevers N, Way K, et al. Reactivation of koi herpesvirus infections in common carp *Cyprinus carpio*. Dis Aquat Org 2005;67:15–23.

54. Szignarowitz BA. Update on koi herpesvirus. Exotic DVM 2005;7(3):92–5.

55. Haramoto E, Kitajima M, Katayama H, et al. Detection of koi herpesvirus DNA in river water in Japan. J Fish Dis 2007;30:59–61.

56. Sadler J, Marecaux E, Goodwin AE. Detection of koi herpesvirus (CyHV-3) in goldfish, *Carassius auratus* (L.), exposed to infected koi. J Fish Dis 2008;31:71–2.

57. Yanong RP. Emerging viral diseases of fish. Talk at Western Veterinary Conference 2009; 2009; Las Vegas (NV). Available at: http://www.vin.com/Members/Proceedings/Proceedings.plx?CID=wvc2009&PID=pr51233&O=VIN. Accessed October 24, 2010.

58. Weber ES, Waltzek TB, Young DA, et al. Systemic iridovirus infection in the Banggai cardinalfish (*Pterapogon kauderni* Koumans 1933). J Vet Diagn Invest 2009; 21:306–20.

59. Khoo L. Fungal diseases in fish. Semin Avian Exot Pet Med 2000;9:102–11.
60. Yanong RPE. Fungal diseases of fish. Vet Clin North Am Exot Anim Pract 2003;6: 377–400.
61. Noga EJ. Problems 1-9. In: Noga EJ, editor. Fish disease: diagnosis and treatment. St Louis (MO): Mosby; 1996. p. 55–74.
62. Roberts HE, Palmeiro BP. Toxicology of aquarium fish. Vet Clin North Am Exot Anim Pract 2008;11:359–74.
63. Mahjoor AA, Loh R. Some histopathological aspects of chlorine toxicity in rainbow trout (Oncorhynchus mykiss). Asian J Anim Vet Adv 2008;3(5):303–6.
64. Noga EJ. Problems 79-88. In: Noga EJ, editor. Fish disease: diagnosis and treatment. St Louis (MO): Mosby; 1996. p. 221–43.
65. Yonkos LT, Fisher DJ, Wright DA, et al. Pathology of fathead minnows (Pimephales promelas) exposed to chlorine dioxide and chlorite. Mar Environ Res 2000;50:267–71.
66. Karges RG, Woodward B. Development of lamellar epithelial hyperplasia in gills of pantothenic acid-deficient rainbow trout, Salmo gairdneri (Richardson). J Fish Biol 1984;25:57–62.
67. Wilson RP, Bowser PR, Poe WE. Dietary pantothenic acid requirement of fingerling channel catfish. J Nutr 1983;113(10):2124–8.
68. Sahoo PK, Mukherjee SC, Nayak SK, et al. Acute and subchronic toxicity of aflatoxin B1 to rohu, Labeo rohita (Hamilton). Indian J Exp Biol 2001;39(5):453–8.
69. Groff JM. Neoplasia in fishes. Vet Clin North Am Exot Anim Pract 2004;7:705–56.
70. Reavill DR. Neoplasia in fish. In: Roberts HE, editor. Fundamentals of ornamental fish health. Ames (IA): Wiley-Blackwell; 2009. p. 204–13.
71. Fracalossi DM, Allen ME, Nichols DK, et al. Oscars, Astronotus ocellatus, have a dietary requirement for vitamin C. J Nutr 1998;128:1745–51.
72. Al-Harbi AH. Skeletal deformities in cultured common carp Cyprinus carpio L. Asian Fish Sci 2001;14:247–54.
73. Govett PD, Rotstein DS, Lewbart GA. Gill metaplasia in a goldfish, Carassius auratus auratus (L). J Fish Dis 2004;27:419–23.
74. Mashima T, Lewbart GA. Pet fish formulary. Vet Clin North Am Exot Anim Pract 2000;3(1):117–30.
75. Carpenter JW. Fish. In: Exotic animal formulary. 2nd edition. Philadelphia: WB Saunders; 2001. p. 1–21.
76. Lewbart GA, Butkus D, Papich M, et al. Evaluation of a method of intracoelomic catheterization in koi. J Am Vet Med Assoc 2005;226:784–8.
77. Lewbart GA, Papich MG, Whitt-Smith D. Pharmacokinetics of florfenicol in the red pacu (Paractus brachypomus) after single dose intramuscular administration. J Vet Pharmacol Ther 2005;28:317–9.
78. Lewbart GA, Vaden S, Deen J, et al. Pharmacokinetics of enrofloxacin in the red pacu (Colossoma brachypomum) after intramuscular, oral and bath administration. J Vet Pharmacol Ther 1997;20:124–8.
79. Yanong RP, Curtis EW, Simmons R, et al. Pharmacokinetic studies of florfenicol in koi carp and threespot gourami Trichogaster trichopterus after oral and intramuscular treatment. J Aqua Anim Health 2005;17:129–37.
80. Federal Drug Administration (FDA). List of approved drugs in aquaculture. Available at: http://www.fda.gov/AnimalVeterinary/DevelopmentApprovalProcess/Aquaculture/ucm132954.htm. Accessed September 23, 2010.
81. 35% Perox-Aid [Package drug insert]. Western Chemical Inc. Available at: http://www.wchemical.com/Assets/File/35peroxAid_instructions.pdf. Accessed September 23, 2010.

82. Yanong R. Use of antibiotics in ornamental fish aquaculture. VM-84. Florida Cooperative Extension Service, UF-IFAS 2006. Available at: http://edis.ifas.ufl.edu/fa084. Accessed September 23, 2010.

83. Doi AM, Stoskopf MK, Lewbart GA. Pharmacokinetics of oxytetracycline in the red pacu following different routes of administration. J Vet Pharmacol Ther 1998;21:364–8.

84. Durborow R, Francis-Floyd R. Medicated feed for food fish. SRAC-473, Southeast Regional Aquaculture Center 1996. Available at: http://aquanic.org/publicat/usda_rac/efs/srac/473fs.pdf. Accessed September 23, 2010.

85. Parasite-S [Package drug insert]. Available at: http://www.wchemical.com/Assets/file/Parasite-S_Insert2009.pdf. Accessed October 1, 2010.

86. Wildgoose WH, Lewbart GA. Therapeutics. In: Wildgoose WH, editor. BSAVA manual of ornamental fish health. 2nd edition. Gloucester (UK): BSAVA; 2001. p. 237–58.

87. Holliman A. Fungal diseases and harmful algae. In: Wildgoose WH, editor. BSAVA manual of ornamental fish health. 2nd edition. Gloucester (UK): BSAVA; 2001. p. 195–200.

Respiratory Medicine of Reptiles

Juergen Schumacher, Dr. Med. Vet., DACZM, DECZM (Herpetology)

KEYWORDS

- Respiratory disease • Reptile • Treatment • Diagnosis
- Tortoise • Lizard • Snake

Respiratory tract disease is commonly diagnosed in captive reptiles and, in most cases, should be considered a multifactorial disease. Often pet reptiles are kept in suboptimal environmental conditions (eg, inadequate humidity and temperature), resulting in an immunocompromised animal being highly susceptible to a variety of respiratory pathogens. The absence of a quarantine program also allows introduction of infectious agents into an established collection of reptiles. Infectious agents associated with respiratory tract disease in reptiles include viral, bacterial, fungal, and parasitic organisms. Noninfectious causes may include trauma, foreign bodies, inhalation of toxic fumes, and neoplasia. In many cases, clinical signs of respiratory tract disease are initially subtle, slow to develop, and may not be recognized by the owner. Therefore, most reptiles are presented with chronic upper and/or lower respiratory tract disease. However, acute respiratory distress does occur and presents an emergency situation. To provide effective therapy, identification and correction of the underlying cause is essential.

The veterinary practitioner should have a good knowledge and understanding of the reptilian respiratory anatomy and physiology. Respiratory disease may be the primary disease or may have developed secondary to other disease processes such as stomatitis. In reptiles, the initial approach in the diagnosis of respiratory disease follows the same principles known from domestic animals. However, diagnostic investigations such as advanced imaging modalities, interpretation of diagnostic tests, as well as treatment protocols often need to be modified in reptiles. The pathophysiology of respiratory tract disease differs considerably from mammals. Reptiles commonly respond differently to therapeutic regimens, including drugs, compared with mammals. As in domestic species, it is essential to determine the causative agent(s) for respiratory disease in order to design an effective treatment protocol. If indicated, environmental inadequacies need to be corrected to ensure optimal response to treatment of the patient.

Preventive measures are a key factor to reduce the development of respiratory disease in reptiles. Adequate environmental conditions should be provided, including

Avian and Zoological Medicine Service, Department of Small Animal Clinical Sciences, College of Veterinary Medicine, The University of Tennessee, Knoxville, TN 37996-4544, USA
E-mail address: jschumacher@utk.ekdu

Vet Clin Exot Anim 14 (2011) 207–224
doi:10.1016/j.cvex.2011.03.010
1094-9194/11/$ – see front matter © 2011 Elsevier Inc. All rights reserved.

appropriate temperature, humidity, and nutrition. An effective quarantine protocol is essential to prevent introduction of sick or carrier animals into an established collection. During quarantine, which should last minimally 90 days, every reptile should have a thorough physical examination, including collection of a venous blood sample for hematologic and plasma biochemical determinations and fecal screens. Apparently sick animals should never be introduced into an established collection.

Pulmonary anatomy and function may differ considerably between orders of reptiles as well as between genus and family.[1–3] Reviews are available on reptile respiratory tract disease and information on diagnostic techniques and therapeutics has been published.[4–10] This article outlines anatomic and physiologic characteristics of the reptilian respiratory tract, and presents common causes, clinical signs, diagnostic procedures, and treatment of respiratory tract disease in reptiles. Future investigations are needed to clearly understand normal respiratory physiology as well as the pathophysiology of respiratory tract disease in common reptile species. In addition, drugs and dosage regimens need to be established for the effective and safe treatment of reptiles diagnosed with respiratory tract disease.

ANATOMY AND PHYSIOLOGY OF THE RESPIRATORY TRACT

Reptile respiratory anatomy and physiology differ considerably from mammalian and avian species. Differences in the morphology and function of the respiratory system are found between orders of reptiles and have also been described between species from the same order.[2,3] The unique reptilian respiratory anatomy and physiology has been reviewed previously.[7,9,10] Although anatomic differences of the reptilian respiratory system have been described, the terminology used for the description of pulmonary structures is inconsistent.[2] These differences have to be accounted for in order to design an appropriate diagnostic work-up as well as to formulate an effective treatment protocol.

Reptiles lack a diaphragm and therefore the force to move air during inspiration and expiration comes from movement of respiratory muscles such as the intercostal, pectoral, and abdominal musculature causing changes in intrapulmonary pressure. Comparable with mammalian and avian species, the reptile respiratory tract is divided into an upper and a lower part.

In snakes, air passes through the external nares, the nasal sinuses, the internal nares, and enters the glottis from the buccal cavity.[11] The rostral position of the glottis ensures respiration while swallowing large prey items. The trachea consists of incomplete cartilaginous rings and bifurcates into short bronchi at the level of the heart. Some snake species have a tracheal lung consisting of vascularized respiratory tissue.[11] The lungs are elongated, saclike structures. In most snake species, the left lung is either absent or vestigial. Boid snakes have a left and right lung; however, the left lung is smaller. The right lung is lined with respiratory epithelium that caudally changes into a nonrespiratory epithelium and functions as an air sac. In contrast with terrestrial species, the lungs of aquatic snakes are most developed, facilitating efficient gas exchange during prolonged periods of apnea during dives.

In chelonians, air enters through the nares and passes through the nasal cavities, which are lined by olfactory and mucosal epithelium.[8,12] The glottis of chelonians is located at the base of the tongue and is difficult to visualize in an awake animal. In contrast with snakes and lizards, the trachea is short, consists of complete tracheal rings, and bifurcates into a left and right intrapulmonary bronchus at the level of the thoracic inlet. Chelonians have multichambered lungs located underneath the carapace. The lungs are rigid and may extend caudally to the cranial pole of the kidneys.

In lizards, the glottis is located more rostrally in carnivorous species, whereas, in herbivorous animals, it is located caudally at the base of the tongue. Lizards have incomplete tracheal rings and, similar to snakes, the trachea bifurcates approximately at the base of the heart. The lungs of most lizard species are saclike, single-chambered structures and may extend caudally into an avascular airsac, occupying a major portion of the coelomic cavity. Iguanids have a short intrapulmonary bronchus and possess multichambered lungs consisting of a small anterior chamber and a large posterior chamber. Agamid lizards lack an intrapulmonary bronchus.[2]

In crocodilians, the glottis is located behind the epiglottal flap, which seals the oral cavity while the animal is submerged, thus allowing the animal to open the mouth while being underwater. The complex, well-developed lungs of crocodilians are multichambered and the bronchi branch into multiple internal lobes.

Respiratory physiology of reptiles differs considerably between orders and species, and the most pronounced differences are found between terrestrial and aquatic species. The major organ for gas exchange is the lung, but species such as aquatic snakes and turtles are also capable of gas exchange across pharyngeal and cloacal mucosa, and the skin. Studies have shown that cutaneous gas exchange is most important in the elimination of CO_2 rather than the uptake of O_2. Some species of sea snakes (*Pelamis platurus*) eliminate approximately 74% of CO_2 via cutaneous gas exchange.[3] Reptiles, especially aquatic species, are capable of converting to anaerobic metabolism during prolonged periods of apnea.

In comparison with mammals, reptiles have larger lung volumes independent of their structural type,[2] whereas the surface area for gas exchange is approximately 20% of a mammal of comparative body mass. Although reptilian lungs have high compliance values, the work of breathing is lower and therefore reptiles increase their minute volume by increasing their respiratory rate.

Control of ventilation in reptiles is different from mammalian and avian species. In contrast with mammalian respiratory physiology, in which high carbon dioxide concentrations stimulate respiration, reptilian respiration is controlled by hypoxia and hypercapnia, as well as environmental temperature. Many species differences exist, depending on their environmental adaptations. Different receptors cause an increase in ventilation during periods of low O_2 and high CO_2. In tortoises, respiratory rate increases during hypercapnia but decreases during hypoxia.[3] In most reptile species, hypercapnia causes increases in tidal volume, whereas periods of hypoxia increase respiratory rate. The stimulus to breath in reptiles comes from low oxygen concentrations. The higher demand for oxygen during increased temperature or following prolonged dives in aquatic species is met by increasing the tidal volume and not the respiratory rate. Exposure of a reptile to high concentrations of inspired oxygen decreases ventilation, including a decrease in respiratory rate and tidal volume. As mentioned earlier, reptiles have the ability to tolerate varying degrees of hypoxia and are capable of converting to anaerobic metabolism. Intrapulmonary shunts, representing the portion of pulmonary blood bypassing gas exchange, have been observed in reptiles. Shunts are most developed in Testudines and sea snakes, and increases with reduced lung volumes. Large intrapulmonary shunts reduce the efficiency of gas exchange in the lungs and consequently result in a reduction of arterial Po_2 concentrations.[3]

CAUSES

Both infectious and noninfectious causes have been associated with respiratory tract disease in reptiles.[7,9] In many patients, respiratory tract disease is multifactorial and environmental inadequacies as well as mixed infectious causes have to be considered. Bacterial organisms, especially gram-negative bacteria commonly isolated from reptiles with acute or chronic respiratory disease, are often opportunistic bacteria also found in healthy animals. However, in certain conditions, especially in an immunocompromised reptile, these organisms become primary pathogens. Signs of respiratory disease and compromise may also be caused by obesity, cardiac disease, coelomic effusions, as well as organomegaly.[7]

Noninfectious Diseases

Penetrating injuries to the lungs are often seen in lizards and snakes caused by bite wounds from other pets. Fractures of the carapace and subsequent injury to the underlying lung parenchyma are commonly found in chelonians hit by cars and lawn mowers as well as bite wounds.

In ball pythons (*Python regius*), cartilaginous granulomas have been reported originating from the tracheal cartilage rings.[13] Signs of respiratory distress including open-mouth breathing as well as anorexia have been reported in affected snakes. For diagnosis, radiography or endoscopic examination of the trachea should be performed.

Neoplasia within the major airways and the lungs has been reported infrequently. Its presence results in respiratory compromise depending on their size and location. Lymphoma has been described in snakes, lizards, and chelonians and is commonly associated with oral tissues and the lung.[14] Radiography, endoscopy, and advanced imaging modalities such as computed tomography (CT) are the most useful tools in the detection of space-occupying masses.

Foreign bodies are most commonly seen in lizards, especially in green iguanas (*Iguana iguana*) as well as in chelonians. Plastic objects may accidentally become lodged within the oropharynx, causing acute respiratory distress. Free-ranging aquatic turtles often present with a fishhook embedded within the oral cavity or the oropharynx. Trauma and inflammation of the surrounding tissue may result in a partial obstruction of the tracheal opening and severe respiratory compromise.

Infectious Diseases

Infectious agents play an important role in the causes of respiratory tract disease in reptiles. Viruses, bacteria, fungi, and parasites have been detected and associated with primary respiratory disease in reptiles.[4,5,8] Secondary bacterial infections may complicate the diagnosis of a primary viral pneumonia. A viral cause should be suspected in those patients who continue to exhibit signs of respiratory disease despite appropriate antimicrobial therapy. Serology, histopathology of biopsy specimen, viral isolation, or electron microscopy is indicated in these cases. As mentioned earlier, reptiles are often diagnosed with mixed infections of the respiratory tract such as bacterial and fungal pneumonia.

Viral

Herpesvirus infections causing upper or lower respiratory tract disease are commonly seen in chelonians. Chelonians diagnosed with herpesvirus infections include terrestrial and aquatic species, including marine turtles. Lung, eye, and trachea (LET) disease associated with a herpesvirus has been described in juvenile green sea turtles (*Chelonia mydas*).[15] European tortoises commonly infected with herpesvirus are Mediterranean (*Testudo graeca*) and Hermann (*Testudo hermanni*) tortoises.[16,17] Infected animals have been diagnosed in both Europe and the United States. Clinical signs of infected tortoises include stomatitis, rhinitis, tracheitis, and pneumonia.[8] In many tortoises, serous to purulent nasal and ocular discharge may be present. Infected tortoises are commonly anorectic and caseous, and necrotizing lesions are located within the oral cavity and the trachea. A diagnosis can be made by demonstration of intranuclear inclusions in cytologic or biopsy specimen, collected from oral lesions.

Ophidian paramyxovirus infection (OPMV) of snakes primarily affects viperid snakes, but nonviperid snakes have also been diagnosed with OPMV. Investigations in Europe and the United States have detailed the epidemiology, clinical and patho-logic findings, as well as viral characteristics.[18] Transmission of the virus is via respi-ratory secretions of infected snakes. Clinical signs are variable and include signs of respiratory tract disease such as stomatitis, open-mouth breathing, and nasal discharge. Purulent tracheal discharge may also be present. In advanced stages of the disease, signs of central nervous system disease may be seen. An interstitial pneu-monia and proliferation of lining epithelial cells are the most significant histologic find-ings. Serology is available to determine exposure of a snake to OPMV; however, no specific treatment is known.[18] Treatment should include supportive care such as anti-microbial therapy against secondary bacterial infections, fluid therapy, and nutritional support. Most importantly, preventative measures such as an effective quarantine program, screening of all incoming snakes, and isolation of infected and exposed animals is indicated to prevent introduction and transmission of OPMV through a collection.

Imported caiman lizards (*Dracaena guianensis*), have been diagnosed with prolifer-ative pneumonia associated with members of the Paramyxoviridae.[19] Clinical signs of infected caimans include anorexia, dehydration, and possible respiratory distress.

Inclusion body disease (IBD) of boid snakes is primarily associated with clinical signs of regurgitation, chronic wasting, and central nervous system disease. However, some snakes also exhibit signs of respiratory tract disease caused by secondary bacterial infections. Both upper and lower respiratory tract disease may be seen in infected snakes. An interstitial pneumonia with the presence of typical eosinophilic intracytoplasmic inclusion bodies in epithelial cells has been described in infected snakes.[20] There is no specific treatment of IBD, and isolation of infected and exposed snakes is recommended. Prevention is the most important factor and all new arrivals should be quarantined for at least 90 days and carefully screened before introduction into an established collection of boid snakes.

Bacterial

In reptiles, respiratory tract disease commonly has a bacterial cause. Bacterial organ-isms often isolated from reptiles with respiratory tract disease are gram-negative and part of the normal flora and the environment. Frequently isolated organisms include *Pseudomonas* spp, *Klebsiella* spp, *Proteus* spp, *Aeromonas* spp, *Salmonella* spp and *Staphylococcus* spp. Although these organisms can be part of the normal flora in a healthy reptile, isolation of these bacteria from a tracheal wash of a reptile with respiratory disease is an indication of a bacterial cause. Few bacterial organisms have been associated with primary respiratory infection; however, *Pasteurella testu-dines* has been isolated from desert tortoises (*Gopherus agassizii*) with pneumonia.[21] Anaerobic bacteria are rarely the primary cause for respiratory disease although *Fusobacterium* spp, *Clostridium* spp, and *Bacteroides* spp have been isolated from reptiles.[22] In some cases, both aerobic and anaerobic bacteria can be implicated for the development of respiratory disease.

Mycoplasmosis is an upper respiratory tract disease that has been described in captive and free-ranging populations of tortoises, especially California desert tortoises (*G agassizii*) and Florida gopher tortoises (*Gopherus polyphemus*).[8,12] A variety of other chelonian species, including pet reptiles as well as animals from large private and zoologic collections, have also been diagnosed with mycoplasma infection. Clinical signs of mycoplasmosis include conjunctivitis and serous to purulent nasal discharge. In chronic cases, erosive changes of the nares may be seen. Severely affected tortoises can be seen open-mouth breathing and are often anorectic. In captive tortoises, clinical signs seem to be more apparent in periods of stress caused by shipping, seasonal changes, or suboptimal husbandry. Supportive care measures include nutritional support, fluid therapy, as well as systemic and local administration of effective antimicrobial agents. Mycoplasmosis is a chronic infection and elimination of the organism may not be possible. Treatment of infected tortoises reduces or eliminates clinical symptoms, but infected animals should be considered carriers of the disease.

Fungal

Mycosis in reptiles is a common finding and the integument, gastrointestinal tract, and respiratory tract are most often infected. Fungal disease may be seen as a focal infection, such as cutaneous fungal granuloma, or as a systemic mycosis.[23] Systemic mycosis is often characterized by disseminated granulomas or pneumonia. Chelonians in particular seem to be more susceptible to the development of systemic mycosis.[23,24] Clinical findings include caseous, firm masses within the lung parenchyma of infected reptiles. In snakes, disseminated fungal disease including pneumonia is most often seen. Few reports have identified fungal organisms as a primary cause of respiratory disease in reptiles. Fungal elements are commonly isolated from sick reptiles and, in some cases, seem to be secondary invaders following bacterial infections. Improper husbandry practices such as too high or too low environmental temperature, high humidity levels within the enclosure, and chronic stress promote growth of fungal organisms. As mentioned earlier, chelonians seem to be more susceptible to fungal infections than other orders of reptiles and *Candida* spp, *Aspergillus* spp, and *Penicillium* spp have been isolated from chelonians with respiratory disease.[6,24] To confirm a diagnosis of fungal pneumonia, collection of a tracheal wash for cytology and culture, or endoscopy and collection of biopsies and specimen for culture are indicated. Demonstration of fungal hyphae or spores and culture of a fungal organism indicates fungal pneumonia.

Parasitic

Parasites can cause primary respiratory tract disease and are commonly accompanied by bacterial and fungal infections. Pentastomids have been described in wild and captive reptiles, especially in snakes.[25] Increased respiratory efforts can be seen, including open-mouth breathing and severe respiratory compromise caused by obstruction of major air passageways. To confirm a diagnosis, a tracheal wash and demonstration of ova or bronchoscopy are indicated. Because there is no effective chemical treatment, surgical removal of the worms is required. The zoonotic potential of this infection should also be considered before treatment.

High parasite loads of ascarids may also cause respiratory tract disease and confirmation of typical eggs within fecal material is diagnostic. *Kalicephalus* spp migrate through lung tissue, resulting in irritation of pulmonary tissue and subsequent secondary bacterial infections. *Rhabdias* spp, especially *Rhabdias fuscovenosa*, are found in the lung of infected snakes and their direct lifecycle results in high parasite loads if left untreated. Secondary bacterial infections as well as severe inflammatory responses result in pneumonia. Hookworm and lungworm infections are diagnosed by detection of larvae in a fecal or tracheal wash specimens.

CLINICAL SIGNS

In early stages of respiratory disease, clinical signs are often difficult to detect. Nonspecific signs such as lethargy, anorexia, and weight loss are often not recognized by owners. As mentioned earlier, respiratory tract disease in reptiles often has multifactorial causes. In some cases, signs of other organ disease may be more pronounced. Consequently, respiratory tract disease may not be diagnosed initially and treatment focuses on other organ systems. Respiratory disease may develop slowly in reptiles and many patients are presented with signs of chronic disease. Infected animals may be in severe respiratory distress, multiple organ systems may be affected, and the reptile may have developed septicemia.

In lizards, clinical signs of respiratory disease include nasal and ocular discharge, accompanied by rhinitis, conjunctivitis, and stomatitis. Bacterial oral abscesses may cause displacement of the glottis and severe dyspnea. Sneezing along with serous to mucoid discharge may also be present. In severe cases of pneumonia, increased respiratory efforts are often present.

In snakes, common clinical signs include serous to purulent nasal discharge, wheezing, accumulation of respiratory secretions within the oral cavity, and stomatitis. In severe cases, increased respiratory efforts and dyspnea are also present. Because snakes lack the mechanism to expel respiratory secretions from the trachea because of the lack of a functioning diaphragm, the presence of fluid within the trachea results in a decreased diameter of the tracheal lumen. Affected snakes can be seen open-mouth breathing and the front half of the body is extended to facilitate movement of air through the trachea.

In chelonians, nasal and ocular discharge, rhinitis, and conjunctivitis are often signs of upper respiratory disease. Tortoises with chronic upper respiratory tract disease often exhibit cutaneous erosion and depigmentation around the nares. Rhinitis in tortoises is often multifactorial and caused by a variety of gram-negative organisms.[26] Stomatitis, with the presence of necrotizing lesions and abscesses, may be present with both upper and lower respiratory tract disease. In severe and chronic cases, especially with obstructive processes as well as hypertrophy of upper respiratory tract epithelium, open-mouth breathing may be present. In aquatic species buoyancy problems and the inability of infected animals to dive may be observed. These signs are typically caused by unilateral or bilateral gas pockets within the lungs or consolidation of large areas of the lung parenchyma.

Many reptiles are presented with chronic respiratory tract disease and, at the time of presentation, additional diagnostic tests are required to fully elucidate the extent of respiratory disease, as well as other organ system function. In the author's opinion, septicemia is often not diagnosed in reptiles, resulting in incomplete treatment of the patient. A presumptive diagnosis of septicemia can be made by physical findings, whereas collection of a venous blood sample is required for culture and sensitivity testing for confirmation. In some cases, it is indicated to treat the animal with broad-spectrum antimicrobial agents for a suspected septicemia while laboratory results are pending.

CLINICAL EVALUATION AND DIAGNOSTIC TESTS

Clinical evaluation of any sick reptile should include a detailed history and thorough review of husbandry practices. If available, information on hygiene procedures and onset of clinical signs should be recorded. For larger reptile collections, quarantine procedures should also be reviewed. These measures should be followed by a visual examination and thorough physical examination. Particular attention should be paid to the respiratory tract.

A visual examination should assess overall body condition, mental status, and body posture, and particular attention should be paid to the respiratory status of the reptile. Mild signs of respiratory disease may include nasal and oral discharge as well as ocular discharge and conjunctivitis. Evidence of respiratory distress such as increased resting respiratory rate, labored breathing, and open-mouth breathing should be noted. A physical examination with attention to the respiratory tract should also include evaluation of other major organ systems. Nasal and ocular discharges, if present, should be evaluated and submitted for diagnostic testing such as cytology and culture. The nares and the oral cavity should be examined for signs of infection and obstructive processes. Sterile swabs can be used to collect samples for cytology and culture from these areas; however, some of the organisms isolated from a swab sample may present contaminants and may not be the disease-causing agents. Mucous membrane color should be evaluated as well as signs of cyanosis. Auscultation of the lungs is difficult in reptiles and often does not give the desired information. However, the pattern of respiration may be of diagnostic value in localizing the underlying cause. Collection of a venous blood sample for hematology and plasma biochemistries is recommended to identify organ system disease and to initiate effective supportive care measures including fluid therapy, nutritional support, and antimicrobial therapy. Appropriate diagnostic tests such as cytology, culture, radiography, endoscopy, and other advanced imaging modalities should be performed if indicated.

Imaging

In most patients, radiography is the initial imaging modality of choice for the detection of respiratory tract disease, especially in tortoises and lizards.[27,28] Radiography is required for the diagnosis and treatment of pulmonary disorders such as parenchymal disease and evaluation of masses. As indicated earlier, the morphology of the reptilian lung is different from mammalian lungs, therefore radiographic appearance is also different in reptiles. Especially in snakes and lizards, the lungs have more homogeneous radiopacity compared with mammalian lungs.[28] Dorsoventral views are often of limited diagnostic value because visualization of the lungs is commonly obscured by coelomic organs.[28] In lizards and snakes, standard views should be obtained, including a lateral and dorsoventral view. In snakes, radiography is of only limited value to assess the respiratory tract, unless severe pulmonary changes such as bacterial granulomas or neoplasia are present. In snakes, the lateral projection is most useful to identify areas of increased pulmonary opacities. In chelonians, 3 views are recommended to evaluate the respiratory tract, including a lateral, dorsoventral, and craniocaudal view (**Fig. 1**). The craniocaudal view allows for visualization of both lung fields, and interstitial and alveolar opacities can best be shown with this projection (**Fig. 2**). For all imaging modalities, it is essential to be familiar with the normal anatomy of the species evaluated, including location of the lungs and extent of the air sacs, to identify any abnormalities.

Ultrasonography is a useful adjunct to radiography and aids in the detection of discrete pulmonary masses. Ultrasonography offers the ability to noninvasively evaluate the morphology and extent of focal pulmonary changes such as granulomas and neoplasia. Diagnostic specimens such as aspirates and biopsies can be collected for cytology and culture with ultrasound guidance.

CT provides thin, cross-sectional images and the technique is noninvasive. Although scans are usually done in transverse directions, computer programs are capable of creating three-dimensional models of the images. CT has been used to

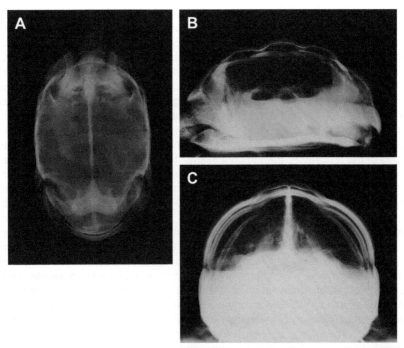

Fig. 1. Whole body radiographs of a clinically normal Burmese star tortoise (*Geochelone platynota*). Standard views include a dorsoventral (*A*), lateral (*B*), and anterior-posterior (*C*) projection. The anterior-posterior projection (*C*) allows visualization of both lung fields while the dorsoventral view (*A*) is of limited diagnostic value in the evaluation of the lower respiratory tract.

obtain images of reptilian respiratory organs.[29] In reptiles, CT scans can be collected from the upper respiratory tract to diagnose acute or chronic conditions within the nasal cavities and sinuses. CT can also be applied to diagnose pathologic conditions of the lung such as pneumonia and masses. However, more information is needed to clearly describe the normal anatomy of various organs including the respiratory tract in reptiles and their appearance in CT. A study in Indian pythons (*Python molurus*) evaluated the use of CT in snakes with and without signs of respiratory tract disease.[30] CT

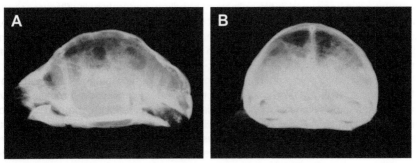

Fig. 2. Northern spider tortoise (*Pyxis arachnoides brygooi*) with pneumonia. Pulmonary opacities are visible on both the lateral (*A*) and craniocaudal (*B*) projections.

was capable of assessing the lung parenchyma, including thickness and attenuation. Based on the results of this study, reference values were established for the use of CT as a diagnostic tool for pneumonia in snakes. Studies have also been conducted in several boid snakes to describe normal CT appearance of the lung parenchyma.[31] CT can also be used to evaluate the progression of a disease and to stage treatment protocols. CT has been applied in snakes with bacterial pneumonia before and after treatment.[32] Pathologic changes within the lung parenchyma were assessed before treatment and improvement of lesions were noted following therapy.

Magnetic resonance imaging (MRI) has been applied in reptiles and is useful for visualization of soft tissues and fluids.[33] MRI has also been used to identify pathologic changes of the respiratory tract in chelonians.[34] MRI offers an advantage compared with other imaging techniques in that soft tissue contrast is improved. The trachea and lung fields, including pulmonary septae, can readily be identified. Pulmonary changes such as edema, inflammatory conditions, and interstitial changes can also be detected with this imaging modality.

Endoscopy is a minimally invasive imaging modality commonly used in reptile medicine. Endoscopy has been successfully used to evaluate coelomic structures, collect diagnostic samples such as biopsy specimens, and has also become increasingly popular to perform a variety of surgical procedures such as ovariectomies. In reptiles, endoscopy facilitates examination of the upper and lower respiratory tract of even small reptile species.[7,35,36] Endoscopic equipment is available to examine the smallest reptile patients. Selection of the instruments depends on the size and the species to be examined. The nares, trachea, bronchi, lungs, and air sacs can be visualized with small, rigid, as well as flexible endoscopes. In reptiles, endoscopy may be the most suitable diagnostic modality to fully assess and characterize pathologic changes of the respiratory tract and facilitate collection of diagnostic samples. Via endoscopy, diagnostic samples such as biopsies and washes can be collected and should be submitted for cytology, histology, and culture. Endoscopy is also a useful tool for detection and evaluation of focal changes such as granulomas. In chelonians, endoscopic techniques to evaluate the lower respiratory tract using a carapacial and prefemoral approach have been described.[7,35] Before these procedures, it is essential to accurately localize the pulmonary lesions via radiography.

Diagnostic Samples and Tests

The principles of collecting and handling diagnostic samples are similar between domestic animals and reptiles. Most importantly, the sample should be collected from the infected organ system or the infected anatomic location. For correct interpretation of results and in order to make an accurate diagnosis, it is essential that sterile techniques have been used in the collection, handling, and transport of the specimen. It is also recommended to establish contact with the diagnostic laboratory and receive guidelines for the handling, including shipment, of collected samples. It is best to use a laboratory specializing and experienced in the handling and interpretation of reptilian samples. As part of the diagnostic work-up, a venous blood sample should be collected for hematologic and plasma biochemical determinations. Few serologic tests are available for the diagnosis of infectious disease processes in reptiles. Exposure of snakes to ophidian paramyxovirus can be determined with a hemagglutination inhibition (HI) assay.[18] An enzyme-linked immunosorbent assay (ELISA) has been developed to detect antibodies to *Mycoplasma agassizii* in tortoises.[37] A polymerase chain reaction (PCR) test is available for the detection of mycoplasma DNA in secretions of suspected tortoises.[38] For culture, mycoplasma organisms require specific media and are slow to grow. For isolation, samples collected for culture, such as swabs from nasal secretions or flushes of the nasal cavity, may require 4 to 6 weeks of incubation. An ELISA to detect circulating antibodies to herpesvirus has been developed as well as a PCR to show herpesvirus DNA in tissues of infected tortoises.[39,40]

In cases of rhinitis and upper respiratory tract disease, diagnostic samples can either be collected with a sterile swab or by nasal flush. The collected sample should be transferred into an appropriate culture medium for growth, identification of organisms, and sensitivity testing. If lower respiratory tract disease is suspected, such as tracheitis, bronchitis, or pneumonia, a tracheal or lung wash should be performed. Although this procedure can be performed in some species without the need for anesthesia, in order to reduce stress and discomfort for the patient, the reptile should be sedated or anesthetized. In chelonians, the presence of a fleshy tongue often obscures visualization of the glottis and passage of a sterile catheter. It is important to follow aseptic techniques because contamination of the sample with organisms from the oral cavity renders the sample inaccurate, which may lead to inappropriate and ineffective therapy. The trachea of the animal should be intubated with a sterile endotracheal tube and a sterile catheter should be inserted through the endotracheal tube into the trachea. Sterile, physiologic saline (3–5 mL/kg) should be administered followed by repeated gentle aspiration. The collected material should be submitted for cytologic evaluation, parasite screening, bacterial and/or fungal culture, and sensitivity testing. If indicated, samples can also be submitted for viral isolation and electron microscopy. Negative-staining electron microscopy is an excellent and useful diagnostic tool for the detection of viral particles in fluids and secretions. For histopathologic evaluation of the lung parenchyma, biopsy specimens should be collected and can also be submitted for culture and sensitivities. A lung biopsy can be obtained via a standard celiotomy or via endoscopy.[41] Impression smears can be made from lesions or masses and evaluated cytologically. Techniques for both procedures have been described previously. For endoscopic collection of lung biopsy specimens, rigid or flexible fiberscopes can be used.

THERAPY

Respiratory tract disease in reptiles is commonly a multifactorial, chronic disease that requires long-term, aggressive therapy including correction of suboptimal environmental conditions. As in mammals, maintenance of a patent airway is of most importance and may require tracheal intubation or a tracheostomy. In reptiles with pronounced laryngeal and pharyngeal edema and inflammation, administration of glucocorticoids (dexamethasone 0.2 mg/kg intravenous or intramuscular [IM]) may assist in reducing these signs. For obstructive processes of the lower airway, administration of bronchodilators such as terbutaline (0.01–0.02 mg/kg IM) may reduce bronchospasm. Environmental deficiencies need to be corrected in order to ensure proper drug metabolism and immune system function. Systemic and local antimicrobial and/or antifungal treatment should be accompanied by supportive care measures such as nutritional support and fluid therapy.

Treatment of pneumonia requires administration of broad-spectrum antimicrobial agents while results of culture and sensitivity are pending. Treatment of bacterial infections with antimicrobial agents can be challenging in some reptile species because pharmacokinetic data are often lacking. Effective and safe drugs and therapeutic levels are commonly unknown even for popular reptile species such as bearded dragons and green iguanas. Therefore, in some cases, broad-spectrum antimicrobials effective against known reptilian bacterial pathogens are administered. Bacterial culture and sensitivity testing is recommended to ensure appropriate antimicrobial therapy.

Broad-spectrum antimicrobials commonly used for the treatment of reptile respiratory disease include amikacin, enrofloxacin, ceftazidime, and piperacillin. Anaerobic infections are most often treated with metronidazole (**Table 1**). A combination of antimicrobials (eg, amikacin and ceftazidime) may also be administered to effectively treat several gram-negative isolates based on culture and sensitivity testing.

Antifungal therapy in reptiles presents some challenges because of the lack of pharmacokinetic data. Several antifungal agents have been used in reptiles, but the success of treatment has been variable. Before therapy, it is important to determine whether a mixed bacterial/fungal infection is present requiring both antimicrobial as well as antifungal therapy. Pulmonary mycoses should be treated with long-term, aggressive, systemic antifungal therapy. Antifungal agents most commonly used in reptiles include itraconazole, ketoconazole, and amphotericin-B (see **Table 1**). Amphotericin-B can also be administered by aerosol therapy. In reptiles, it is common to find fungal granulomas that may require surgical removal for successful therapy. Long-term systemic antifungal therapy combined with aerosol therapy offers the best prognosis. In chelonians with severe granulomatous pneumonia, a technique for placement of an intrapneumonic catheter for direct administration of antimicrobials and antifungal agents has been described.[42]

Parasitic infections should be treated with appropriate antiparasitic agents. Ivermectin, fenbendazole, and metronidazole are most commonly used (see **Table 1**). Many reptiles diagnosed with parasitic infection also have secondary bacterial infections that should be treated concurrently. Successful antiparasitic therapy requires

Table 1
Antimicrobial, antifungal, and antiparasitic agents commonly used for the treatment of respiratory tract infections in reptiles

Drug	Dosage (mg/kg)	Route of Administration	Frequency (h)
Amphotericin-B	1	IT	24
	1 mg/mL saline	Aerosol	12
Ampicillin	50	SC, IM	12
Amikacin	5 then 2.5	IM	72
	5 mg/mL saline	Aerosol	4–6
Ceftazidime	20	IM	24–72
Cephalexin	20–40	PO	12–24
Doxycycline	25–50	IM	72
Enrofloxacin	5–10	IM, PO	12–48
Fenbendazole	50–100	PO	Repeat in 14 d
Itraconazole	10–20	PO	24
Ivermectin	0.2–0.4	IM, SC	Repeat in 14 d
Ketoconazole	15–30	PO	24
Metronidazole	20	PO	48
Praziquantel	8	IM, PO	Repeat in 14 d
Piperacillin	100–200	IM	24
	10 mg/mL saline	Aerosol	4–6
Trimethoprim-sulfadiazine	30	IM, SC, PO	24–48

For more information on drugs and dosages see: Funk RS, Diethelm G. Reptile formulary. In: Mader DR, editors. Reptile medicine and surgery. 2nd edition. St Louis (MO); Saunders Elsevier; p. 1119–39.

Abbreviations: IM, intramuscular; IT, intratracheal; IV, intravenous; PO, by mouth; SC, subcutaneous.

knowledge of the life cycle of the parasites, and husbandry practices should be evaluated and corrected.

Reptiles diagnosed with upper respiratory tract disease are most effectively treated with systemic administration of antimicrobial agents accompanied by local treatment of affected areas. Systemic antimicrobial treatment with enrofloxacin accompanied by flushes of the nasal cavities with a 1:10 solution of enrofloxacin and saline is recommended. A small-gauge catheter can be inserted into the nares and the solution should be administered twice daily for 10 days. If no improvement of clinical signs is noted after several days of treatment, antimicrobial selection should be reevaluated. In addition to systemic antimicrobials, bacterial stomatitis should be treated by debridement and removal of abscess material. Radiographic evaluation might be necessary to determine involvement of bony structures such as the mandible or maxilla.

Corrective and supportive care measures accompanying antimicrobial or antifungal treatment include provision of species-specific environmental conditions, as well as supplemental oxygen in cases of respiratory distress. Mucolytic agents often aid in the elimination of exudates.

Traumatic, penetrating injuries to the carapace are commonly inflicted to chelonians by cars or by predators. In severe cases, the underlying lung tissue may be exposed and contaminated with potential pathogens. In addition to diagnostic procedures to fully elucidate the extent of the shell fracture (eg, radiography, CT), breathing status of the animal should be carefully evaluated. Repair of the shell should be accompanied by supportive care measures such as appropriate analgesic therapy and long-term antimicrobial therapy to prevent secondary bacterial infections. The prognosis in some cases is guarded, depending on the severity of the injury.

For the successful treatment of the reptile presented with respiratory tract disease, it is essential to frequently monitor success of therapy, such as improved breathing pattern and decreased nasal discharge. In contrast with mammals, evaluation of respiratory performance via blood gas analysis is challenging in reptiles. Access to a peripheral artery is often limited and requires a cut-down procedure for most species. Normal values for venous and arterial blood gas parameters have not been established for reptiles, making interpretation difficult. Imaging modalities such as radiography and CT also aid in monitoring improvement of pulmonary lesions.

Aerosol therapy is indicated in reptiles with severe, chronic respiratory disease in order to facilitate delivery of antimicrobials/antifungals, and/or saline and water directly to the respiratory surface. Administration of antimicrobial or antifungal agents by aerosol in conjunction with systemic antibiotic or antifungal therapy improves delivery of the agent to the source of infection. Culture and sensitivity testing is recommended to select an effective antimicrobial or antifungal agent. Aerosol therapy with saline and water alone results in loosening of viscous respiratory secretions and more efficient elimination of necrotic debris. In severe cases, suctioning of the trachea following aerosol therapy is indicated for removal of secretions. Aerosols are most effectively delivered by nebulizers, which can be installed in an incubator. Aerosol therapy should be administered 3 to 4 times daily for approximately 20 to 30 minutes. Prolonged aerosol therapy should be avoided because it has been shown to negatively affect pulmonary function, including bronchospasm and pulmonary shunting.[43]

In addition to antimicrobials and saline, mucolytic and proteolytic agents can be administered; however, data on the effectiveness of these drugs in reptiles are lacking. Administration of bronchodilators should be exercised with caution because of potential side-effects on the cardiovascular system. Selective β2-agonists such as salbutamol and terbutaline are preferred, rather than nonselective sympathomimetic agents such as epinephrine and ephedrine.

Respiratory Support and Monitoring

Reptiles presented in stages of advanced or chronic respiratory disease require intensive supportive care including support of respiratory function. Basic principles known from small animal respiratory medicine also apply to reptile patients.[44] Patients with impaired pulmonary function, such as pneumonia, pulmonary edema, and suspected hypoxia, benefit from oxygen therapy. In mammals, arterial blood gas analysis is the most accurate means of determining the need for oxygen therapy; however, this is impractical in most reptile species. A major limitation of the accuracy of blood gas analysis in reptiles is the calibration of analyzers based on the human oxygen hemoglobin dissociation curve. Calculated values may therefore be inaccurate and may lead to inappropriate, ineffective, or even improper therapy. The presence of cardiac shunts in reptiles may indicate that arterial blood gas analysis may not reflect lung gas composition. Cardiac shunting may regulate arterial blood gas composition independently from pulmonary ventilation.[3] Clinical signs such as dyspnea and tachycardia often indicate the need for supplemental oxygen. The clinical response of the reptile to higher inspired oxygen concentrations assists in the diagnosis of hypoxemia. Techniques for effective administration of oxygen to the reptilian patient are similar to domestic animals. The size and temperament of the reptile often dictates the most effective and safe way to administer oxygen therapy. The severity of clinical signs, the size of the reptile, and available equipment dictate therapy. For prolonged therapy, the animal should be placed in an oxygen-enriched environment such as an incubator. An incubator facilitates provision of appropriate temperature and humidity levels. More efficient means of oxygen administration are the use of a face mask or placement of a nasal catheter and O_2 insufflation. A face mask can be used in all reptile species and is indicated for short-term administration of oxygen or in emergency situations. In larger reptiles, a nasal catheter can be used for prolonged administration of oxygen. The flow rate of oxygen for smaller reptiles (<10 kg body weight) should be 1 to 2 L/min, whereas larger species (>10 kg body weight) require flow rates up to 5 L/min. To prevent drying and irritation of the nasal mucosa, inspired oxygen should be humidified using a bubble humidifier, and the humidity within the cage should be increased. In emergency situations such as obstructive processes, endotracheal intubation and positive pressure ventilation may be indicated. Clinical signs of hypoxemia such as dyspnea, tachycardia, and cyanosis should resolve during effective oxygen therapy.

Respiratory Emergencies

Reptiles presented in respiratory distress are often challenging to treat. Although therapy for respiratory emergencies in reptiles follows the same principles known from small animal emergency medicine,[45] few data have been established in reptiles for effective treatment, including safe and effective drugs and adequate monitoring of the patient. Effective therapy for acute respiratory distress includes accurate localization of the disorder. As in mammals, upper and lower airway obstruction, pulmonary parenchymal and vascular disease, as well as abdominal distension such as coelomic effusion may result in severe respiratory compromise. Obstructive processes of the upper airway may be diagnosed via physical examination; however, those affecting the lower respiratory tract require advanced diagnostic techniques such as imaging modalities. Supplemental administration of oxygen via a face mask is of short-term benefit and establishment of a patent airway via endotracheal intubation or placement of a tracheostomy tube is indicated. Tracheal suctioning is required in reptiles with large amounts of fluid present in the tracheal lumen.

Pathologic conditions within the nasal cavity are usually not considered a respiratory emergency. However, obstructive processes within the oropharynx interfering with the movement of air through the glottis are considered emergencies. Commonly, abscesses or large amounts of purulent material may impair respiration if they cause displacement or occlusion of the glottis. Foreign bodies such as plastic or wood may also displace or occlude the glottis. Establishment of a patent airway is indicated, by either endotracheal intubation or tracheostomy followed by debridement of the abscess and removal of the foreign body.

Clinical signs of obstructive processes of the lower respiratory tract include expiratory dyspnea. Obstructive lesions of the trachea and the major airways are often caused by the presence of foreign bodies, bacterial/fungal granulomas, and, more rarely, neoplastic masses. Additional causes of lower airway obstruction include bronchoconstriction and exudate within the lumen of the bronchi. Pneumonia and interstitial lung disease often lead to signs of acute respiratory compromise. A diagnosis should be made based on radiography and/or endoscopy of the lower respiratory tract. Endoscopy is a useful tool for removal of foreign material, whereas most masses such as granulomas or neoplasia require surgical intervention.

Respiratory distress, especially on inspiration, can also be caused by distension of the coelomic cavity. Common causes in reptiles include organomegaly and pregnancy. In gravid chelonians and lizards especially, follicles and eggs may occupy a large portion of the coelomic cavity, resulting in respiratory compromise. Coelomic effusion associated with a ruptured follicle is seen in female reptiles presented with an acute onset of respiratory compromise. Accumulation of intracoelomic fluid and displacement of the lungs dorsally often results in signs of severe respiratory impairment. Radiography, endoscopy, and ultrasonography are the most useful diagnostic tools to identify the presence of coelomic fluid. Respiratory support such as endotracheal intubation and intermittent positive pressure ventilation (IPPV) should be initiated depending on the severity of respiratory compromise. Further diagnostics and treatment should include aspiration and characterization of the fluid. Following stabilization of the patient, surgical intervention is recommended.

SUMMARY

Reptiles presented with chronic pneumonia and severe impairment of pulmonary function require intensive care, advanced diagnostics, and lengthy hospitalization. Physical examination, evaluation of hematologic and plasma biochemical parameters, collection of appropriate diagnostic samples such as tracheal washes for cytology and culture, as well as imaging modalities eg radiography are essential to fully elucidate the severity of pulmonary compromise and dysfunction. In severe, chronic cases, systemic antimicrobial therapy should be accompanied by nebulization and frequent aspiration of respiratory secretions from the trachea.

ACKNOWLEDGMENTS

Sections of this article have been taken/modified from: Schumacher J. Reptile respiratory medicine. Vet Clin North Am Exot Anim Pract 2003;6(1):213–31; with permission.

REFERENCES

1. Murray MJ. Cardiopulmonary anatomy and physiology. In: Mader DR, editor. Reptile medicine and surgery 2nd edition. St Louis (MO): Saunders Elsevier; 2006. p. 124–34.

2. Perry SF. Lungs: comparative anatomy, functional morphology, and evolution. Morphology G Visceral Organs. In: Gans C, Gaunt AS, editors, Biology of the reptilia, vol. 19. St Louis (MO): Society for the Study of Amphibians and Reptiles; 1998. p. 1–92.
3. Wang T, Smits AW, Burggren WW. Pulmonary function in reptiles. Morphology G Visceral Organs. In: Gans C, Gaunt AS, editors, Biology of the reptilia, vol. 19. St Louis (MO): Society for the Study of Amphibians and Reptiles; 1998. p. 297–374.
4. Coke RL. Respiratory biology and diseases of captive lizards (Sauria). Vet Clin North Am Exot Anim Pract 2000;3:531–6.
5. Driggers T. Respiratory diseases, diagnostics, and therapy in snakes. Vet Clin North Am Exot Anim Pract 2000;3:519–30.
6. Jacobson ER. Diseases of the respiratory system in reptiles. Vet Med (Sm Anim Clin) 1978;73:1169–75.
7. Murray MJ. Pneumonia and lower respiratory tract disease. In: Mader DR, editor. Reptile medicine and surgery 2nd edition. St Louis (MO): Saunders Elsevier; 2006. p. 865–77.
8. Origgi FC, Jacobson ER. Diseases of the respiratory tract of chelonians. Vet Clin North Am Exot Anim Pract 2000;3:537–49.
9. Schumacher J. Respiratory diseases of reptiles. Semin Avian Exotic Pet Med 1997;6:209–15.
10. Schumacher J. Reptile respiratory medicine. Vet Clin North Am Exot Anim Pract 2003;6(1):213–31, viii.
11. Wallach V. The lungs of snakes. Morphology G Visceral Organs. In: Gans C, Gaunt AS, editors, Biology of the reptilia, vol. 19. St Louis (MO): Society for the Study of Amphibians and Reptiles; 1998. p. 93–295.
12. Jacobson ER, Gaskin JM, Brown MB, et al. Chronic upper respiratory tract disease of free-ranging desert tortoises, Xerobates agassizii. J Wildl Dis 1991; 27:296.
13. Greenacre CB, Ritchie BW, Latimer KS. Treatment of cartilaginous hyperplasia in ball pythons. Comp Cont Ed Pract Vet 1999;21:633–7.
14. Garner MM, Raymond JT. Lymphoma in reptiles with special emphasis on oral manifestation. Proc Assoc Rept Amp Vet 2001;165–9.
15. Jacobson ER, Gaskin JM, Roelke M, et al. Conjunctivitis, tracheitis and pneumonia associated with herpes-virus infection in Green Sea Turtles. J Am Vet Med Assoc 1986;189:1020–3.
16. Marschang RE, Gravendyck M, Kaleta EF. Herpes virus in tortoises: Investigation into virus isolation and the treatment of viral stomatitis in T. hermanni and T. graeca. J Vet Med 1997;44:385.
17. Mueller M, Sachse W, Zangger N. Herpesvirus-epidemie bei der griechischen (Testudo hermanni) und der maurischen Landschildkroete (Testudo graeca) in der Schweiz. Schweiz Arch Tierheilkd 1990;132:199.
18. Jacobson ER, Gaskin JM, Wells S, et al. Epizootic of ophidian paramyxovirus in a zoological collection: pathological, microbiological and serological findings. J Zoo Wildl Med 1992;23:318–27.
19. Jacobson ER, Origgi F, Pessier AP, et al. Paramyxovirus infection in caiman lizards (Draecena guianensis). J Vet Diagn Invest 2001;13:143–51.
20. Schumacher J, Jacobson ER, Homer BL, et al. Inclusion body disease in boid snakes. J Zoo Wildl Med 1994;25:511–24.
21. Snipes KP, Biberstein EL. Pasteurella testudinis sp. nov: a parasite of desert tortoises. Int J Sus Bact 1982;32:201.

22. Stewart JS. Anaerobic bacterial infections in reptiles. J Zoo Wildl Med 1990;21: 180–4.
23. Pare JA, Sigler L, Rosenthal KL, et al. Microbiology: Fungal and bacterial diseases of reptiles. In: Mader DR, editor. Reptile medicine and surgery 2nd edition. St Louis (MO): Saunders Elsevier; 2006. p. 217–38.
24. Hernandez-Divers SJ. Pulmonary candidiasis caused by *Candida albicans* in a Greek tortoise (*Testudo graeca*) and treatment using intrapulmonary amphotericin B. J Zoo Wildl Med 2001;32(3):352–9.
25. Hendrix CM, Blagburn BL. Reptilian pentastomiasis: a possible emerging zoonosis. Comp Cont Educ 1988;10:46–51.
26. Stoakes LC. Respiratory system. In: Lawton PC, Cooper JE, editors. Manual of reptiles. British small animal veterinary Association. Ames (IA): Iowa State University Press; 1992. p. 88–100.
27. Schumacher J, Toal RL. Advanced radiography and ultrasonography in reptiles. Semin Avian Exotic Pet Med 2001;10:162–8.
28. Silverman S. Diagnostic imaging. In: Mader DR, editor. Reptile medicine and surgery 2nd edition. St Louis (MO): Saunders Elsevier; 2006. p. 471–89.
29. Gumpenberger M, Henninger W. The use of computed tomography in avian and reptile medicine. Semin Avian Exotic Pet Med 2001;10(4):174–80.
30. Pees MC, Kiefer I, Ludewig EW, et al. Computed tomography of the lungs of Indian pythons (*Python molurus*). AJVR 2007;68(4):428–34.
31. Pees MC, Kiefer I, Thielebein J, et al. Computed tomography of the lung of healthy snakes of the species *Python regius*, BOA constrictor, *Python reticulates*, *Morelia viridis*, *Epicrates cenchria*, and *Morelia spilota*. Vet Radiol Ultrasound 2009;50(5):487–91.
32. Pees MC, Kiefer I, Krautwald-Junghanns ME. Computed tomography for the diagnosis and treatment monitoring of bacterial pneumonia in Indian pythons (*Python molurus*). Vet Rec 2008;163(5):152–6.
33. Wyneken J. Computed tomography and magnetic resonance imaging anatomy of reptiles. In: Mader DR, editor. Reptile medicine and surgery 2nd edition. St Louis (MO): Saunders Elsevier; 2006. p. 1088–95.
34. Straub J, Jurina K. Magnetic resonance imaging in chelonians. Semin Avian Exotic Pet Med 2001;10(4):181–6.
35. Divers SJ, Lawton MP. Two techniques for endoscopic evaluation of the chelonian lung. Proc Assoc Rept Amp Vet 2000;123–5.
36. Schildger B, Wicker R. Endoskopie bei Reptilien und Amphibien-Indikationen, Methoden, Befunde. Praktische Tierarzt 1992;73:516–26.
37. Schumacher IM, Brown MB, Jacobson ER, et al. Detection of antibodies to a pathogenic *Mycoplasma* in the desert tortoise (*Gopherus agassizii*). J Clin Microbiol 1993;31:1454.
38. Brown DR, Crenshaw BC, McLaughlin GS, et al. Taxonomic analysis of the tortoise *Mycoplasmas*, *M. agassizii* and *M. testudines* by 16S rRNA gene sequence comparison. Int J Syst Bacteriol 1995;45:348.
39. Origgi F, Jacobson ER, Romero CH, et al. Diagnostic tools for herpesvirus detection in chelonians. Proc Assoc Rept Amp Vet 2000;127–9.
40. Origgi F, Jacobson ER, Romero CH, et al. Tortoise herpesvirus and stomatitis-rhinitis in tortoises. Proc Assoc Rept Amp Vet 2001;101–2.
41. Hernandez-Divers SJ. Diagnostic techniques. In: Mader DR, editor. Reptile medicine and surgery. 2nd edition. St Louis (MO): Saunders Elsevier; 2006. p. 490–532.
42. Lewis W. How to place intrapneumonic catheters in chelonians. Exotic DVM 2001; 3.5:16–7.

43. Malik SK, Jenkins DE. Alteration in airway dynamics following inhalation of ultrasonic mist. Chest 1972;62:660–4.

44. Court MH. Respiratory support of the critically ill small animal patient. In: Murtaugh RJ, Kaplan PM, editors. Veterinary emergency and critical care medicine. St Louis (MO): Mosby-Year Book; 1992. p. 575–92.

45. Gibbons G. Respiratory emergencies. In: Murtaugh RJ, Kaplan PM, editors. Veterinary emergency and critical care medicine. St Louis (MO): Mosby-Year Book; 1992. p. 399–419.

The Chelonian Respiratory System

Tracy Bennett, DVM, DABVP (Avian)

KEYWORDS

• Turtle • Tortoise • Chelonian • Respiratory • Disease
• Oxygen • Mycoplasma • Herpesvirus • Iridovirus

This article reviews anatomy, physiology, diagnostic techniques, and specific disease syndromes of the chelonian respiratory system. Respiratory disease is common in chelonians and is a cause of significant morbidity and mortality in these animals. Mycoplasma, herpesvirus, and iridovirus are reviewed in depth.

ANATOMY AND PHYSIOLOGY

Chelonians and other reptiles have distinct anatomic features of the respiratory tract that distinguish them from other vertebrates. They have an unbranched interpulmonary bronchus and, therefore, no bronchial tree and they lack the alveoli that are present in mammals. The gas exchange sites in reptiles are called ediculi and faveoli, and consist of small crypts instead of alveolar sacs.[1]

Due to the presence of the bony shell, chelonian lungs have limited expansion capabilities. Chelonians breathe through the nares. Open mouth breathing is abnormal and a sign of respiratory distress. The glottis is positioned at the base of the tongue and caudally in the oropharynx. The air passes from the nares to the glottis, then through the trachea and into the paired bronchi where it enters the lungs. Chelonians possess complete tracheal rings and the trachea is short and flexible to allow retraction of the head into the shell.

The lungs in chelonians are multicameral (multichambered) and attached to the ventral carapace and the vertebral column by the pulmonary ligament (**Fig. 1**).[2] A layer of connective tissue forms the border of the lungs and also attaches to the viscera.[3] A distinct reticular pattern is visible when examining the sac-like lungs. As with other reptiles and birds, no muscular diaphragm is present. Ventilation is achieved through movement of the inguinal, axial, and shoulder muscles creating a pressure change in the pleuroperitoneal cavity (**Fig. 2**). Movement of the limbs can be seen during normal respiration. Chelonians can exhibit a movement of the ventral mandibular area called "gular pumping." In amphibians, gular pumping is part of normal respiration but in

The author has nothing to disclose and received no funding.
Bird and Exotic Clinic of Seattle, 4019 Aurora Avenue North, Seattle, WA 98103, USA
E-mail address: daniel.tracy@comcast.net

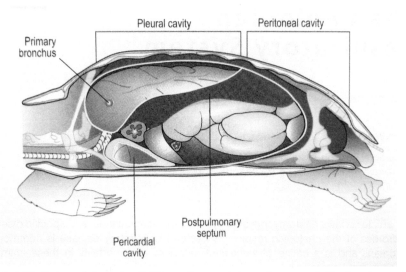

Fig. 1. Lateral view of chelonian (left lung, liver, and stomach removed). The heart occupies a cranial position because the lungs are restricted to the dorsal thorax. (*Reprinted from* O'Malley, B. Clinical anatomy and physiology of exotic species. Structure and function of mammals, birds, reptiles, and amphibians. Elsevier; 2005. p. 50; with permission.)

chelonians it assists in olfaction rather than ventilation and is not a sign of respiratory distress.[4]

Respiration is driven by low partial pressures of oxygen, elevated partial pressures of carbon dioxide, acid-base balance, and lung stretch receptors. Hypoxia increases breathing frequency and hypercapnia causes an increase in the tidal volume by suppressing lung stretch receptors.[5] Chelonians employ positive pressure ventilation, which allows them to continue to breathe normally even when the shell is compromised.[6]

DIAGNOSTICS
Physical Exam

The bony shell of chelonians presents certain diagnostic challenges to the clinician. If a limb or the head can be grasped and manually extended, it prevents the patient from retreating into the shell and examination and sampling can proceed. Large chelonians may require sedation. A thorough history must be taken before examination of the patient. The diet, environment, location of purchase or adoption, exposure to other chelonians, and medical history are all crucial considerations to proper treatment (**Fig. 3**). Most problems encountered by the clinician can be traced to improper husbandry.

During the physical examination, the nares should be observed to determine patency, erosive lesions, and the presence of any discharge. The palpebrae are often inflamed in cases of upper respiratory disease. The oral cavity can be examined using a soft spatula or metal speculum to hold the mouth open. The oral cavity should be examined for the presence of mucus, blood, caseous debris, ulcerations, or other abnormalities. The glottis can also be observed. Open mouth and audible breathing are considered abnormal but these findings may be absent even in cases of severe lower respiratory disease. Chelonians move their limbs minimally during normal

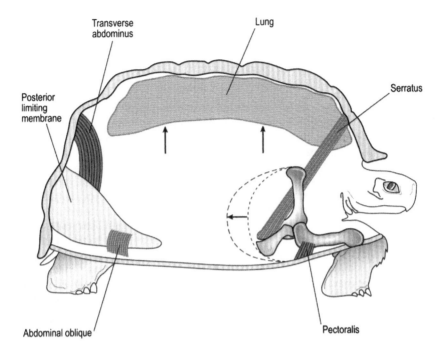

Red = Inspiratory muscles
Gray = Expiratory muscles

Fig. 2. Lateral view of tortoise showing lungs and demonstrating inspiratory and expiratory muscles of respiration. (*Reprinted from* O'Malley, B. Clinical anatomy and physiology of exotic species. Structure and function of mammals, birds, reptiles, and amphibians. Elsevier; 2005. p. 52; with permission.)

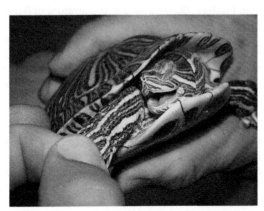

Fig. 3. Conjunctivitis in a red-eared slider secondary to a bacterial upper respiratory infection and poor husbandry. (*Courtesy of* Marc H. Kramer, DVM, Miami, FL.)

respiration and excessive movement can be a sign of dyspnea. A Doppler probe or an electronic stethoscope can be used to aid auscultation of the heart and lungs. Aquatic turtles with respiratory disease may exhibit abnormalities while swimming, such as listing to one side in the water or the inability to submerge.

Hematology

A complete blood count aids in determination of the presence of infectious disease in chelonians. Phlebotomy can be performed using the jugular vein, subcarapacial vein, dorsal coccygeal vein, occipital sinus, or the brachial vein. The jugular vein is the site least likely to be contaminated with lymph but restraint can be difficult.[7] In uncooperative patients the subcarapacial vein may be preferred.[8] This site can be accessed by pushing the head into the shell, which is more easily accomplished in some animals than extending the head for jugular venipuncture. The vein is supravertebral and ventral to the carapace on the midline. An appropriately sized needle is directed toward the dorsal midline. Lymph contamination is possible when using the subcarapacial vein and samples for hematology should be discarded if lymph is obtained during venipuncture. Samples for hematology should include fresh blood films and whole blood preserved in heparin as EDTA can cause lysis of chelonian erythrocytes.[9] Chelonian leukocyte values can vary by species, gender, and time of year among other factors. Monocytosis is a common finding in sick individuals and is usually indicative of a response to bacterial or parasitic infection.[7]

Culture and Cytology

Cultures and cytologic samples can be obtained from chelonians in a number of ways. Samples can be obtained from ocular or nasal discharge and the oral cavity but may be contaminated with the normal flora present in these areas. For oral sampling, the beak can be opened with a rubber spatula or metal oral speculum after the head is restrained. A culture swab can be used to swab the pharynx and the glottis. Mini-tip culture swab are useful in small patients or those that allow limited access to the oral cavity and glottis. Large chelonians often must be sedated to obtain samples. Examination of cytologic stains can aid in determining appropriate preliminary treatment while awaiting culture and sensitivity results.

For sampling the lower respiratory tract, a transtracheal wash can be performed. Sedation or anesthesia is recommended for this procedure. To avoid contamination from the oral microflora, a sterile catheter is carefully placed directly into the glottis and advanced into the trachea. Sterile saline in the amount of 0.5 to 1 mL per 100 g body weight is introduced into the lungs.[10] The fluid is aspirated repeatedly while gently rotating the patient slightly to facilitate recovery of the saline. Aerobic, anaerobic, fungal, and, occasionally, viral cultures can be obtained in this way. Calcium alginate swabs must be used when *Mycoplasma* sp is suspected. Viral cultures require specific media and the clinician should discuss transport of the sample with the laboratory being used.

Imaging

Radiology generally requires a higher milliampere seconds (mAs) setting than a similarly sized nonchelonian patient due to difficulty penetrating the bony shell. High detail film with rare earth screens or digital radiography is recommended. Positioning is important as the shell creates a barrier that causes many areas to be indistinct radiographically. The three important routine radiographic views are dorsoventral, lateral (**Fig. 4**), and craniocaudal (**Fig. 5**). Unilateral lung disease is common and the craniocaudal view is the only view that allows comparison of the both lung fields. Horizontal

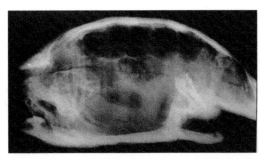

Fig. 4. Lateral radiograph (horizontal beam) showing lung fields. (*Reprinted from* O'Malley, B. Clinical anatomy and physiology of exotic species. Structure and function of mammals, birds, reptiles, and amphibians. Elsevier; 2005. p. 51; with permission.)

beam projections are easily accomplished with minimal restraint but, when necessary, passive restraint using tape or sand bags works well for most patients.[11]

A CT scan allows excellent detail of the internal structures of chelonians and is the preferred method of imaging the respiratory system when available. Most chelonians can be imaged using CT without sedation using passive restraint. The slow respiratory rate of chelonians and the rapid scanning capabilities of modern CT scan machines allow detailed images of the lungs. The patient can be taped onto a solid block and placed in a human cervical immobilization device, or the limbs can simply be taped into the shell. The patient should be placed in ventral recumbency to avoid compression of the lungs by the viscera.[12] MRI is also an excellent imaging modality for chelonians and, where available, is an asset to diagnosis.[13]

Biopsy

Lung biopsies are best obtained by endoscopy either through a prefemoral approach or by creating a temporary osteotomy in the carapace directly above the lungs. The area of interest should be determined by imaging studies before performing a carapacial osteotomy. This allows an opening made directly above the lesion. The

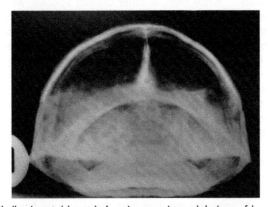

Fig. 5. Radiograph (horizontal beam) showing craniocaudal view of lungs – the best view for assessing the lungs for pneumonia. (*Reprinted from* O'Malley, B. Clinical anatomy and physiology of exotic species. Structure and function of mammals, birds, reptiles, and amphibians. Elsevier; 2005. p. 51; with permission.)

endoscope can then be advanced into the lung and the area visualized and biopsied. After the procedure, the lesion can be closed using an epoxy or acrylic patch. Endoscopic lung biopsies can also be obtained through a prefemoral approach. The entry incision is made in the craniodorsal area of the prefemoral fossa. To allow identification of the lung, the coelomic membrane may need to be perforated. An incision is made in the poorly vascular portion of the lung allowing entrance by the endoscope. Examination of the lung can then be performed and biopsies taken of the desired area. The lung must be sutured before closure of the skin incision.[14]

INFECTIOUS DISEASE
Bacterial

Bacterial infections of the respiratory tract are common in chelonians. Poor water quality, inadequate heat, and poor nutrition are often predisposing factors. Most bacterial pathogens in chelonians are gram-negative organisms such as *Klebsiella* sp, *Pseudomonas* sp, and *Aeromonas* sp.[15] All reptiles have gram-negative organisms as part of the normal flora of their gastrointestinal tract and consideration must be given to the species of bacteria grown and the location that was cultured. Initial treatment should target gram-negative organisms until culture and sensitivity results can be obtained. Many common reptile pathogens such as *Pseudomonas* sp can have multidrug resistance.

Mycobacterium species are occasionally found on cytology or histology in wild chelonians but the occurrence is rare in captive animals. Mycobacterium does not normally cause primary respiratory disease but can affect the lungs if it spreads from another location.[16] Diagnosis requires sampling of the lesion and acid-fast or Ziehl-Neelsen staining for confirmation. A polymerase chain reaction (PCR) test has also been used to detect the organism in tissues.[17]

Mycoplasma sp is a major pathogen of captive and wild tortoises. Mycoplasmal disease has been documented in tortoises in Europe and the United States. A major decline of *Gopherus agassazii* in the Mojave Desert in the 1980s has been at least partly attributed to the disease.[18] The presence of *Mycoplasma* sp has been documented in association with upper respiratory tract disease (URTD) in many of these tortoises. A new *Mycoplasma* species was isolated at that time and was designated *Mycoplasma agassazii*.[19] Since then, another distinct species, *M testudineum*, has also been found to cause URTD in *Gopherus agassazii*.[20] An additional species of *Mycoplasma*, *M testudinis*, has been isolated from tortoises but has not been shown to cause respiratory disease.[21] *M agassazii* has been used to experimentally induce characteristic URTD in previously clinically normal individuals. Mycoplasmas have been isolated from almost every species of tortoise common in the pet trade including *Geochelone sulcata*, *G carbonaria*, *Testudo graeca*, and *T horsfieldii*.[22] It has also been isolated in box turtles (*Terrapene carolina carolina*).[23]

The clinical presentation of mycoplasmal disease varies depending of the chronicity. In the acute form, rhinitis, conjunctivitis, nasal, and ocular discharge are common. Edema of the palpebral, periocular, and conjunctival tissues is also common. In the chronic form of the disease, depigmentation of the nares as well as vertical erosions ventral to the nares are often noted. Differential diagnoses include herpes viral infection, iridovirus, other bacterial agents, or fungal infection.[24] Three diagnostic tests for *M agassazii* are available; these include bacterial culture, PCR, and an ELISA antibody test (University of Florida, Gainesville, FL, USA). Bacterial culture can be unrewarding as the organism lacks a cell wall and is fastidious and slow growing. An ELISA test is available to measure antibodies to *M agassazii* and can be performed on serum or plasma.[25,26] A positive titer indicates exposure to the disease. Paired titers should be run 6 to 8 weeks apart to determine if the infection is acute. A very sensitive PCR test is also available but is less specific than the ELISA test. The samples for the PCR test can be obtained from swabs taken from the nasal cavity or other upper respiratory sites.[27]

Transmission is usually through direct contact with a clinically ill individual. Environmental transmission might occur in the pet trade where individuals are overcrowded and contaminated material accumulates in the environment. The incubation period can be as little as 2 weeks.[22] Affected individuals shed intermittently and chronic subclinical cases do occur. Several antibiotics have been used anecdotally with resolution of clinical signs. Antibiotics that have shown to be effective in treating mycoplasmal infections in other animal species have been used. Historically, fluoroquinolones and macrolides have been good choices. Clearance of the organism may occur subsequent to antibiotic therapy but has been difficult to document. Individuals may appear to recover then relapse later.

Viral

Herpes is the most prevalent viral infection documented in captive and free-ranging chelonians. Many nonspecific clinical signs are associated with herpes viral infections. These include anorexia, lethargy, rhinitis, conjunctivitis, and stomatitis. Oral herpes lesions may occlude the pharynx and cause dyspnea. Clinical signs are similar to mycoplasmal infections and the two can occur simultaneously.[28] Another finding associated with herpesviral infection in tortoises is the development of diphtheritic oral plaques in some individuals.[29] These lesions can occur and resolve in a cyclic manner. Herpes infection has also been associated with many nonrespiratory presentations, sometimes affecting the liver, shell or skin, nervous system, and gastrointestinal tract. Respiratory disease attributable to herpesvirus has been found primarily in tortoises and aquatic turtles. Herpesvirus has been associated with fibropapillomatosis disease in sea turtles. This syndrome primarily has a cutaneous distribution, but pulmonary and oropharygeal lesions have been reported.[30] Fibropapillomatosis disease is a major cause of morbidity and mortality in sea turtles worldwide.[31] Another herpesviral-associated disease in sea turtles is termed lung-eye-trachea disease and is also a concern for sea turtle populations.[32] In clinical practice, herpes is most commonly seen in tortoises with URTD. Although all tortoises are potentially susceptible to herpesviral infection, *Testudo* sp appear to be the most commonly infected. One study on exposure of tortoises to herpesvirus found that 42.5% of Greek tortoises and 18.5% of Hermann's tortoises were seropositive.[33]

The exact mechanism of herpesviral transmission is unknown. Experimentally, tortoises have been infected by both intranasal and intramuscular routes.[34] The phrase "herpes is forever" should be considered valid in chelonians as in other animals and individuals that have been previously infected likely will remain latently infected. Additionally, apparently asymptomatic tortoises may have subclinical disease. Vertical transmission is possible but has not been documented.

All infected individuals should be isolated immediately from uninfected animals. Disinfection of holding facilities with a solution consisting of one-half cup bleach and 1 gallon of water has been recommended.[35] A study designed to test the persistence of tortoise viruses in the environment found herpesvirus to be the most easily inactivated of the viruses studied. Inactivation was highly dependent on temperature. At 23°C it took 63 days for herpesvirus to achieve a reduction of three $\log_{10}$ units in soil.[36] Two antibody tests are available for detection of herpesviral antibodies in tortoises. The first is a serum neutralization (SN) test developed in 1997.[37] A newer test using ELISA technology is available for detection of antibodies to herpesvirus in tortoises and can be read more rapidly than the SN test (Veterinary Medical Teaching Hospital, Gainesville, FL, USA). The accuracy of these tests does not appear to be significantly different.[38] Tests based on indirect and direct immunoperoxidase techniques have also been developed for detecting herpesviral antigen and antiherpes immunoglobulin in serum and tissues.[39] Additionally, there are several PCR tests available for detection of even minute quantities of herpesvirus present in tissues or swabs taken from infected animals.[40–43] A review of the various diagnostic tests was published and concluded that PCR diagnostics are most appropriate in cases where an acute outbreak is occurring and antibodies may not be present at that stage of disease. A 6-month quarantine was recommended with two antibody tests performed at the beginning and end of the quarantine period before the introduction of naïve individuals into an existing population. PCR testing is also recommended during this time to detect both acutely and chronically infected individuals.[44] Likewise, using both types of tests would be beneficial for herpesvirus surveillance in established populations. All deceased individuals should be necropsied and submitted for histology. Eosinophilic intranuclear inclusions are characteristic of the disease. Also, syncytial giant cells and bacterial granulomas are often described in infected individuals. PCR is used to detect the virus in tissues if histologic examination is inconclusive.

Very little has been published on methods of treatment of infected tortoises. One study suggested ganciclovir and acyclovir prevented viral replication in tortoise cells in vitro.[38] No obvious positive effects with acyclovir treatment were noted in a study involving URTD in *Testudo horsfieldii* posthibernation.[45] A single dose pharmacokinetic study in marginated tortoises treated with acyclovir concluded that the standard dose of 80 mg/kg may be too low for therapeutic benefit.[46] Anecdotally, many investigators still recommend the use of acyclovir during herpesviral outbreaks but no studies have been performed to support this practice. Supportive care of effected animals is essential and should include fluid therapy, assisted feeding, antibiotics for secondary bacterial infections, and cleaning and debridement of oral lesions.[47]

Iridoviruses

Iridoviruses are large nonenveloped double-stranded DNA viruses. *Ranavirus* is a genus in the family Iridoviridae.[48] *Ranavirus* historically has been known to infect invertebrates, fish, and amphibians. *Ranavirus* has been documented to cause infections in reptiles and several cases of URTD in chelonians have been attributed to ranaviral infection. The presenting clinical signs are very similar to mycoplasmal and herpesviral URTD and have included nasal and ocular discharge, conjunctivitis, palpebral edema, and caseous plaques in the oral cavity. The presence of *Ranavirus* has been documented in several species of chelonians, including a free-ranging gopher tortoise (*Gopherus polyphemus*), captive eastern box turtles (*Terrapene carolina carolina*), farm-raised, soft-shelled turtles (*Trionyx sinensis*), a Hermann's tortoise (*Testudo hermanni*), and captive Burmese star tortoises (*Geochelone platynota*).[49–53] Johnson and colleagues[54] documented five additional cases of *Ranavirus* infection in chelonians between 2003 and 2005 in a variety of species, including a free-ranging gopher tortoise (*Gopherus polyphemus*), free-ranging eastern box turtles (*Terrapene carolina carolina*), a Florida box turtle (*Terrepene carolina bauri*), and captive Burmese star tortoises (*Geochelone platynota*). Experimentally, red-eared sliders (*Trachemys scripta*) have developed URTD after intramuscular and oral inoculation with a *Ranavirus* isolated from a Burmese star tortoise, thereby fulfilling Koch's postulates for *Ranavirus* as a causative agent of URTD disease in chelonians.[55] Molecular studies have suggested that *Ranavirus* isolated from chelonians is amphibian in origin and that amphibians may serve as a reservoir host for susceptible chelonians.[54,56,57] PCR and virus neutralization tests are available.[49] Ranavirus is a major disease threat to amphibians worldwide and appears to be an emerging disease in chelonians. No treatment other than supportive care has been described.

Fungal

Mycotic infections of the respiratory tract are more common in chelonians than in other reptiles. In most cases, fungal infections involving the respiratory tract are due to opportunistic saprophytic fungi that are ubiquitous in soil and other organic debris. Fungal infections in chelonians are often secondary to a primary cause of disease such as traumatic shell lesions or bacterial infections. Husbandry failure is the major factor in development of mycotic disease. Improper temperature, humidity, nutrition, and excessive stress have all been linked to fungal disease in chelonians. *Candida* sp, *Aspergillus* sp, and *Penicillium* sp have been found in chelonians with respiratory disease.[58] An epizootic of pneumonia in captive-bred green sea turtles (*Chelonia mydas*) was found to be caused by a mixed mycoses, including *Sporotrichum* sp, *Cladosporium* sp, and *Paecilomyces* sp.[59] *Paecilomyces* sp have been found as causative agents of pulmonary granulomatous disease in aquatic turtles.[60,61]

When culturing lesions of the respiratory tract it is advisable to routinely request fungal culture in addition to anaerobic and aerobic bacterial cultures. Granulomas should be biopsied and sent for histopathology and cytology when possible. A guarded prognosis is associated with granulomatous fungal disease involving the lungs as systemic fungal infections are normally seen in severely debilitated patients. Treatment for mycotic disease will depend on the location in the respiratory tract and the condition of the patient. Pharmacologic studies have been conducted with several azole antifungals in chelonians.[62] A dose for ketoconazole of 15 mg/kg by mouth every 24 hours for 2 to 4 weeks was found to achieve therapeutic drug levels in gopher tortoises.[63] Itraconazole at a dose of 5 mg/kg by mouth every 24 hours or 15 mg/kg by mouth every 72 hours in sea turtles has also been described.[64] Therapeutic levels have been achieved with fluconazole at 21 mg/kg subcutaneously once, then 10 mg/kg subcutaneously 5 days later, in healthy sea turtles. A single dose trial of voriconazole in red-eared sliders used 5 mg/kg subcutaneously and found the drug was absorbed well initially but appeared to be rapidly metabolized with therapeutic levels detected only at 1 and 2 hours postinjection.[65] Amphotericin B was used safely in a Greek tortoise with pulmonary candidiasis. In this case, the drug was delivered directly to the affected lung via a carapacial osteotomy.[66] In some cases the surgical removal of granulomas is recommended.

Parasitic

Primary parasitic disease of the respiratory tract is rare in chelonians and usually found only as part of a systemic process. Disseminated intranuclear coccidiosis has been reported in several species of chelonians.[67] Examination of the lungs of systemically affected individuals often reveals *Coccidia*. The organisms can be present in the nuclei of the pneumocytes and associated with pneumocyte hypertrophy. Another report described intranuclear coccidiosis of the nasal cavity in Sulawesi tortoises (*Indotestudo forstenii*).[68] No treatment has been described for pulmonary intranuclear coccidiosis. Diagnosis was originally made by observation of the organisms in histologic samples. A PCR test has been developed to detect intranuclear coccidiosis in tortoises.[67] It is unknown if sulfa drugs that have been used to treat gastrointestinal coccidiosis would be efficacious in cases of disseminated intranuclear coccidiosis affecting the lungs. Spirorchid flukes can infect wild marine and freshwater turtles.

These turtles are the definitive hosts. The disease is often disseminated, with adults inhabiting the heart and cardiac vessels. When the eggs are released, they can cause a severe granulomatous reaction in the lungs.[69] Spirorchid infection can be diagnosed by the presence of fluke eggs on fecal direct smears or sedimentation.[70] Praziquantel has been used for the treatment of spirorchids in loggerhead sea turtles. A dose of 25 mg/kg three times every 3 hours was recommended.[71] Ascarid larval migration can affect the lungs in infected chelonians. Primary lesions from the larval migration may not cause morbidity by themselves but can be an underlying cause of secondary bacterial pneumonia.[16]

NONINFECTIOUS CAUSES OF RESPIRATORY DISEASE
Hypovitaminosis A

Hypovitaminosis A is epidemic in aquatic and semiaquatic turtles adapted to wild diets high in vitamin A. This syndrome was first described in aquatic turtles in 1967.[72] Clinical signs of this disease are attributable to squamous metaplasia and immune suppression. Mild cases usually present with bilateral periorbital swelling. Secondary bacterial respiratory infections are common in more severely affected individuals (**Fig. 6**). Aural abscesses and caseous debris covering the cornea are also commonly noted. Hypovitaminosis A is very rare in tortoises.

Affected turtles can be given two injections of vitamin A subcutaneously at 500 to 5000 IU/kg 14 days apart.[73] Overdose of vitamin A, particularly water soluble preparations, can cause sloughing of the skin. Dietary correction is essential for long-term treatment. Liquid cod liver oil is widely available at human pharmacies, very high in vitamin A, and readily accepted by most turtles on food. Secondary bacterial infections can be treated based on culture and sensitivity.

Trauma

As stated earlier, trauma to the carapace often usually causes little or no respiratory problems in chelonians. However, pulmonary contusions and hemorrhage secondary to the injury can cause severe respiratory compromise and mortality. Additionally, if secondary infections are not controlled, many individuals will eventually succumb to bacterial or even fungal pneumonia. Flushing the wound with sterile saline is recommended to remove any foreign material. Antibiotics should be started immediately

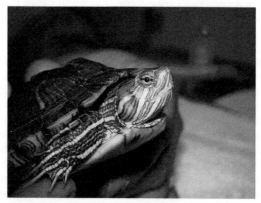

Fig. 6. An aural abscess in a red-eared slider secondary to hypovitaminosis A. (*Courtesy of* Marc H. Kramer, DVM, Miami, FL.)

while awaiting culture and sensitivity results. Fresh wounds can be repaired quickly. Older wounds should only be permanently repaired after antibiotic therapy and topical disinfection have eliminated any existing infection.[74]

Therapeutics

Treatment for respiratory disease depends on the cause of disease and the condition of the patient. Husbandry correction is imperative in all cases. Very ill patients should receive supportive care in addition to treatment for specific pathologies. Fluids, assisted feeding, oxygen therapy, heat, and nutritional correction may all be used. The daily maintenance fluid requirement for reptiles has been estimated to be between 15 and 25 mL/kg.[75] Desert-adapted species will fall on the lower end of the range. Dehydration is common in sick chelonians and can be estimated on physical examination by the sunken appearance of the eyes and the turgor of the jugular vein.

Many debilitated and dehydrated chelonians experience lactic acidosis. The clearance of lactate is slow in compromised reptiles with hypoperfusion of the liver or liver disease making administration of lactated fluids controversial. A crystalloid with an osmolality (mOsm) of 250 to 290 mOsm/L is ideal for routine fluid replacement in reptiles.[76] Fluids containing 0.45% saline and 2.5% dextrose are commercially available and have an osmolality of 280 mOsm/L. Fluids should be warmed to match the preferred optimum temperature zone of the patient. Assisted feeding is indicated if the patient is chronically anorectic. An esophagostomy tube can be placed to deliver food, fluids, vitamins, and oral medications in these individuals. For patients exhibiting respiratory distress, oxygen may be administered by face mask. In severe cases, endotracheal intubation and intermittent positive pressure ventilation may be necessary. Generally, 2 to 6 breaths per minute are recommended for reptiles.[77] Care must be taken not to overinflate the chelonian lungs, which are restricted by the carapace. Antimicrobials have been discussed under specific diseases and many antibiotic, antifungal, and antiparasitic drug doses are available for chelonians.[78,79] Nebulization therapy can be used in addition to parenteral medications. Anecdotally, it has been reported that chelonians with acute respiratory disease respond to nebulization therapy with aminophylline at 2.5 mg/ml combined with sterile saline followed by nebulization with antimicrobials every 12 hours.[77] Antibiotics that have been used for nebulization include: amikacin 5 mg per10 mL saline for 30 minutes every 24 hours, cefotaxime 100mg per 10 mL saline every 24 hours, and piperacillin 100 mg per10 mL saline every 24 hours. Amikacin should only be used in patients with normal renal function that are receiving supplemental fluid therapy.[16]

REFERENCES

1. Wyneken J. Respiratory anatomy—form and function in reptiles. Exotic DVM 2001;3:17–22.
2. Wyneken J. The structure of cardiopulmonary systems of turtles. In: Wyneken J, Godfrey MH, Bels V, editors. Biology of turtles. Boca Raton (FL): CRC Press; 2008. p. 916–8.
3. Heard DJ. Reptile anesthesia. Vet Clin North Am Exot Anim 2001;4:83–117.
4. Boyer TH, Boyer DM. Turtles, tortoises and terrapins. In: Mader D, editor. Reptile medicine and surgery. Philadelphia: WB Saunders; 1996. p. 61–78.
5. Hernandez-Divers SJ, Read M. Reptile respiration and controlled ventilation during anesthesia. Proc Assoc Rep Amphib Vet 2002;145–7.
6. Bennett RA. Anesthesia. In: Bennett RA, editor. Reptile medicine and surgery. Philadelphia: WB Saunders; 1996. p. 241–7.

7. Sykes IV, Klaphake E. Reptile hematology. Vet Clin North Am Exot Anim 2008;11: 481–500.
8. Hernandez-Divers SJ, Hernandez-Divers SM, Wyneken J. Clinical applications of a supravertebral (subcarapacial) vein in chelonians. Proc Assoc Rep Amphib Vet 2001;7–12.
9. Campbell TW, Ellis CK. Hematology of reptiles. In: Avian and exotic animal hematology and cytology. Ames (IA): Blackwell Publishing; 2007. p. 51–81.
10. Hernandes-Divers SJ. Diagnostic techniques. In: Mader D, editor. Reptile medicine and surgery. 2nd edition. St Louis (MO): Elsevier; 2006. p. 490–532.
11. Bennett T. Tips for selected clinical techniques in anurans and chelonians. Exotic DVM 2010;12:3–6.
12. Gumpenberger M. Computed tomography in chelonians. Proc Assoc Rep Amphib Vet 2002;41–3.
13. Straub J, Jurina K. Magnetic resonance imaging in chelonians. Semin Avian Exotic Pet Med 2002;10:181–6.
14. Divers SJ. Reptile diagnostic endoscopy and endosurgery. Vet Clin North Am Exot Anim Pract 2010;13:217–42.
15. Chinnadurai SK, DeVoe RS. Selected infectious diseases of reptiles. Vet Clin North Am Exot Anim Pract 2009;12:583–96.
16. Murray M. Pneumonia and lower respiratory tract disease. In: Mader D, editor. Reptile medicine and surgery. 2nd edition. St Louis (MO): Elsevier; 2006. p. 865–77.
17. Soldati G, Lu ZH, Vaughan L, et al. Detection of mycobacteria and chlamydiae in granulomatous inflammation of retiles: a retrospective study. Vet Pathol 2004;41: 388–97.
18. Jacobsen ER, Gaskin JM, Brown MB, et al. Chronic upper respiratory tract disease of free ranging desert tortoises (Xerobates agassazii). J Wildl Dis 1991;27:296–316.
19. Brown MB, Schumacher IM, Klein PA, et al. Mycoplasma agassizii causes upper respiratory disease in the desert tortoise. Infect Immun 1994;62:4580–5.
20. Brown DR, Merritt JL, Jacobson ER, et al. Mycoplasma testudineum sp. nov., from a desert tortoise (Gopherus agassizii) with upper respiratory tract disease. Int J Syst Evol Microbiol 2004;54:1527–9.
21. Hill AC. Mycoplasma testudinis a new species isolated from a tortoise. Int J Syst Bacteriol 1985;35:489–92.
22. Soares JF, Chalker VJ, Erles K, et al. Prevalence of Mycoplasma agassizii and chelonian herpesvirus in captive tortoises (Testudo sp) in the United Kingdom. J Zoo Wildl Med 2004;35:25–33.
23. Feldman SF, Wimsatt J, Marchang RE, et al. A novel mycoplasma detected in association with upper respiratory tract disease syndrome in free-ranging eastern box turtles (Terrapene carolina carolina) in Virginia. J Wildl Dis 2006;42:279–89.
24. Wendland LD, Brown DR, Klein PA, et al. Upper respiratory tract disease (Mycoplasma) in tortoises. In: Mader D, editor. Reptile medicine and surgery. 2nd edition. St Louis (MO): Elsevier; 2006. p. 931–8.
25. Schumacher IM, Brown MB, Jacobson ER, et al. Detection of antibodies to a pathogenic mycoplasma in desert tortoises (Gopherus agassizii) with upper respiratory tract disease. J Clin Microbiol 1993;31:1454–60.
26. Wendland LD, Zacher LA, Klein PA, et al. Improved enzyme-linked immunosorbent assay to reveal Mycoplasma agassizii exposure: a valuable tool in the management of environmentally sensitive tortoise populations. Clin Vaccine Immunol 2007;14:1190–5.

27. Brown DR, Schumacher IM, McLaughlin GS, et al. Application of diagnostic tests for mycoplasmal infections of desert and gopher tortoises, with management recommendations. Chelonian Conserv Biol 2002;4:497–507.
28. Johnson AJ, Morafka DJ, Jacobson ER. Seroprevalence of *Mycoplasma agassizii* and tortoise herpes virus in captive desert tortoises (*Gopherus agassizii*) from the greater Barstow area of the Mojave Desert. Cal J Arid Environ 2006;67:199–201.
29. Biermann RH, Blahak S. First isolation of a herpesvirus from tortoises with diphtheroid-necrotizing stomatitis. Second World Congress of Herpetology. Abstr 1994;6:27.
30. Herbst LH, Jacobsen ER, Klein PA, et al. Comparative pathology and pathogenesis of spontaneous and experimentally induced fibropapillomas of green turtles (*Chelonia mydas*). Vet Pathol 1999;36:551–64.
31. Jacobson ER, Buergelt C, Williams B, et al. Herpesvirus in cutaneous fibropapillomas of the green turtle (*Chelonia mydas*). Dis Aquat Org 1991;12:1–6.
32. Jacobsen ER, Gaskin JM, Roelke M, et al. Conjuctivitis, tracheitis and pneumonia associated with herpesvirus infection of green sea turtles. J Am Vet Med Assoc 1986;189:1020–3.
33. Frost JW, Schmidt A. Serological evidence for susceptibility of various species of tortoises to infections by herpesvirus. Verh ber Erkrg Zootiere 1997;38:25–8.
34. Origgi FC, Romero CH, Bloom DC, et al. Experimental transmission of a herpesvirus in Greek tortoises (*Testudo graeca*). Vet Pathol 2004;41:50–61.
35. McKeown S. General husbandry and management. In: Mader D, editor. Reptile medicine and surgery. Philadelphia: WB Saunders; 1996. p. 9–19.
36. Reinauer S, Reinhard B, Marschang RE. Inactivation of tortoise viruses in the environment. J Herp Med Surg 2005;15:10–5.
37. Marschang RE, Gravendyck M, Kaleta EF, et al. Investigation into virus isolation and the treatment of viral stomatitis in *T. Hermanni* and *T. Graeca*. J Vet Med Series 1997;44:385–94.
38. Origgi FC. Herpesvirus in tortoises. In: Mader D, editor. Reptile medicine and surgery. 2nd edition. St Louis (MO): Elsevier; 2006. p. 814–21.
39. Origgi FC, Klein PA, Tucker SJ, et al. Application of immunoperoxidase-based techniques to detect herpesvirus infection in tortoises. J Vet Diagn Invest 2003; 15:133–40.
40. Teifke JP, Löhr CV, Marschang RE, et al. Detection of chelonid herpesvirus DNA by nonradioactive in situ hybridization in tissues from tortoises suffering from stomatitis-rhinitis complex in Europe and North America. Vet Pathol 2000;37: 377–85.
41. Murakami M, Matsuba C, Une Y, et al. Development of species-specific PCR techniques for the detection of tortoise herpesvirus. J Vet Diagn Invest 2001; 13:513–6.
42. Johnson AJ, Norton TM, Wellehan JF, et al. Iridovirus outbreak in captive Burmese star tortoises (*Geochelone platynota*). Proc Assoc Rep Amphib Vet 2004;143–4.
43. VanDevanter DR, Warrener P, Bennett L, et al. Detection and analysis of diverse herpesviral species by consensus primer PCR. J Clin Microbiol 1996;34:1666–71.
44. Marschang RE, Origgi FC. Diagnosis of herpesvirus infections in tortoises— a review. Verh Ber Erkrg Zootiere 2003;41:1–8.
45. McArthur SD. An acyclovir trial in *Testudo* sp. Proc BVZS Spring Meet 2000.
46. Gaio C, Rossi T, Villa R, et al. Pharmacokinetics of acyclovir after single dose oral administration in marginated tortoises, *Testudo marginata*. J Herp Med Surg 2007;17:8–11.

47. McArthur S. Chelonian herpesvirus roundtable discussion. J Herp Med Surg 2002;12:14–31.
48. Wellehan JF, Johnson AJ. Reptile virology. Vet Clin Exot Anim 2005;8:27–52.
49. Westhouse RA, Jacobson ER, Harris RK, et al. Respiratory and pharyngo–esophageal iridovirus infection in a gopher tortoise (Gopherus polyphemus). J Wildl Dis 1996;32:682–6.
50. DeVoe RK, Geissler S, Elmore D, et al. Ranavirus-associated morbidity and mortality in a group of captive eastern box turtles (Terrapene carolina carolina). J Zoo Wildl Med 2004;35:534–43.
51. Chen ZX, Zheng JC, Jiang YL. A new iridovirus isolated from soft-shelled turtle. Virus Res 1999;63:147–51.
52. Marschang RE, Becher P, Posthaus H, et al. Isolation and characterization of an iridovirus from Hermann's tortoises (Testudo hermanni). Arch Virol 1999;144: 1909–22.
53. Johnson AJ, Norton TM, Wellehan JFX, et al. Iridovirus outbreak in captive Burmese star tortoises (Geochelone platynota). Proc Assoc Rep Amphib Vet 2004;143–4.
54. Johnson AJ, Pessier AP, Wellehan JF, et al. Ranavirus infection of free-ranging and captive box turtles and tortoises in the United States. J Wildl Dis 2008;44:851–63.
55. Johnson AJ, Pessier AP, Jacobsen ER. Experimental transmission and induction of ranaviral disease in western ornate box turtles (Terrapene ornata ornata) and red-eared sliders (Trachemys scripta elegans). Vet Pathol 2007;44:285–97.
56. Huang Y, Huang X, Liu H, et al. Complete sequence determination of a novel reptile iridovirus isolated from soft-shelled turtle and evolutionary analysis of Iridoviridae. BMC Genomics 2009;10:224.
57. Schumacher J. Fungal diseases of reptiles. Vet Clin North Am Exot Anim 2003;327–35.
58. Schumacher J. Reptile respiratory medicine. Vet Clin North Am Exot Anim 2003;6: 213–31.
59. Jacobsen ER, Gaskin JM, Shields RP, et al. Mycotic pneumonia in mariculture-reared green sea turtles. J Am Vet Med Assoc 1979;175:929–33.
60. Hernandez-Divers SJ, Norton T, Hernandez-Divers S, et al. Endoscopic diagnosis of pulmonary granulomas due to Paecilomyces in a juvenile loggerhead sea turtle (Caretta caretta). Proc Assoc Rep Amphib Vet 2002;3–4.
61. Gámez VS, García MLJ, Osorio SD, et al. Pathology in the Olive Ridley turtles (Lepidochelys olivacea) that arrived to the shores of Cuyutlan, Colima, Mexico. Vet Mex 2009;40:69–78.
62. Jacobsen ER, Cheatwood JL, Maxwell LK. Mycotic diseases of reptiles. Semin Avian Exot Pet Med 2000;9:94–101.
63. Page CD, Mautino M, Derendorf H, et al. Multiple-dose pharmokinetics of ketoconazole administered orally to gopher tortoises (Gopherus polyphemus). J Zoo Wildl Med 1991;22:191–8.
64. Manire CA, Rhinehart HI, Pennick GL, et al. Steady state plasma concentrations of itraconazole after oral administration in Kemp's Ridley sea turtles, Lepidochelys kempi. J Zoo Wildl Med 2003;43:171–8.
65. Innis C, Young D, Wetzlich S, et al. Plasma voriconazole concentrations in four red-eared slider turtles (Trachemys scripta elegans) after a single cutaneous injection. Proc Assoc Rep Amphib Vet 2008;72.
66. Divers SJ. Pulmonary candidiasis caused by Candida albicans in a Greek tortoise (Testudo graeca) and treatment with intrapulmonary amphotericin B. J Zoo Wildl Med 2001;32:352–9.

67. Garner MM, Gardiner CH, Wellehan JFX, et al. Intranuclear coccidiosis in tortoises: nine cases. Vet Pathol 2006;43:311–20.
68. Innis CJ, Garner MM, Johnson AJ, et al. Antemortem diagnosis and characterization of nasal intranuclear coccidiosis in Sulawesi tortoises (*Indotestudo forsteni*). J Vet Diagn Invest 2007;19:670–7.
69. Jacobsen ER. Parasites and parasitic diseases of reptiles. In: Jacobsen ER, editor. Infectious diseases and pathology of reptiles: color atlas and text. Boca Raton (FL): CRC Press; 2007. p. 571–615.
70. Reavill DR, Schmidt RE, Stevenson R. Review of spirorchid flukes (Digenea: *Spirorchidae*) and three cases in freshwater turtles. Proc Assoc Rep Amphib Vet 2004;139–42.
71. Jacobsen ER, Harman G, Laille E, et al. Plasma concentrations of praziquantel in loggerhead sea turtles (*Caretta caretta*), following oral administration of single and multiple doses. Proc Assoc Rep Amphib Vet 2002;37–9.
72. Elkan E, Zwart P. The ocular disease of young terrapins caused by vitamin A deficiency. Pathol Vet 1967;4:201–22.
73. Boyer TH. Hypovitaminosis A and hypervitaminosis A. In: Mader D, editor. Reptile medicine and surgery. 2nd edition. St Louis (MO): Elsevier; 2006. p. 831–5.
74. Barten SL. Shell damage. In: Mader D, editor. Reptile medicine and surgery. 2nd edition. St Louis (MO): Elsevier; 2006. p. 893–9.
75. Boyer TH. Emergency care of reptiles. Vet Clin North Am Exot Anim 1998;1: 191–206.
76. Martinez-Jimenez D, Hernandez-Divers SJ. Emergency care of reptiles. Vet Clin North Am Exot Anim 2007;10:557–85.
77. Raiti P. Administration of aerosolized antibiotics to reptiles. Proc Assoc Rep Amphib Vet 2002;119–23.
78. Carpenter JW. Exotic animal formulary. 3rd edition. St Louis (MO): Elsevier; 2005. p. 55–131.
79. Funk RS, Diethelm G. Reptile formulary. In: Mader D, editor. Reptile medicine and surgery. 2nd edition. St Louis (MO): Elsevier; 2006. p. 119–39.

Avian Respiratory Distress: Etiology, Diagnosis, and Treatment

Susan E. Orosz, PhD, DVM, DABVP (Avian), DECZM (Avian)[a],*,
Marla Lichtenberger, DVM, DACVECC[b]

KEYWORDS

- Respiratory distress • Avian • Anatomy and physiology
- Infraobital sinus • Upper respiratory infection
- Paleopulmonic respiratory system
- Neopulmonic respiratory system

Respiratory distress is usually a life-threatening emergency in any species and this is particularly important in avian species because of their unique anatomy and physiology. In the emergency room, observation of breathing patterns, respiratory sounds, and a brief physical examination are the most important tools for the diagnosis and treatment of respiratory distress in avian patients.[1–5] These tools will help the clinician localize the lesion, which will facilitate immediate steps to stabilize patients. This discussion focuses on the 5 anatomic divisions of the respiratory system and provides clinically important anatomic and physiologic principles and diagnosis and treatment protocols for the common diseases occurring in each part.

Every bird with breathing difficulties requires immediate stabilization in a warmed incubator with oxygen flow at 5 L/min, delivering oxygen concentrations at 78% to 85% in a Lyon cage (Lyon Technologies Inc, Chula Vista, CA, USA). A bronchial dilator, terbutaline (eg, 0.01 mg/kg intramuscularly [IM] every 6–8 hours; Brethine), and an anti-anxiety analgesic, butorphanol (1–2 mg/kg IM every 2–3 hours; Torbutrol), are usually given to birds in respiratory distress before placing in the oxygen-enriched incubator.

FIVE AREAS OF THE RESPIRATORY SYSTEM
Upper Airway and Infraorbital Sinus

Anatomy and physiology
The cere is the area around the most dorsal surface of the maxillary rhamphotheca or upper bill. It may be feathered or unfeathered in various species of birds. In adult male

The authors have nothing to disclose.
[a] Bird and Exotic Pet Wellness Center, 5166 Monroe Street, Suite 305, Toledo, OH 43623, USA
[b] Milwaukee Emergency Medicine Center for Animals, 3670 South 108th Street, Greenfield, WI 53228, USA
* Corresponding author.
E-mail address: drsusanorosz@aol.com

budgerigars, the cere is usually blue (**Fig. 1**); in adult females it is usually brownish pink. Changes in the normal color pattern of the cere are suggestive of gonadal tumors in this species. Each species has a characteristic size and shape and any variation should be noted on the physical examination.

The nares or nostrils are located dorsally within the area of the cere in psittacine birds. The openings may be shaped abnormally as a result of chronic upper respiratory infection and should be noted on the physical examination (**Fig. 2**). Air moves through the nares into the nasal cavity. In Amazon parrots and Galliformes, a rounded, keratinized structure called the operculum is found in the rostral-most extent of the nasal cavity. It acts as a baffle to deflect and prevent inhalation of foreign bodies.

In most species, the nasal cavity is divided by a nasal septum. Within the lateral walls of the cavity are highly vascularized nasal conchae (**Fig. 3**). Most birds have 3 conchae: the rostral, middle, and caudal nasal conchae. The middle nasal concha is the largest. A clinically important anatomic feature is the relationship of this concha to the openings of the infraorbital sinus, the only true paranasal sinus of birds. This sinus opens dorsally into both the middle and caudal nasal conchae. The caudal nasal concha drains only into the nasal cavity by its dorsal opening into the infraorbital sinus. As a result, the only passageway for drainage of mucopurulent material in the infraorbital sinus is the caudal nasal concha up through the dorsal opening, or over the middle nasal concha into the nasal cavity. Pus collects in the sinus and can distend it around the eye.

The infraorbital sinus is located ventromedial to the orbit and has numerous diverticuli. A rostral diverticulum extends into the maxillary rostrum or bill, a preorbital diverticulum lies rostral to the orbit, a postorbital diverticulum may be subdivided to surround the opening of the ear, and a mandibular diverticulum extends into the mandibulary rostrum. In addition to its communication with the nasal conchae, the infraorbital sinus also communicates with the cervicocephalic air sac at its caudal-most extent. Knowledge of the relationship of this sinus and air sac with the bones of the skull is important during examination of the upper respiratory system and during irrigation and surgical drainage procedures.

History
The owner will often describe nasal discharge, redness or swelling of a portion of the infraorbital sinus and particularly around the eye (**Fig. 4**), feather loss on the head and ocular discharge, and some birds will rub their beak on the perch or scratch the sides of their head.

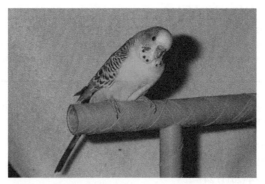

Fig. 1. Blue cere in a male budgerigar (*Melopsittacus undulatus*). Males typically have a blue cere at the base of the beak, whereas females have a brownish pink one.

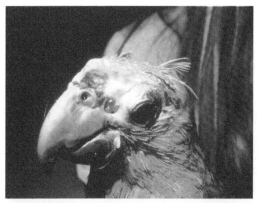

Fig. 2. Severe upper respiratory tract infection, double yellow-headed Amazon parrot (*Amazona oratrix*). The feathers are missing from head rubbing in an attempt to reduce pressure within the infraorbital sinus. Excoriated areas just distal to cere indicate where the rostral portion of the infraorbital sinus is now exposed.

Pattern of breathing, respiratory sounds, and physical examination
There will be a soft nasal sound with open beak breathing only with complete, bilateral nasal obstruction. There will be an increased respiratory rate without an increased effort.

Etiology
The differential diagnoses for a URI are a secondary response to hypovitaminosis A; other nutritional deficiencies; squamous metaplasia; altered immunocompetence; infections from predominantly gram-negative bacteria, mycobacteria, mycoplasma,

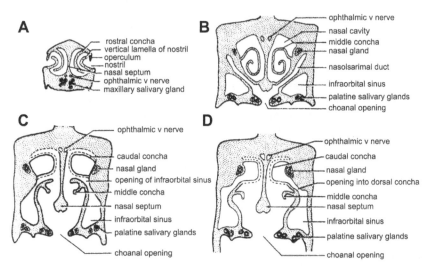

Fig. 3. Cross-sectional anatomy of the nasal conchae and infraorbital sinus in fowl, from (*A*) (rostral) to (*D*) (caudal). The anatomic plan is similar among species. Note the only connection between the nasal cavity and infraorbital sinus is dorsal over the middle nasal conchae. (*Reprinted from* King AS, McLelland J. Birds: their structure and function. 2nd edition. Bath (United Kingdom): Bailliere Tindall; 1984. p. 111; with permission.)

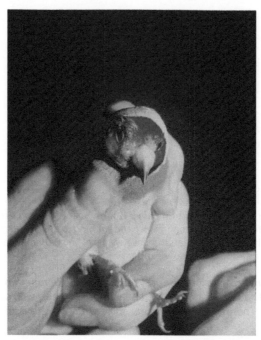

Fig. 4. Gouldian finch (*Erythrura gouldiae*) with an infraorbital sinusitis. Pus collects in the infraorbital sinus and distends it laterally, making the periorbital area swollen.

and fungal elements (such as *Aspergillus* sp or yeast); viral infections, including avipox virus,[6] and *Chlamydophila*; and parasitic infections, such as trichomonads, *Capillaria*, nematode cysts, and *Knemidokoptes*. The clinician should examine the choanal slit in the roof of the oropharynx (**Fig. 5**). Blunting of the papillae is associated with disease processes or hypovitaminosis A in those species with papillae.

Although passerines with conjunctivitis and other symptoms of upper respiratory tract infections are associated with mycoplasma, psittacines can also be affected. Diagnosis is often based on polymerase chain reaction (PCR) samples taken from swabs of the conjunctiva or fluid from flushes of the nasal cavity. Isolation and culture is often difficult.[7] Common serotypes of paramyxovirus (PMV) of passerines include PMV-1, 2, and 3 and these can produce respiratory signs in passerines and other avian species. Often the birds show respiratory signs along with gastrointestinal (GI) and neurologic signs, but can die acutely.

Noninfectious causes may include airborne toxins, cigarette smoke, polytetrafluoro-ethylene, allergies, foreign-body inhalation, and subcutaneous swellings of unknown etiology.

Diagnostic tests
A nasal flush (**Fig. 6**) or infraorbital sinus aspiration should be performed. The fluid obtained can be gram stained, a cytology performed, or culture and sensitivity done. Endoscopy of the choanal area and biopsy of any lesions could be considered as the next diagnostic procedure for those that are nonresponsive to initial treatment. Radiographs of the head and computed tomographic scans of sinuses may be useful. Various PCR tests may be used based on the differential diagnoses.

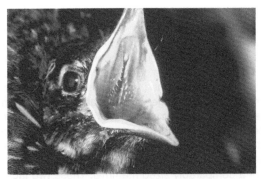

Fig. 5. Choanal slit from a robin (*Turdus migratorius*). The clinician should examine the roof of the oropharynx. Many species have caudally directed papillae normally. Blunting is associated with hypovitaminosis A and a variety of diseases.

Treatment
Many times a nasal flush will help remove mucous and discharge so that the bird can breathe easier. Initial cytology and gram stains of the fluid can help the clinician decide on treatment (antibiotics, antifungals) pending cultures and sensitivity results.

Large Airway (Glottis, Trachea to the Syrinx)

Anatomy and physiology
The larynx is composed of 4 mostly ossified cartilages with an overlying mucosa or laryngeal mound. The larynx is not involved in sound production in birds. The rima glottis represents the laryngeal opening into the trachea and is not covered by an epiglottis as it is in mammals. The rima glottis and trachea are larger in diameter on a per weight basis than they are in mammals. This principle provides one reason

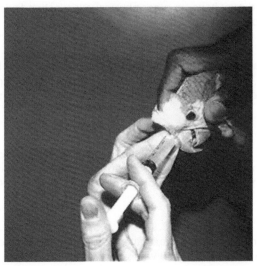

Fig. 6. Nasal flush of an orange-winged Amazon (*Amazona amazonica*). Holding the bird in this position allows the flush to move from the nostril through the rostral portion of the nasal cavity and out the choanal slit without aspirating the bird. Use pH-balanced saline.

why it is easier to intubate birds than mammals. This increased diameter directly reflects one physiologic adaptation of birds: the use of their beaks for the manipulation of objects. The increased length of the trachea is part of an adaptation in birds whereby the increased length of their necks allows use of their beak to manipulate objects. However, the increase in length causes an increased air resistance. A wider rima glottis, as well as a wider trachea, is necessary to reduce this resistance. To compensate for the wider and longer trachea and its corresponding increase in dead space, the respiratory rate of birds is less than that of mammals, with a larger tidal volume. These anatomic and physiologic differences are important when selecting endotracheal tubes for anesthetic procedures. In addition, the tracheal rings of birds are complete. They are shaped like a signet ring and overlap to form a more rigid trachea than that of a comparably sized mammal. These two facts are important to reduce the possibility of tracheal kinking when moving the neck. Overinflation of a cuffed endotracheal tube is potentially easier in a bird because of the less expansive nature of the trachea. Overinflation can lead to mucosal edema and difficulty breathing. Whenever possible, uncuffed endotracheal tubes should be used.

The trachea often bifurcates immediately after entering the thoracic inlet. At this bifurcation is the syrinx (**Fig. 7**), which represents the voice box of birds. The syrinx is highly variable among species but represents several cartilages, which may be ossified, and syringeal muscles and membranes. Most syringeal muscles are external to the tracheal bifurcation. Depending on the species, birds may also have internal syringeal muscles within the space of the trachea or bronchi. This narrowed internal diameter of the syrinx is a common site for tracheal granulomas and foreign bodies.

History
The bird may have demonstrated inspiratory stridor that has increased in intensity or the respiratory distress could be acute because of complete obstruction.

Pattern of breathing, respiratory sounds, and physical examination
There is a loud inspiratory stridor. There is an increase rate and effort with open beak breathing. The bird may have no other physical examination findings. The bird will present gasping for air if there is a complete obstruction.

Etiology
Causes of large airway disease include obstruction by a foreign body (ie, seed in cockatiels), mass, *Aspergillus* granuloma (**Fig. 8**A) or oropharyngeal granulomas, *Mycobacterium genavense* infection causing a granuloma,[8] and tracheal fibrinous seal.[9]

Diagnostic tests
Radiographs (see **Fig. 8**B), complete blood count (CBC) and a biochemical profile, transtracheal wash, and endoscopy can help to diagnose the cause of airway obstruction. Material removed by endoscopy can be submitted for PCR, culture, and cytology.

Treatment
Large airway obstruction requires rapid anesthetic induction with sevoflurane/isoflurane anesthesia, rapid intubation and ventilation with 100% oxygen. If there is a total upper airway obstruction, emergency air sac tube placement is performed. The bird will relax and breathe easier under inhalant anesthesia. Endoscopy can be used to remove an obstruction as a granuloma or seed caught at the syrinx.

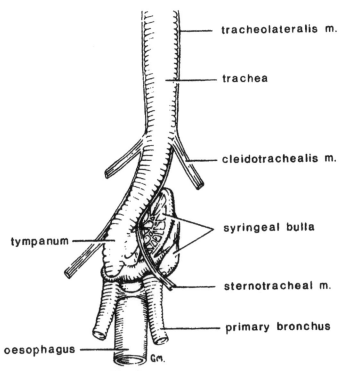

Fig. 7. Ventral view of the tracheal bifurcation and syrinx from a tufted duck. Ducks often have a syringeal bulla that is a diverticulum to enhance sound production. Psittacine birds do not have one; however, sound is produced at the tracheal bifurcation in birds, not at the tracheal opening (larynx) as in mammals. (*Reprinted from* King AS, McLelland J. Birds: their structure and function. 2nd edition. Bath (United Kingdom): Bailliere Tindall; 1984. p. 119; with permission.)

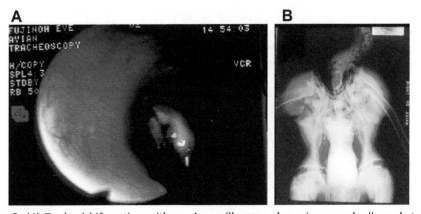

Fig. 8. (*A*) Tracheal bifurcation with an *Aspergillus* granuloma in an umbrella cockatoo (*Cacatua alba*) using a rigid endoscope. Note the narrowing of the trachea opening. The cockatoo presented with open mouth breathing, inspiratory stridor, and labored abdominal effort in breathing. (*B*) Ventrodorsal radiograph of a bald eagle (*Haliaeetus leucocephalus*). There is thickening of the caudal thoracic air sac membrane, an opacity in the abdominal air sac, and increased opacity of the parabronchi.

Small Airway

Anatomy and physiology

The mainstem or primary bronchi (**Fig. 9**) represent the continuation of the syrinx. Each perforates the septal surface of the lung and continues into the lung parenchyma as the intrapulmonary primary bronchus. The portion of the bronchus is long as it continues to the caudal extremity of the lung. Its diameter is variable among species but is widest at its entrance into the lung tissue and then tapers progressively. The epithelium of the primary bronchus is pseudostratified with goblet cells and there are areas with ridges carrying cilia. There are 4 groups of secondary bronchi that arise from the primary bronchus. Their anatomy is described with the description of the lung parenchyma.

History

A blue and gold macaw will present with the history of periodic respiratory distress and is commonly raised with a cockatoo or African gray. The offending toxin, such as smoke, aerosol, or cigarettes, will be identified on history. Bird may appear open mouthed with increased abdominal effort on expiration.

Pattern of breathing, respiratory sounds, and physical examination

There will be a soft (heard by placing ear next to birds beak) expiratory wheeze. The bird will be in extreme respiratory distress with open beak breathing and may even fall on its side gasping.

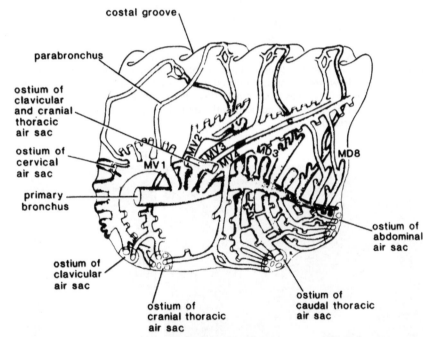

Fig. 9. The septal surface of the right lung of the domestic fowl, which shows the anatomic arrangement of the medioventral (MV-arising dorsally) and the lateroventral (LV-arising ventrally) secondary bronchi as they arise from the primary bronchus. Also shown are the mediodorsal (MD) secondary bronchi. The direction of origin of the secondary bronchi and the termination of the primary bronchus into the abdominal air sac explains opacities that can be observed radiographically. (*Reprinted from* King AS, McLelland J. Birds: their structure and function. 2nd edition. Bath (United Kingdom): Bailliere Tindall; 1984. p. 122; with permission.)

Etiology
Small airway disease includes inhalant respiratory irritants, such as smoke, polytetrafluoro-ethylene toxicity, aerosols, cigarette smoke, candles, heated polytetrafluoroethylene,[10] and overheated microwave.[11] Granulomas in the small airways may also cause this expiratory distress.

Diagnostic tests
Stabilize the bird for 12 to 24 hours with bronchodilators and oxygen. Radiographs, CBC, and chemistry profile should be performed to rule out an infectious disease. Birds with aspergillosis often have high white counts with total protein levels of approximately 7.

Treatment
The most effective bronchodilators are pharmaceutical agents that stimulate β-adrenergic receptors in bronchial smooth muscle and promote smooth muscle relaxation. For this reason they have become the authors' first line of treatment for bronchoconstriction causing acute respiratory distress. These β-receptor agonists are most effective and least toxic when they are given as an aerosol that is inhaled. β-agonists, such as terbutaline, can be given IM in birds (0.01 mg/kg every 6–8 hours) initially and then continued by nebulization.

Nebulizers are designed to convert liquids to appropriately sized aerosol particles for inhalation. The nebulizer consists of a disposable or reusable nebulizer and a pressurized gas (air or oxygen) source. A small volume of medication and a larger volume of diluent are placed into the nebulizer chamber.

Ultrasonic nebulizers generate an aerosol through ultrahigh-frequency vibration of a piezoelectric crystal at the bottom of a liquid. The advantages of using an ultrasonic nebulizer include faster nebulization time, longer product life, smaller particle size, and quieter operation compared with a jet nebulizer. The veterinarian nebulizer used most commonly is an ultrasonic nebulizer (DVM pharmaceuticals, Inc, IVAX Corp, Miami, FL, USA), which costs about $150, delivers particle size of 2 to 7 μm, and can be used by an owner in the home. It is not known if the particle size will reach the atria of the lung, but use of this nebulizer will deliver particles to the bronchi for treatment of bronchoconstriction.

Coelomic Cavity Disease (Mass, Fluid, or Organomegaly)

Anatomy and physiology
The coelomic cavities of birds are similar between species and in general there are 16 distinct and separate cavities in the adult bird. Eight of the cavities are air sacs and the remaining 8 are cavities of the coelom proper with 5 as peritoneal cavities and the remaining 3 also represented in mammals. The mammalian cavities include the right and left pleural cavities and the pericardial cavity. The 5 peritoneal cavities of birds include the left and right ventral hepatic peritoneal cavities, the left and right dorsal hepatic cavities, and the intestinal peritoneal cavity.

History
The bird will likely have a history of lethargy, decreased appetite, and not doing well before the respiratory distress.

Pattern of breathing, respiratory sounds, and physical examination
The bird will have increased respiratory rate and effort, which will become extreme dyspnea with open beak breathing on handling. There will be no respiratory sounds. A distended abdominal lift will be found on physical examination.

Etiology

Causes of coelom space disease include fluid accumulation heart disease, hypoalbu-
minemia, liver disease, egg-related peritonitis,[12] organomegaly (hepatic lipidosis), and
mass (neoplasia, abscess, egg).

Diagnostic Tests and Treatment

Ascites

Ascites causing coelomic distension will require immediate coelomocentesis. Coelomocentesis is done in the right lateral coelom just cranial to the cloaca. Use a 25- to
22-gauge needle or a 24-g angiocatheter and 1-, 3-, 5- to 12-mL syringe. The angiocatheter introduces a plastic tube into the coelom and potentially reduces trauma to
the surrounding organs if the bird moves. The smaller birds require a smaller syringe
as it provides lower pressure when aspirating. Often, ultrasound can help guide
coelomic centesis if the fluid is loculated and difficult to aspirate.

Save any fluid recovered for culture/sensitivity, PCR, or cytology. A transudate is
characterized by a clear to pale yellow color, with a low specific gravity (<1.020),
low protein (1 g/dL), and a low cellularity. The most common causes of a transudate
are liver failure (eg, cirrhosis) or heart failure. Exudate is characterized by a high
specific gravity (>1.020), a high protein content (>3 g/dL), and presence of inflammatory cells and mesothelial cells. Septic exudates may contain intracellular bacteria.
Septic peritonitis can be distinguished from a nonseptic peritonitis by the presence
of a lower coelomic glucose than serum glucose in septic peritonitis.

Turbid yellow, green, or brown yolky fluid or aspiration of inspissated yolk material in
the coelomic cavity is indicative of an ectopic ovulation of yolk or a ruptured oviduct.
Cytology reveals yolk material and fat particles. Free yolk in the abdomen may be
absorbed and inflammation is treated with nonsteroidal antiinflammatory drugs. If
bacteria are found on cytology of the yolk, antibiotics are used systemically. Often
antibiotics that include an anaerobic spectrum should be included in the treatment
plan. There can also be a fungal coelomitis so that cytology and gram stains of the
exudates and possible aerobic and anaerobic culture should be part of the diagnostic
plan.

With neoplasia, bloody fluid is often obtained on cystocentesis. Occasionally, exfo-
liated neoplastic cells can be observed on cytology. Abdominal ultrasound is
performed to identify the presence of an abdominal mass. A 22-gauge needle is
used for ultrasound-guided aspiration of the mass and cytology evaluation can then
be performed.

Organomegaly, egg binding, or mass lesions

Organomegaly, egg binding, or a mass lesion is suspected when the coelom is firm on
palpation. Ultrasonography is useful for identification of the egg (eg, laminated egg,
ectopic egg, or normal egg) or ultrasound-guided aspiration of the mass. Endoscopy
may be used to biopsy the mass or liver. Medical management of an abnormal egg
should be attempted using fluids, subcutaneous (SQ) or oral, and calcium administered by IM or SQ injection. Patients should be placed in a warmed incubator with
moisture added to help in the passage of the egg. Surgical exploratory may be
required if the egg does not pass in 24 hours or if the egg is within the coelomic cavity.

Parenchymal Disease (Lungs or Air Sacs)

Anatomy and physiology

The lungs are paired and attached firmly to the ribs and dorsal body wall. They appear
spongy with a honeycombed appearance on radiographs and are best visualized

using a lateral view. The mainstem bronchi divide into secondary bronchi. These bronchi subsequently divide into parabronchi. All parabronchi anastomose freely with other parabronchi and have expansions within their walls, called atria, which allows for gas exchange. Parabronchi (**Fig. 10**) maintain a constant mean diameter within a species.

The mediodorsal and medioventral secondary bronchi connect to form a functional unit. These bronchi terminate at the cranial pulmonary air sacs and form the basis of the paleopulmonic respiratory system (**Fig. 11**). The parabronchi of the lateroventral secondary bronchi connect with the laterodorsal secondary bronchi. The cranial pulmonary air sacs are expandable sacs that are connected to the lungs by these bronchial arrangements and include the cervical, clavicular, and cranial thoracic air sacs. The lateroventral bronchi are connected with the caudal pulmonary air sacs of the lungs. These caudal air sacs are the caudal thoracic and abdominal air sac. This latter arrangement represents the neopulmonic respiratory system. Air sacs, in general, are histologically similar to a peritoneum, with squamous to columnar epithelium, a basement membrane, and an underlying connective tissue support. Only in the area immediately surrounding an opening of a parabronchus does the tissue change to ciliated columnar epithelium. The paleopulmonic and neopulmonic systems are best defined physiologically rather than anatomically.

Birds do not have a diaphragm and therefore rely on changes in pressure between their air sacs relative to the atmospheric pressure to move air through a nonexpandable lung. The pressure changes within the air sacs are the result of volume changes in the thoracoabdominal cavity. On inspiration, the ribs move cranioventrally, thereby increasing the thoracoabdominal space. This action results in a lowering of the pressure in the air sacs. On expiration, the ribs move caudodorsally, thereby reducing the space in the chest and increasing the pressure in the air sacs. Expiration is also an active process requiring skeletal muscle contraction. For this reason, it is extremely

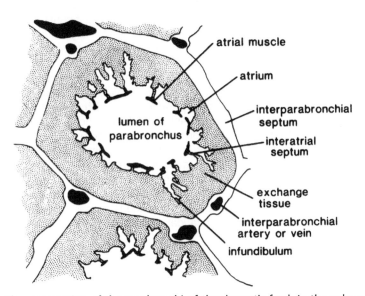

Fig. 10. The cross section of the parabronchi of the domestic fowl. In the paleopulmonic portion of the lungs, the parabronchi form a series of parallel tubes with the lung parenchyma between. (*Reprinted from* King AS, McLelland J. Birds: their structure and function. 2nd edition. Bath (United Kingdom): Bailliere Tindall; 1984. p. 125; with permission.)

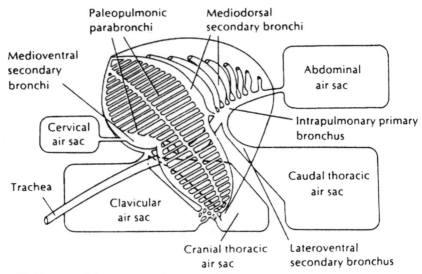

Fig. 11. Diagram of the lower respiratory tract after Fedde. The paleopulmonic system has the parallel parabronchi that connect with the cervical, clavicular, and cranial thoracic air sacs. This system, through aerodynamic valving, moves air in one direction. The neopulmonic system moves air in and out of the same parabronchial tubes bilaterally. The neopulmonic system includes the caudal thoracic and abdominal air sacs.

important when holding a bird that the sternum can move freely or the bird will suffocate.

Gas exchange occurs in the walls of the parabronchi, the atria, and more importantly in the air capillaries, which are the avian equivalent of alveoli (**Fig. 12**). The blood-gas barrier of birds is similar to that of mammals in that it consists of an endothelial capillary cell, a common basal lamina, and an air capillary epithelium of squamous cells. The difference is that the blood-gas barrier is much thinner in birds than in mammals. The diameter of the air capillaries of birds is much smaller than that of a mammalian alveolus, allowing for a much larger number of air capillaries in a given space when compared with mammals. For this reason, fluid can accumulate in the air capillary faster than an alveolus. Clinically then, birds crash faster than mammals because of their unique anatomy and physiology of the parenchyma of the lungs.

Because of the unidirectional continuous flow of air of the paleopulmonic system, birds are more efficient than mammals in capturing oxygen and removing carbon dioxide. The nonoxygenated blood enters at an approximately 90° angle from the parabronchus. This crosscurrent gas exchange enhances the ability to oxygenate blood.

The epithelial cells of the lung act as fixed macrophages and transfer engulfed material to interstitial macrophages. Air that enters the caudal air sacs is filtered less than that of the cranial air sacs, making the caudal air sacs more susceptible to disease.

History
There is usually a history of not doing well, lethargy, and anorexia.

Pattern of breathing, respiratory sounds, and physical examination
The bird shows signs of an increased respiratory rate or effort. There tends to be no audible respiratory sounds. The bird is usually in poor body condition because of the increased metabolic needs for the required effort to breathe.

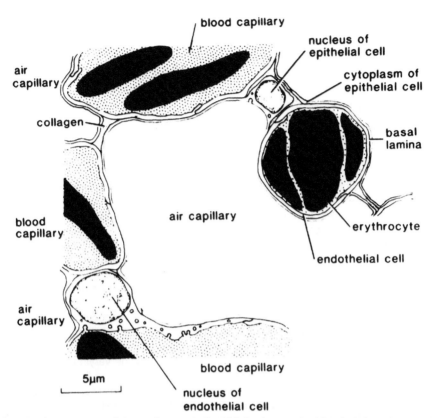

Fig. 12. The anatomy of the exchange surface of the lungs. The blood air barrier is much thinner in birds compared with mammals. It consists of the endothelial blood capillary cell, a common basal lamina, and the squamous epithelial cell of the air capillary. (*Reprinted from* King AS, McLelland J. Birds: their structure and function. 2nd edition. Bath (United Kingdom): Bailliere Tindall; 1984. p. 128; with permission.)

Etiology

Differential diagnoses for lower respiratory tract signs include infectious causes and noninfectious causes. Companion avian patients may have infections that result from a variety of agents and these include bacteria (often gram-negative rods), fungi (*Aspergillus*), viruses pox, Amazon tracheitis virus, Pacheco disease, polyomavirus, reovirus, exotic Newcastle disease, other PMVs, *Chlamydophila*, and parasites (air sac mites, species of *Syngamus*, *Toxoplasma/Atoxoplasma*, *Encephalitozoan*, *Sarcocystis*).

Aspiration is often secondary to crop disorders and may result in bacterial, yeast, or mycelial phase fungal infections. Birds may also aspirate because of foreign bodies in their upper GI tract; a goiter (parakeets) blocking the outflow of the crop, and overfilling of the crop when hand feeding or gavage feeding. Other conditions that cause inflammatory problems for the lower respiratory tree include toxicity (polytetrafluoroethylene, heavily scented products, and cigarette smoke), neoplasia, and a ruptured air sac. Metabolic causes may produce respiratory signs. Allergens are becoming more of a problem and they are suspected in pneumonitis observed in blue and gold macaws. Extrarespiratory causes reduce the available air sac space and do not allow adequate exchange across the blood air barrier. Common reasons for this to happen are ascites and an enlarged abdominal organ.

Diagnostic tests and treatment
Cardiac disease will require blood pressure measurements, radiographs, and an echocardiographic examination. Other diseases on the differential list may require titers, endoscopic biopsies, or cultures.

Parenchymal disease
Parenchymal disease may benefit from use of parental or nebulization of bronchodilators and antibiotics. An air sac tube may partially improve respiration in birds with primary lung and air sac disease.

Careful auscultation is indicated for a heart murmur or gallop or persistent arrhythmia suggestive of cardiogenic edema. If heart failure is suspected, administer furosemide (2–4 mg/kg intravenously) and nitroglycerine ointment on the back and allow the bird to stabilize before further diagnostics.

Birds with a history of regurgitation or vomiting may benefit from broad-spectrum antibiotics (eg, enrofloxacin, trimethoprim sulfadiazine, amoxicillin/clavulanic acid) and bronchodilators when aspiration pneumonia is suspected. Birds administered antibiotics particularly long-term should also be administered an antifungal drug to reduce the incidence of secondary infections.

Birds suspected of aspergillosis (leukocytosis with a monocytosis, increased total protein and pulmonary nodules) should be treated with appropriate antifungal drugs.

Birds suspected of psittacosis (leukocytosis, clinical signs varying from chronic unthriftiness to acute anorexia, diarrhea, respiratory distress, and lime green feces) should be treated with drugs inhibiting the growth of *Chlamydophila* species. Doxycycline is the drug of choice. Most commonly, a real-time PCR test for psittacosis that includes a swab of the conjunctiva, oropharynx, and choanal and cloaca with some whole blood is recommended from a clinical perspective. For further details, see the Compendium of Measures to Control *Chlamydophila psittaci* Infection Among Humans (Psittacosis) and Pet Birds (Avian Chlamydiosis), 2010, issued by the National Association of State Public Health Veterinarians (www.nasphv.org/documentsCompendiaPsittacosis).

REFERENCES

1. Hillyer H. Clinical manifestations of respiratory disorders. In: Altman R, Clubb S, Dorrestein G, Quesenberry K, editors. Avian medicine and surgery. Philadelphia: WB Saunders; 1997. p. 419–54.
2. Rupley A. Critical care of pet birds. Procedures, therapeutics, and patient support. Vet Clin North Am Exotic Anim Pract 1998;1:21–2.
3. Quesenberry K, Hillyer E. Supportive care and emergency therapy. In: Ritchie B, Harrison G, Harrison L, editors. Avian medicine: principles and application. Lake Worth (FL): Wingers Publishing; 1994. p. 406–7.
4. Doneley B, Harrison GJ, Lightfoot TL. Maximizing information from the physical examination. In: Harrison GJ, Lightfoot TL, editors. Clinical avian medicine. 2nd edition. Palm Beach (FL): Spix Publishing; 2006. p. 153–212.
5. Graham JE. Approach to the dyspneic avian patient. Semin Avian Exotic Pet Med 2004;13(3):154–9.
6. McDonald DE, Lowenstine LJ, Ardans AA. Avian pox in blue-fronted Amazon parrots. J Am Vet Med Assoc 1981;179(11):1218–22.

7. Sandmeir P, Coutteel P. In: Harrison GJ, Lightfoot TL, editors, Clinical avian medi-cine. Management of canaries, finches, and mynahs, vol. II. Palm Beach (FL): Spix Publishing; 2006. p. 879–913.
8. Kiehn TE, Hoefer H, Bottger EC, et al. *Mycobacterium genavense* infections in pet animals. J Clin Microbiol 1996;34(7):1840–2.
9. Good DA, Heatley TN, Tully Jr, et al. Anesthesia case of the month. Partial obstruction of the trachea was a differential diagnosis for the bird's respiratory problems. J Am Vet Med Assoc 2001;219(11):1529–31.
10. Wells RE, Slocombe RF, Trapp AL. Acute toxicosis of budgerigars (*Melopsittacus undulates*) caused by pyrolysis products from heated polytetrafluoroethylene: clinical study. Am J Vet Res 1982;43(7):1238–42.
11. Zanen AL, Rietveld AP. Inhalation trauma due to overheating in a microwave oven. Thorax 1993;48(3):300–2.
12. Gorham SL, Akins M, Carter B. Ectopic egg yolk in the abdominal cavity of a cock-atiel. Avian Dis 1992;36(3):816–7.

Rabbit Respiratory System: Clinical Anatomy, Physiology and Disease

Cathy A. Johnson-Delaney, DVM, DABVP (Avian), DABVP (Exotic Companion Mammal)[a],*,

Susan E. Orosz, PhD, DVM, DABVP (Avian), DECZM (Avian)[b]

KEYWORDS

- Rabbit • Respiratory system • Olfactory system
- Pasteurellosis • Staphylococcosis • Neoplasia

The nostrils of rabbits contain sensory pads at the entrance, making the nose very sensitive to touch. For this reason, when inspecting the nostrils and the oral cavity, put fingers lateral to the nasal area. The nostrils are still when totally relaxed, but can twitch at up to 150 twitches per minute. Rabbits have an acute sense of smell due to turbinate bones with a vomeronasal organ and olfactory sensory epithelium.[1]

Rabbits are obligate nose breathers due to their epiglottis positioned rostrally to the soft palate. Any obstruction within the nasal cavity will produce a respiratory wheeze with increased respiratory effort (**Fig. 1**).

Air moves through the nostrils across the alar folds into the nasal cavity. The nasal cavity is divided by the cartilaginous septum into a right side and a left side. Ventrally, the long nasal cavity is separated from the oral cavity by the hard palate cranially and the soft palate caudally. Each portion of the nasal cavity has dorsal and ventral nasal conchae that extend into the cavity from its lateral wall. The nasal conchae are scrolls of cartilaginous tissue covered by mucosa. Additionally, there are openings between the conchae that extend into the maxillary and ethmoid paranasal sinuses.

The epiglottis sits over the caudal portion of the soft palate.[1] This allows for an unobstructed conduit for air to move from the nostrils through the nasal cavity into the rima glottis. When looking into the oral cavity, a wall of tissue covering the opening of the glottis will be observed. To see into the tracheal opening, the soft palate will need to be elevated to drop the epiglottis into view. The mucosa is very sensitive to trauma related to intubation.

The authors have nothing to disclose.
[a] Eastside Avian and Exotic Animal Medical Center, 12930 NE 125th Way, Kirkland, WA 98034, USA
[b] Bird and Exotic Pet Wellness Center, 5166 Monroe Avenue, Suite 305, Toledo, OH 43623, USA
* Corresponding author.
E-mail address: cajddvm@hotmail.com

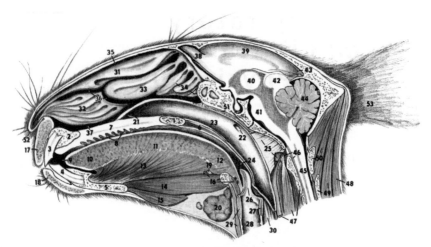

Fig. 1. Paramedian section through the head. Anatomic features with respiratory effect include the soft palate (6), hard palate (7), epiglottis (26), cartilaginous cricoid plate (27), trachea (28), dorsal nasal concha (31), and the ventral nasal concha (32). The epiglottis is positioned rostrally to the soft palate, thus requiring rabbits to be obligate nose breathers. (*Reprinted from* Popesko P, Rajtova V, Horak J. A colour atlas of anatomy of small laboratory animals, vol. 1. Rabbit, guinea pig. London (UK): Elsevier; 1992; with permission.)

The thorax is small in contrast to the size of the abdomen. The thymus persists in the adult and lies ventral to the heart, extending forward into the thoracic inlet (**Fig. 2**).

Both the left and right lungs have cranial, middle, and caudal lobes (**Fig. 3**).[1] However, the right lung has an accessory lobe. The left cranial lobe is smaller than the right due to the presence of the heart. The pleura is thin. There are no septa dividing the lungs into lobules. This accounts for pneumonia being generalized rather than localized. The normal respiratory rate at rest is 30 to 60 breaths per minute. At rest, the diaphragm is used for muscular contractions rather than the intercostal muscles. Open-mouth breathing is not normal and is an indicator of severe respiratory disease or agonal breathing.

DISEASES

Respiratory diseases are a major cause of morbidity and mortality in rabbits.[1–4] Pasteurellosis is the primary respiratory disease, but many other pathogens can play a role in the disease complex. The term snuffles can refer to any upper respiratory disease (URD). Comprehensive studies have shown that rabbits can resist infection even if housed with infected rabbits, spontaneously eliminate *Pasteurella multocida*, become chronic carriers, develop acute disease, develop bacteremia and pneumonia, or develop chronic disease. The pathogenesis depends on host resistance and virulence of the *P multocida* strain. Many rabbits carry *Bordetella bronchiseptica* and *Moraxella catarrhalis* in the nares. The prevalence of *P multocida* infection varies between rabbitries. It increases with the age of rabbits in facilities where the disease is endemic. There is an inverse relationship between *P multocida* and *B bronchiseptica* infections in rabbits. Weanlings have higher infection rates with *B bronchiseptica*, whereas *P multocida* predominates in adults.

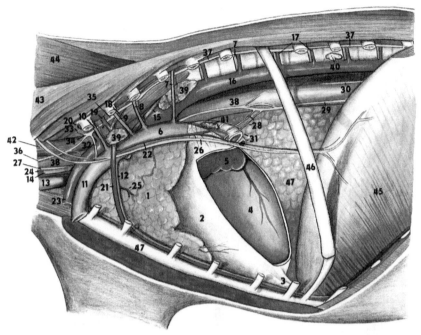

Fig. 2. The left visible lobe of the thymus (1) appears ventral to the heart (4). (*Reprinted from* Popesko P, Rajtova V, Horak J. A colour atlas of anatomy of small laboratory animals, vol. 1. Rabbit, guinea pig. Elsevier; 1992; with permission.)

Pasteurellosis

P multocida is a gram-negative, bipolar, nonmotile asporogenous coccobacillus from the family *Pasteurellaceae*, which includes *Haemophilus*, *Actinobacillus*, and *Pasteurella* species. Different strains require different specialized conditions for growth in the laboratory, which results in many cultures taken for diagnostic purposes failing to grow. *P multocida* can be typed serologically with the use of indirect hemagglutination to identify capsular types (A, B, D, E, or F). The gel diffusion precipitin test has described 16 somatic antigen determinants of the capsule lipopolysaccharide. Antibiotic sensitivities are varied depending on the strain. Generally, *P multocida* strains isolated from rabbits are sensitive to chloramphenicol, novobiocin, oxytetracycline, penicillin G, nitrofurazone, fluoroquinolones, and trimethoprim-sulfamethoxazole. Choice of antibiotic must be taken in consideration of the rabbit's gastrointestinal flora. Recovery from acute disease and elimination of infection can occur, but spontaneous recovery from chronic infection is unlikely.

Virulence factors of *P multocida* include adhesions, phagocyte resistance, endotoxin (lipopolysaccharide), exotoxin, and iron regulation. Some strains have pili or adhesin proteins on the outer membrane that enhance colonization. Type A strains are more adhesive to respiratory mucosa than are type D strains. Some type D strains resist bactericidal activity of phagocytes. Leukotoxic enzymes may be produced. The availability of iron regulates the growth of some strains. Most strains produce iron-binding outer membrane proteins. *P multocida* can invade and multiply, because the capsule, which is largely hyaluronic acid, inhibits phagocytosis and complement-activated bactericidal activity of serum. Endotoxin enhances resistance and stimulates the release of inflammatory mediators such as interleukin (IL)-1. Free

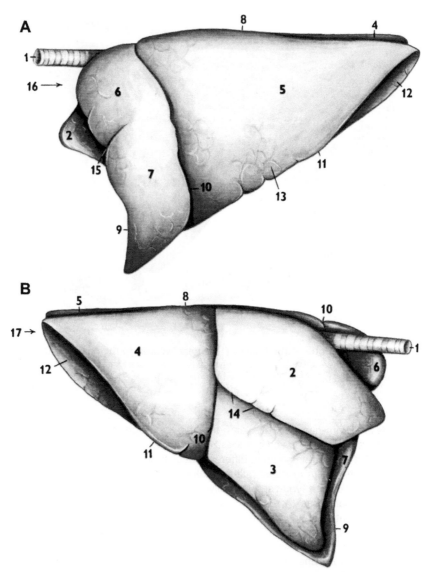

Fig. 3. The left lung (*A*) and right lung (*B*) both have cranial, middle, and caudal lobes, but the right lung also has an accessory lobe. Note the absence of septa and lung lobules. Key features include the trachea (1), cranial, and medial lobes of the right lung (2, 3), right caudal lobe (4), left caudal lobe (5), and the cranial and caudal parts of the left cranial lobe (6, 7). (*Reprinted from* Popesko P, Rajtova V, Horak J. A colour atlas of anatomy of small laboratory animals, vol. 1. Rabbit, guinea pig. Elsevier; 1992.)

endotoxin in the plasma during bacteremia causes fever, causes depression, and can induce shock. Some strains produce an exotoxin. The dermonecrotic toxin termed *P multocida* toxin of some type D strains is similar to the toxin that causes atrophic rhinitis in pigs. A toxin has also been demonstrated for type A strains. Purified *P multocida* toxin induces pneumonia, pleuritis, lymphoid atrophy, and possibly osteoclastic bone resorption in rabbits. Most *Pasteurellaceae* are commensal organisms on mucous membranes. Pathogenicity occurs under conditions of immunodeficiency and stress.

Research into the role of the humoral immune response has shown that while immunization may protect the rabbit from the development of severe disease, infection was not prevented by antibody formation. Antibodies to antigens of *P multocida* and other cross-reacting antigens of gram-negative bacteria, notably other *Pasteurella* species, *Yersinia* species, and *Moraxella* species, could enhance opsonization and phagocytosis. Rabbits that have chronic or severe infections usually have high titers of immunoglobulin G (IgG) to *P multocida*. Secretory immunoglobulin (IgA) does not protect against nasal infection, but may play a role in limiting the spread. Cell-mediated immunity may play a role, as depressed T lymphocyte function has resulted in severe disease in infected rabbits. Several antigens associated with virulence have been identified, and in research studies, have been recognized consistently by infected rabbits.

The clinical signs of pasteurellosis include URD (rhinitis, sinusitis, conjunctivitis, dacryocystitis), otitis, pleuropneumonia, bacteremia, and abscesses (subcutaneous tissues, organs, bones, joints, genitalia). Pasteurellosis may also be involved in tooth root abscesses and resulting malocclusions or osteomyelitis. A serous nasal discharge precedes the typical white or yellowish mucopurulent discharge. Exudate adheres to the fur around the nares. The medial aspects of the forepaws will become matted and yellow–gray from grooming. Affected rabbits may make audible sonorous noises and have bouts of sneezing with discharge. The nasolacrimal duct can be infected and thereby involve the conjunctiva (**Fig. 4**). Exudate occluding the duct may lead to excessive tearing, scalding of the face, alopecia, and pyoderma (**Fig. 5**).

In many rabbits, the signs of rhinitis subside or disappear as the infection continues into the paranasal sinuses or middle ear canals. Acute infection of the nares is accompanied by hyperemia and edema of the mucosa. Rabbits may present dyspneic and visibly cyanotic if the occlusion is significant. Mucosal erosion and nasoturbinate atrophy occur with chronic infection. Otitis media can be asymptomatic or if the inner ear is affected, torticollis, nystagmus, and ataxia can develop. The tympanic membrane may rupture. The rabbit may scratch persistently at the base of the ear. Radiographs may show an increased soft tissue density within the bulla with bone thickening.

Pet rabbits, however, presenting with URD, otitis, or abscesses, are less likely than those from rabbitries, to have *P multocida* as the causative agent. For pet rabbits, infections with *Bordetella bronchiseptica* or *Staphylococcus* species are more likely

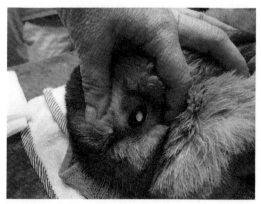

Fig. 4. Rabbit with cataracts, chronic conjunctivitis, and ocular discharge.

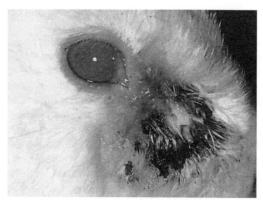

Fig. 5. Obstructed lacrimal ducts may present as facial abscesses and may be part of upper respiratory disease. This may also be seen with nasal abscesses or tooth root abscesses.

differential diagnoses. Chronic infection in the thoracic cavity may be subclinical long after the acute phase of the infection. If caused by *P multocida* or *Staphylococcus* species, pleuropneumonia, pericarditis, and abscessation around/in the lungs and heart may occur (**Fig. 6**). The rabbit may present with nonspecific signs such as anorexia, weight loss, depression, and fatigue. Dyspnea may only be noticeable upon exertion. Lung sounds may be absent due to consolidation or abscess. Rales must be differentiated from sounds heard from the upper respiratory tract (**Fig. 7**). Radiography is needed to determine the extent of the disease process. Side-stream capnography done using face mask may be clinically helpful to determine extant oxygenation/CO_2 levels. SpO_2 levels with pulse oximetry may also help evaluate response to treatment.

The main routes of transmission are by direct contact, airborne spread, and fomites. It occurs more readily from rabbits with acute infections than from rabbits with chronic infections. Venereal transmission occurs if genital infection is present. Kits can be infected at birth from a doe with genital infection. The incubation period is difficult to assess, because many rabbits are subclinically infected. Once *P multocida* is established in the nasal tissues, infection spreads to contiguous tissues including the paranasal sinuses, nasolacrimal ducts, conjunctiva, eustachian tubes, middle ears,

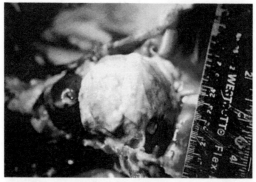

Fig. 6. *Pasteurella* infections in the thorax in addition to lung lesions may cause pericarditis and adhesions of the pericardium to the lung.

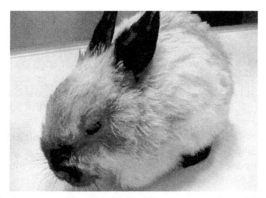

Fig. 7. Rabbit with dyspnea and conjunctivitis. Note posture. This rabbit had audible rales and blepharospasm, evidence of ocular discharge.

trachea, bronchi, and lungs (**Fig. 8**). Hematogenous spread may also reach the middle ears, lungs, and internal organs.

Complications of treatment of *Pasteurella* osteomyelitis or rhinitis or associated with dental abscesses are often associated with the inability of the drug to reach the site of infection due to the capsule produced and the inflammation of the area.

Bordetellosis

Bordetella bronchiseptica is a common inhabitant of the respiratory tract of rabbits. The nares and bronchi become colonized. Usually respiratory disease is not associated with infection, but predominant recovery of this organism in a rabbit with URD points to it as the causative agent. The organism adheres to ciliated mucosa and resists respiratory clearance. It induces ciliostasis, reduced macrophage adherence, and phagocytosis. Some strains are cytotoxic and enhance colonization by toxigenic *P multocida*. *B bronchiseptica* can be considered a copathogen or a predisposing factor in *P multocida* infections. Clinical signs often include nasal discharge, sneezing, or dyspnea, but there may be no signs with this commensal organism. The trachea, bronchi and lungs, nares, and paranasal sinuses are the most common sites of infection; the middle ears are less commonly affected. Most rabbits are infected with *B bronchiseptica* at an early age.[4]

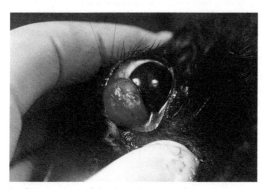

Fig. 8. Infection and inflammation of the lymph tissue of the glans nictitans in a rabbit with chronic *Pasteurella* conjunctivitis.

Staphylococcosis

Staphylococcus aureus and *S albus* are frequently isolated from the nares of both healthy and ill rabbits. *Staphylococcus* species infection can increase the inflammation of already compromised mucosa. Pathogenicity depends on host susceptibility and bacterial virulence. *S aureus* produces toxins lethal for rabbit neutrophils as well as protein A that binds the Fc portion of IgG, blocking host bactericidal mechanisms. Otitis media, fibrinous pneumonia, or abscesses in the lungs or heart have been caused by disseminated staphylococcosis. Grossly, the abscesses appear similar to ones caused by *P multocida*. Antibiotic resistance is encountered more frequently with *S aureus* than with *P multocida*. Many commercial laboratories are now determining type of *S aureus*, closely looking for instances of methicillin-resistant *S aureus* (MRSA), which pose a public health concern. Although culture and sensitivity testing are ideal, the abscess may be inaccessible. Blood culture may be helpful.[5] (Several clinical laboratories are noted in **Box 1**). Antibiotics of choice when a culture cannot be obtained include the fluoroquinolones, chloramphenicol, or trimethoprim-sulfamethoxazole.

Other Bacterial Pathogens

Moraxella catarrhalis (formerly *Micrococcus*, *Neisseria*, or *Branhamella catarrhalis*) is common in the normal nasal flora. It can be isolated from clinical cases of rhinitis or conjunctivitis. If it is isolated in pure culture from a symptomatic rabbit, it is implicated as the disease agent. However, it is more likely an opportunist on unhealthy mucosa. Treatment should be initiated only if there is clinical disease. One of the authors (CAJD)

Box 1
Diagnostic laboratories with experience in rabbit polymerase chain reaction, serology, parasitology, histopathology, microbiology, or necropsy

BioReliance Corporation, Laboratory Animal Diagnostic Service, Rockville (MD), USA,1-800-804-3586, www.bioreliance.com. Available testing: polymerase chain reaction (PCR), serology, parasitology, histopathology, clinical pathology, microbiology

Charles River Laboratories, Incorporated. Research Animal Diagnostic Services, Wilmington (MA) and San Diego (CA), USA, 1-800-338-9680, www.criver.com. Available testing: PCR, serology, parasitology, histopathology, necropsy, microbiology

Division of Laboratory Animal Medicine, Louisiana State University School of Veterinary Medicine, Baton Rouge (LA), USA, 225-578-9643. Available testing: rodent serology

University of Miami Comparative Pathology Laboratory, Miami (FL), USA, 1-800-596-7390, http://pathology.med.miami.edu. Available testing: serology, histopathology, necropsy, microbiology, parasitology

Research Animal Diagnostic Laboratory, University of Missouri, Columbia (MO), USA, 1-800-669-0825, www.radil.missouri.edu. Available testing: PCR, serology, necropsy, histopathology, microbiology, clinical pathology, parasitology

Zoologix, Incorporated, Chatsworth (CA), USA, 1-818-717-8880, www.zoologix.com. Available testing: PCR

Sound Diagnostics, Woodinville (WA), USA, 1-206-363-0787, www.sounddiagnosticsinc.com. Available testing: rabbit serology

Veterinary Molecular Diagnostics, Milford (OH), USA, 1-513-576-1808, www.vmdlabs.com. Available testing: small mammal PCR

has associated episodes of sneezing and epistaxis clinically with this organism in rabbits as well as other species.

Mycobacterium species (*M avium*, *M bovis*, *M tuberculosis*) have been isolated from cases of pneumonia in rabbits. *Moraxella bovis* and *Pseudomonas aeruginosa* have also been documented. *Pasteurella aeruginosa* can also cause abscesses similar to those of *P multocida* as well as septicemia. *Francisella paratuberculosis* (pseudotuber-culosis) and *F tularensis* (tularemia) are rare in domestic rabbits but can occur in feral rabbits. Both will cause bacteremia, multiorgan fibrinopurulent disease, and pneumonia. Due to the zoonotic potential, caution should be taken when doing necropsies of wild or feral rabbits. Domestic rabbits housed in outdoor hutches in contact with wild rodents are most commonly affected. *Chlamydophila* species (formerly *Chlamydia* species) have been isolated from the lungs of domestic rabbits with pneumonia. Cilia-associated respiratory (CAR) bacillus has been recently characterized, and appears to be closely related to *Helicobacter* species. This is not the same organism called CAR bacillus of rats, which appears related to gliding bacteria of phylum *Flavobacterium*. Rabbit CAR bacillus is an opportunistic infection with organisms found between the cilia of the respiratory epithelium. Natural infections may show slight nasal discharge, although histologically the lesions include slight hypertrophy and hyperplasia of the laryngeal, tracheal, and bronchial epithelium. Treatment efficacy has not been evaluated.

Other Etiologies of Respiratory Disease

Viral diseases associated with primary respiratory disease have not been identified. Rhinitis and chronic bronchitis from exposure to allergens are seen commonly in pet rabbits. Identifying and eliminating the allergen may be difficult. Air filters are helpful during the spring pollen season in rabbits housed indoors. The differential diagnosis of pathogenic agents must be ruled out. Symptomatic treatment with antihistamines and limited use of ophthalmic corticosteroids may be helpful. Thorough dental examination and radiographs must always be included, as many upper respiratory symptoms may be secondary to deep-seated tooth root abscesses.

Neoplasia

Adenocarcinoma of the nasal turbinates should be a differential of URD.[5] It progresses relatively rapidly and causes cavitation of the turbinates, which is visible radiographically. Thymomas have been diagnosed in both young and old rabbits (**Fig. 9**). Clinical signs may include tachypnea and moderate-to-severe dyspnea. Bilateral exophthalmos

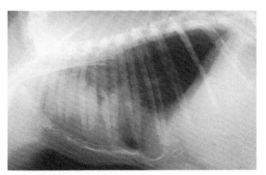

Fig. 9. Lateral radiograph of a rabbit that presented with dyspnea and nasal discharge. The dyspnea was a consequence of a thymoma.

due to the interference of vascular return to the heart is also seen with thymoma. The mass is visible radiographically. Treatment may include surgical removal or chemotherapy. Lymphoma and thymoma may both cause dyspnea, lower respiratory rales, and cyanosis on exertion. Lymphocytosis is usually present. Radiography and a chest tap with cytology will be useful to differentiate neoplasia from abscessation/infectious disease. The author (CAJD) has found that ultrasound-guided biopsy of suspected thymomas or granulomas may provide diagnoses to guide treatment.

REFERENCES

1. Hrapkiewicz K, Medina L, Holmes D. Rabbits. In: Clinical laboratory animal medicine: an introduction. 3rd edition. Ames (IA): Blackwell Publishing; 2007. p. 198–238.
2. Deeb BJ. Respiratory disease and pasteurellosis. In: Quesenberry KE, Carpenter JW, editors. Ferrets, rabbits, and rodents: clinical medicine and surgery. 2nd edition. St Louis (MO): Saunders; 2004. p. 172–82.
3. Percy DH, Barthold SW. Pathology of laboratory rodents and rabbits. 3rd edition. Ames (IA): Blackwell Publishing; 2007.
4. Deeb BJ, DiGiacomo RF, Bernard BL, et al. *Pasteurella mutocida* and *Bordetella bronchiseptica* infections in rabbits. J Clin Microbiol 1990;28(1):70–5.
5. Jenkins JR. Rabbit diagnostic testing. J Exotic Pet Med 2008;17:4–15.

Hedgehogs and Sugar Gliders: Respiratory Anatomy, Physiology, and Disease

Dan H. Johnson, DVM, DABVP (Exotic Companion Mammal)

KEYWORDS

- Pneumonia • Cardiomyopathy • Hibernation • Torpor
- Marsupial

This article discusses the respiratory anatomy, physiology, and disease of African pygmy hedgehogs (*Atelerix albiventris*) and sugar gliders (*Petaurus breviceps*), two species commonly seen in exotic animal practice. Where appropriate, information from closely related species is mentioned because cross-susceptibility is likely and because these additional species may also be encountered in practice. Hedgehogs and sugar gliders, like most mammals, are susceptible to respiratory disease caused by infection, neoplasia, and trauma. As with other exotic animals, many problems encountered with hedgehogs and sugar gliders are at least partially related to improper diet and husbandry. Although this article emphasizes the respiratory system, other body systems and processes are discussed insofar as they relate to or affect respiratory function. Although some topics, such as special senses, hibernation, or vocalization, may seem out of place, in each case the information relates back to respiration in some important way.

RESPIRATORY ANATOMY AND PHYSIOLOGY

Hedgehog

The hedgehog body plan is considered primitive and unspecialized.[1,2] The airways and lungs of the hedgehog are similar to that of other small mammals. The snout is elongate and blunt, and the nose is normally moist and active.[3,4] Hedgehogs have relatively small eyes and poor eyesight but well developed senses of smell and hearing. They rely on olfactory and auditory cues for communication.[2,5] A hedgehog's keen sense of smell is essential for locating food, predator detection, orientation, navigation, sexual behavior, maternal behavior, and intraspecific communication.[1,5]

Olfactory stimuli are also responsible for initiating self-anointing, or anting, a behavior exhibited by all hedgehog species.[3,5] This strange behavior is usually initiated by

---

The author has nothing to disclose.
Avian and Exotic Animal Care, 8711 Fidelity Boulevard, Raleigh, NC 27617, USA
E-mail address: drdan@avianandexotic.com

a period of intense olfactory stimulation by strong or unusual odors.[1,3] Self-anointing may be triggered by anesthetic gasses, perfume, cigarettes, glue, leather, wool, creosote, fish, cat food, plants, vegetables, and many other substances.[1,3,5] Direct contact with a substance is not necessary to elicit the behavior.[5] The hedgehog begins to hypersalivate, producing copious, foamy saliva that is then slathered onto the spines of the flank and back with its tongue. Self-anointing may be used to mark the individual or its home range with distinctive odor.[1,3] Hedgehogs have a well-developed and functional Jacobson (vomeronasal) organ that is used during self-anointing behavior. The Jacobson organ is an olfactory structure present in the palate of many vertebrates. Nerves from its sensory cells run separately from those of the nasal olfactory organ, and link to parts of the brain associated with reproductive physiology and behavior.[1]

Hedgehogs normally produce a wide variety of vocalizations including grunts, squeals, snuffling, and sneezing.[1,6] Respiration is normally silent, except in the frightened or aggressive animal, in which forceful expulsion of air through the nose creates a distinctive hissing sound.[3] It is important not to confuse these noises with abnormalities of the respiratory tract, which might require treatment.[7,8]

All hedgehogs are capable of undergoing hibernation. Hedgehog body temperature is normally 95.7°F to 98.6°F (37.4°C–36°C).[3] However, under cold conditions, a hedgehog's body temperature can drop to a level close to that of surrounding air, giving them the ability to reduce energy needs and survive when food is scarce.[2] Hibernation is possible because of energy stored as fat: "white fat" located subcutaneously and intraabdominally, and "brown fat" located around the thorax and along the neck and spine. Ordinary white fat provides a long-term energy supply, whereas brown fat plays a role in thermoregulation. Brown fat has larger mitochondria, smaller fat droplets, and a richer blood supply than white fat, allowing for the rapid production of heat.[1]

Hibernation is characterized by a drastic reduction in overall metabolic rate, resulting in lower body temperature, oxygen consumption, heart rate, and respiration.[1] Hedgehogs may remain dormant for up to 6 weeks but emerge during periods of warm weather.[5] The normal respiratory rate of 25 to 50 breaths per minute can drop to 1 to 8 breaths per minute, and heart rate may fall from 80 to 280 beats per minute while active to only 3 to 20 beats per minute during hibernation.[3,9–11] Hibernation increases blood oxygen affinity and enhances the blood-to-tissue diffusion of oxygen.[12,13] Synthesis of endogenous heparin increases during hibernation, preventing thrombus formation.[8] The European hedgehog (*Erinaceus europaeus*) has been shown to consume less oxygen and exhibit lower heart rate and blood pressure during spontaneous arousal from hibernation than when arousal is induced.[14] The European hedgehog hibernates when temperatures fall below 46.6°F (8°C).[11] Despite claims to the contrary, hedgehogs in southern Africa are known to hibernate from June through September when the weather is cool and dry, remaining torpid for periods of up to 6 weeks, but emerging during warm intervals.[4,8,10] In captivity, the African pygmy hedgehog may enter hibernation if environmental temperature falls below 65°F (18°C).[8,10] Hedgehogs may become immunosuppressed and predisposed to infections during hibernation. There is no need for captive hedgehogs to hibernate, and they do not if kept warm and well fed.[2,8] Therefore, a supplemental heat source (eg, heat lamp or under-tank heater) is recommended for most hedgehog enclosures.[5,15] During prolonged periods of excessive heat, hedgehogs may undergo estivation, the warm-weather equivalent of hibernation.[1]

Sugar Glider

The sugar glider possesses a generalized body plan and a respiratory system similar to that of other small mammals. The metabolic rate of the sugar glider is as much as 45%

below that predicted for a eutherian (placental) mammal of comparable size.[16–18] As a result, the marsupial heart rate is about half that of the eutherian, and for compensatory blood volume the marsupial heart is 30% heavier than the eutherian heart. Additionally, several features of the marsupial heart are considered primitive and closer in form to birds, reptiles, and monotremes than to other mammals.[19] Marsupials are not born with the ability to regulate body temperature. About halfway through life in the pouch they begin to regulate body temperature, and this coincides with the start of thyroid function.[17] Sugar gliders possess a well-developed cecum that uses bacterial fermentation to break down complex polysaccharides contained in gum. However, they do not seem to suffer adverse effects from antibiotic therapy, perhaps because they are omnivores and captive diets provide ample energy without the need for fermentation.[1,20]

Sugar gliders are communal as a species and have a complex communication system based on scents produced by frontal, sternal, and urogenital glands of males, and by pouch and urogenital glands of females. Each animal of a group has its own characteristic smell, which identifies it to other individuals and which is passively spread around the group's territory. In addition, a dominant male actively marks the territory and other members of the group with his scent.[4,21] Sugar gliders make a variety of vocalizations including chirps, barks, hisses, screams, and squeaks. Their alarm call resembles the yapping of a small dog, and when disturbed they make a high-pitched, rattling cry of anger known as "crabbing."[4,21] These unusual sounds should not be mistaken for signs of respiratory disease.[21]

Normal sugar glider respiratory rate is 16 to 40 breaths per minute, and normal heart rate is 200 to 300 beats per minute. Their normal body temperature is 97.3°F (36.3°C). Sugar gliders can tolerate environmental temperatures of 65°F to 90°F (18°C–32°C), although 75°F to 80°F (24°C–27°C) is considered ideal.[18] Therefore, supplemental heat should be provided for animals in captivity.[22,23] The sugar glider's natural range includes habitats that may be cool or tropical, wet or dry. During periods of extreme wet, cold, or food scarcity, sugar gliders conserve energy by huddling, going into torpor (short-term hibernation) for periods lasting between 2 and 23 (average 13) hours per day, and lowering body temperature to as low as 50.7°F (10.4°C).[24,25] Minimization of energy loss seems to be pivotal for their survival in the wild.[25] The oxygen consumption rate of a group of huddling, torpid sugar gliders at an ambient temperature of 46.4°F (8°C) has been shown to be lower than that of a single glider under the same conditions.[24] Despite an apparent lack of functional brown fat, sugar gliders can lower their metabolic rate by about 15% during the winter and at the same time increase their maximum heat production by 20%.[15] Huddling seems to be the most important mechanism for energy conservation for *P breviceps*, whereas torpor is used only to overcome short-term reductions in winter food supplies.[24]

Torpor is not triggered by temperature in the sugar glider; rather, it is triggered by starvation and lack of foraging opportunities (eg, with inclement weather).[25,26] Torpor is not dependent on body condition or weight loss or ambient temperature, it may occur spontaneously throughout the year, and it may occur in gliders that are single or in groups.[26] Evidence suggests that sugar gliders use torpor as an emergency measure rather than a routine energy-saving strategy. Before entering torpor, sugar gliders reduce activity and lower their resting body temperature to lower energy expenditure and perhaps to avoid using torpor.[25,27] Sugar gliders seem to use both anaerobic and aerobic mechanisms of heat production as they arouse from torpor.[24] Patterns of sugar glider activity, thermal physiology, and torpor observed in captivity may differ substantially from those in the wild.[25,28] Gliding may afford the sugar glider yet another strategy for conserving energy.[29]

DIAGNOSIS OF RESPIRATORY DISEASE

The diagnostic approach used in hedgehogs and sugar gliders can be adapted from the methods used in other mammals.[5,19,21,30] In general, the clinician should perform less-invasive, higher-yield diagnostic tests before more-invasive, lower-yield procedures. For this reason, the diagnostics discussed next are presented in roughly the order they might be performed in clinical practice.

A thorough history is likely to reveal dietary, environmental, or other husbandry factors associated with the onset of respiratory disease. Stress may be a predisposing factor.[21] Potential stressors include environmental change; lack of a dark, secure hiding place; fighting; or absence of a companion (sugar gliders). Animals with respiratory disease are likely to exhibit coughing, sneezing, nasal discharge, dyspnea, or increased respiratory rate, but may also exhibit nonspecific signs, such as reduced appetite, anorexia, or even sudden death.[3,15,21]

A careful visual examination before handling may offer the best opportunity for initial evaluation. Observation of respiratory rate and effort, and the color of the nose, lips, and feet, can provide a baseline for comparison with the same after oxygen administration or drug therapy.[19]

Physical examination in hedgehogs is usually difficult because of their shy nature and effective defenses. Auscultation is complicated by their defensive hissing. With patience, it is possible to do a diagnostic physical examination in a socialized hedgehog, although a complete examination usually involves general anesthesia.[5,31] Likewise, physical examination of sugar gliders is complicated by their defensive tendency and loud vocalizations. A complete examination is usually possible with adequate restraint, although anesthesia is occasionally necessary (**Fig. 1**).[21,31] An electronic stethoscope may improve auscultation of cardiac and pulmonary sounds for very small mammals by allowing the user to detect heart and lung sounds that normally may be difficult to auscult.[30] Pulse oximetry can be useful in assessing respiratory function in the awake patient, and may be measured before and after providing supplemental oxygen. In either species, anesthesia may be indicated for examination in debilitated individuals and those that cannot tolerate physical restraint.

Radiography provides valuable, noninvasive supporting evidence for respiratory conditions commonly seen in hedgehogs and sugar gliders.[3,21,32,33] Fractured ribs, diaphragmatic hernias, pneumonia, fluid, and space-occupying lesions can be

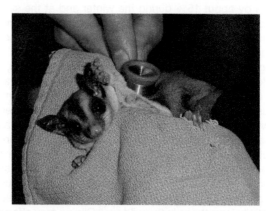

Fig. 1. Auscultation of a sugar glider is often complicated by defensive vocalizations; however, a complete examination is usually possible with proper restraint.

visualized on plain images.[33] Whole-body images in left-lateral, right-lateral, and ventrodorsal projections should be obtained with the legs and body extended. Tabletop techniques are preferred because they eliminate attenuation of the beam and enhance image detail.[30] Detail film–screen combinations improve definition but require greater exposure.[18] Magnification radiography may be used to enhance visualization of areas of special interest (eg, nasal sinuses), but it does so at the expense of image sharpness and spatial resolution, which are inversely proportional to magnification (**Fig. 2**).[30] The spines of a hedgehog may hinder radiographic detail, especially on the dorsoventral view. However, on the lateral view, the mantle and spines may be retracted dorsally away from the area of interest and held in place with a large plastic bag clip (ie, "chip clip") (**Fig. 3**).[3,5] If a female sugar glider has joeys in the pouch that have detached from the teat, the young may be removed from the pouch before taking radiographs.[18] Contrast radiographs may be indicated in the diagnosis of diaphragmatic hernia.[33,34] Anatomic and radiographic atlases with radiographs of both healthy and ill individuals are helpful in image interpretation.[19,34] Radiography in all but the most severely ill patients requires the use of sedation or anesthesia.[18,35]

A minimum database (consisting of complete blood count, blood chemistry panel, fecal examination, and urinalysis) is important in the diagnosis of respiratory and other systemic disease. Hematology and biochemistry are interpreted for hedgehogs and sugar gliders as for other companion animals. Normal parameters for both have been reported.[3,15,21,36] Additionally, serologic testing is possible for many infectious diseases.[33] Manual restraint is not sufficient for blood sample collection or most other procedures; anesthesia with sevoflurane or isoflurane is often recommended.[35] The cranial vena cava may be used for venipuncture in hedgehogs and sugar gliders; however, there is greater risk of cardiac puncture compared with ferrets because of the relatively cranial position of the heart, particularly in hedgehogs.[3,34,35] Fecal examination may reveal ova or larvae of respiratory parasites: nematodes in hedgehogs, pentastomids in sugar gliders.[2,37]

The diagnosis of respiratory disease may be based on analysis of specimens obtained in a variety of ways. Nasal swabs are most applicable to the upper airways, but because of the small size of hedgehogs and sugar gliders, deep nasal swabs are not possible; a nasal flush may be considered as an alternative. Nasal samples are contaminated and do not accurately reflect disease occurring in the lower airways.[32]

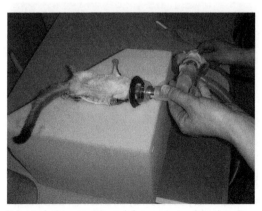

Fig. 2. This sugar glider is being positioned for a ventrodorsal radiograph on a block of foam rubber in order to magnify its image. However, as magnification is increased with technique, image sharpness and spatial resolution are decreased.

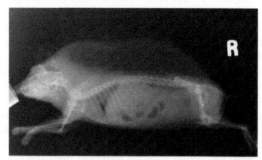

Fig. 3. A lateral radiographic view of the hedgehog typically has greater image detail than the ventrodorsal view, because its mantle and spines are positioned dorsally, away from areas of interest.

In stable patients, a transoral tracheal lavage is preferred.[3,5,21,32] Tracheal lavage may be performed using a technique that minimizes lavage volume while maximizing sample recovery.[38] For patients with advanced respiratory disease, a tracheal swab may be more appropriate (**Fig. 4**).[30] Thoracocentesis may be used to diagnose and treat pleural effusion.[19,21,32] A fine-gauge needle can be placed and fluid collected most efficiently in the ventral third of the fourth to seventh intercostal space.[33] Although rarely used, transthoracic lung lobe aspirate has been used to obtain a pulmonary specimen and seems to be safe and effective in small mammals.[3,39] Ultrasound guidance is likely to improve accuracy and safety for any needle aspirate procedure.[32] Collection of diagnostic specimens from the respiratory system requires sedation or anesthesia in most cases.[19,33]

Standard microbiologic and cytologic techniques are appropriate for hedgehogs and sugar gliders.[3,21,33] Aerobic, anaerobic, bacterial, and fungal cultures should be considered in cases suspected of respiratory infection.[30] Normal respiratory tract microflora for the hedgehog and the sugar glider has not been determined.[18,19] Samples for cytology may be concentrated for examination using sedimentation

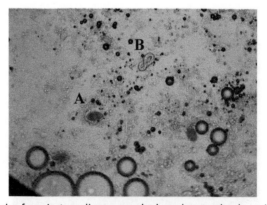

Fig. 4. The diagnosis of respiratory disease may be based on tracheal specimens obtained by lavage or swab. This sputum from a European hedgehog (*Erinaceus europaeus*) contains *Capillaria* ova (*A*) and Crenosoma larvae (*B*) typical of verminous pneumonia. (*Image courtesy of* Emmanuel Risi, DMV.)

techniques or a cytologic centrifuge (Cytospin; Shandon Southern Instruments, Sew-ickley, PA, USA). Wright–Giemsa and Gram staining are recommended for most respiratory specimens.[30] Where mycobacterial infection is suspected, acid-fast staining, mycobacterial culture, enzyme-linked immunosorbent assay testing, or lymphocyte transformation assay may also be indicated.[40]

Endoscopy has multiple uses in the diagnosis of respiratory disease in exotic mammals (eg, evaluation, biopsy, and foreign body retrieval in oral and nasal cavities).[32] However, its application in hedgehogs and sugar gliders is limited based on patient size.[30,32] Potential uses include examination of the oropharynx, glottis, and trachea; assisted orotracheal intubation; and assisted tracheal wash.[30,32,38,41,42]

Ultrasonography is rarely used in respiratory medicine but may aid in the evaluation of pleural effusion, pulmonary pathology, mediastinal masses, and cardiac structures.[32,33] Ultrasound should be used to augment radiographs rather than for primary examination, because radiography helps to localize where ultrasonographic examination should be concentrated.[30] With ultrasound, pleural effusion can be collected by guided thoracocentesis for cytology, protein analysis, or culture and response to treatment can be monitored.[21,30,32] With the patient positioned in ventral recumbency, fluid is dependent and easier to diagnose.[30] Ultrasound may be most useful to determine the type of cardiac dysfunction and the presence of a mass or lung consolidation.[19] In general, small exotic mammals require transducers of higher frequency and smaller contact surface area.[30] Anesthesia is usually required for ultrasound examination of hedgehogs and sugar gliders.[30]

MRI and CT are less commonly used in hedgehogs and sugar gliders, and have limited application for evaluation of the respiratory tract.[32] MRI can be used to evaluate sinuses and pulmonary lesions in small mammals, but gives poor images of lung tissue because of the relative lack of water protons necessary for image formation.[30,43] CT is the best method for evaluating the nasal cavity and sinuses, and can also be useful for locating soft tissue lesions (eg, granulomas and masses) within the respiratory tract.[30,33] To minimize motion artifact during a CT scan, the patient must be still.[33] Sustained positive pressure ventilation is necessary, and the maximal recommended period for this is 1 minute. Helical CT generally allows for the fastest, most practical acquisition of CT images.[30] General anesthesia is required for MRI and CT imaging in most cases.

Necropsy is a final and very valuable diagnostic method for respiratory illness.[32] It allows for a definitive diagnosis of disease processes in many cases, and is especially important where groups of animals are involved and where zoonotic disease is suspected. Necropsy should be performed as soon as possible after death occurs.

RESPIRATORY DISEASE PROCESSES
Hedgehog

Although some references state otherwise, most report that respiratory disease is common in hedgehogs.[5,15,42,44] Pneumonia was reported in 14% of necropsied African pygmy hedgehogs in one retrospective study and in 41% of necropsied European hedgehogs in another.[11,45] Etiologies of respiratory disease include bacterial, viral, fungal, and parasitic infections, and cardiac disease, neoplasia, and trauma. Clinical signs are similar to those in other species: nasal discharge, increased respiratory noise, dyspnea, lethargy, inappetence, and sudden death.[5,15,46] Although some respiratory pathogens are documented in only one species or the other, Erinaceus and Atelerix are closely related and it is assumed that most, if not all, pathogens are contagious to both species of hedgehog.[5,8,47]

Bacterial

Clinical signs of bacterial respiratory infection vary but may include nasal discharge, sneezing, epistaxis, laryngitis, tracheitis, pneumonia, increased respiratory noise, dyspnea, lethargy, anorexia, and sudden death.[3,5,7,15,46,48] Hedgehog respiratory infections have been attributed to *Pasteurella multocida*, *Bordetella bronchiseptica*, and *Corynebacterium* species. Bronchopneumonia with fibrosis, atelectasis, and lung abscesses resulting from *Pasteurella* or *Bordetella* is a common necropsy finding in the European hedgehog.[11] *Bordetella* infection usually occurs secondary to other respiratory infections or diseases.[2] It is often associated with pneumonia and *Crenosoma striatum* lungworm infection in wild European hedgehogs.[48,49] Corynebacterial pneumonia was reported in a pet African pygmy hedgehog that developed necrosuppperative bronchopneumonia with pulmonary abscesses. Clinical signs included anorexia and lethargy for a period of 3 days before death; the hedgehog displayed no respiratory signs.[50] Other bacteria cultured from the respiratory tract of hedgehogs include *Haemophilus*, *Salmonella*, *Staphylococcus*, and hemolytic streptococci.[1,44,51]

Bordetella bronchiseptica seems to have a geographic distribution in the European hedgehog. It was commonly isolated from the respiratory tract of hedgehogs in England but was not isolated from those in New Zealand.[51] *Pasteurella* species and hemolytic streptococci may be considered normal commensals that only become invasive in a hedgehog during stress or captivity.[51] Among wild European hedgehogs in New Zealand, 40% were found to have *Staphylococcus aureus* inhabiting the nostrils.[51] Also in New Zealand, *Mycoplasma* was isolated from the feces and throat of 1 of 15 wild European hedgehogs examined, although the significance of mycoplasmal disease in hedgehogs is unknown.[1]

Free-living European hedgehogs may become infected with *Mycobacterium bovis* and *Mycobacterium avium*.[40,52,53] European hedgehogs likely become infected with *M bovis* through scavenging behavior.[52,54,55] *Mycobacterium marinum* caused systemic infection in a captive European hedgehog. Clinical signs included chronic, progressive cervical lymphadenitis; weight loss; and depression. Numerous granulomatous lesions of the lung were present at necropsy. The source of infection was presumed to be an aquarium in which the animal was initially housed.[56]

Treatment for bacterial infection should include broad-spectrum antibiotics, supportive care, nebulization, oxygen as needed, and correction of husbandry problems.[2,3,46] Because a hedgehog's digestive tract is simple and lacks hindgut fermentation, the antibiotics used to treat respiratory infection can be similar to those used in dogs and cats.[3,5] Predisposing factors for upper and lower respiratory tract infection include suboptimal environmental temperature, dusty or unsanitary bedding, malnutrition, concurrent disease, and other causes of immunocompromise.[2,3,7] By providing the correct diet and environmental conditions, bacterial infections may be minimized or avoided.

Viral

Viral diseases are rare in hedgehogs.[57] Both European and African hedgehogs are susceptible to natural infection with foot-and-mouth disease, a reportable foreign animal disease in the United States, and can transmit it to cattle.[1,5,58] Affected hedgehogs exhibit typical vesicular lesions on the hairless skin of the feet, perineal region, tongue, snout, and lip margins associated with the disease in cattle.[5,51] Symptoms may also include sneezing.[2] The European hedgehog is susceptible to a paramyxovirus closely related to canine distemper virus.[5,59] Reported symptoms were similar to those seen with canine distemper virus in dogs, including neurologic signs, ulceration and hyperkeratosis of the feet, sores on the face, and nasal discharge. Lungs showed consolidated bronchopneumonia and interstitial pneumonia.[59] Cytomegalovirus, a herpesviral disease affecting the respiratory system, has been reported in African pygmy hedgehogs based on microscopic lesions found in the duct epithelium of the salivary glands.[60] However, cytomegalovirus in African hedgehogs has been questioned by Brunnert and coworkers,[61] who determined that the ultrastructural and histochemical findings of cytomegalic cells are more consistent with oncocytes.

Fungal and yeast

Disseminated histoplasmosis has been reported in an African pygmy hedgehog. The liver, kidneys, small intestine, and lungs were multifocally affected by *Histoplasma* yeast and granulomatous infiltrates. The patient showed inappetence, weakness, and lethargy before death. Therefore, histoplasmosis should be a differential diagnosis for vague signs of illness in African pygmy hedgehogs.[62]

Parasitic

A large number of nematodes have been found in the respiratory tract of the European hedgehog.[51] It is particularly susceptible to the lung nematodes *Capillaria aerophila* and *C striatum*.[1–3,5,11,47] Lungworms can also affect African pygmy hedgehogs but are rarely diagnosed in captive-bred individuals.[2,3,5,47] Adult *Capillaria* are found embedded in the mucosa of the trachea, bronchi, and rarely nasal cavities and frontal sinuses of its host.[11,48,63,64] Its other reported hosts include dogs, foxes, coyotes, cat, pine marten, beech marten, wolf, badger, and occasionally humans.[63] The life cycle of *Capillaria* is direct: ova are coughed up and swallowed, passed in the feces, develop in the open, and reach infective stage in about 5 to 7 weeks. Ova may remain infective for over a year under favorable conditions.[63,64] Earthworms, which hedgehogs feed on, can store infective ova and serve as transport hosts.[11,48] Infective larvae do not hatch out of the egg until swallowed by a suitable host. Larvae then penetrate the intestine and migrate in the bloodstream to the lungs in 7 to 10 days, reaching maturity 40 days after infection.[63,64]

Adult *C striatum* resides in the trachea and bronchi of the hedgehog.[11,63] Larvae are produced 3 weeks after infection, coughed up to the pharynx, swallowed, and excreted with the feces.[11] Larvae penetrate the foot of land snails or slugs, which serve as intermediate hosts, and reach infective stage in 16 to 17 days.[11,48,63] Direct (possibly transplacental) transmission may also occur, because *C striatum* may be found in unweaned animals.[48] When snails are eaten by the final host, *Crenosoma* larvae pass by way of the lymphatic glands and hepatic circulation to the lungs. There, they reach maturity in 21 days.[11,63]

Capillaria and *Crenosoma* frequently occur together.[63] Animals with mild infection often show no clinical signs. Severe infections may lead to rhinitis, tracheitis, bronchitis, or bronchopneumonia, often accompanied by secondary *B bronchiseptica* infection. Clinical signs include nasal discharge, tachypnea, dyspnea, coughing, wheezing, and course breathing sounds (**Fig. 5**). Weakness, anemia, and emaciation are also reported.[11,48,63,64] Mortality rate associated with lungworms can be very high.[48,63] Severe lungworm infection is considered to be the most frequent cause of death in European hedgehogs.[48]

Lungworms may be diagnosed by finding bipolar eggs (*C aerophila*) or larvae (*C striatum*) in feces, sputum, or nasal discharge (**Fig. 6**).[2,11,48,63] Infestations can also be diagnosed on histopathology by the finding of parasites and inflammatory changes in the lungs and airways. One study of 53 European hedgehogs found a correlation between the finding of parasites in histologic sections and the detection of eggs in feces; however, neither method seemed completely reliable.[37] Suggested

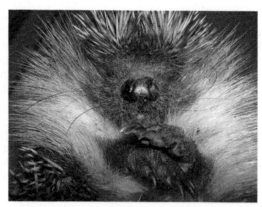

Fig. 5. Mucopurulent and bloody nasal discharge in a wild European hedgehog (*Erinaceus europaeus*) with lungworm infection. (*Image courtesy of* Emmanuel Risi, DMV.)

treatments include ivermectin, levamisole, tetramisol, and fenbendazole.[46,63] Lungworms are prevented by controlling access to infective ova, larvae, and intermediate hosts. Hedgehogs in the United States usually are not affected because they are bred in captivity.[2]

Hedgehogs can be the intermediate hosts for pentastomes. *Armillifer armillatus* larvae have been reported in the African pygmy hedgehog. Pentastomes may be found in the lungs and visualized on radiographs. No effective treatment other than surgery has been reported.[65] Hedgehogs are also susceptible to *Toxoplasmosis* and may acquire infection by eating raw meat.[2]

Neoplasia

African pygmy hedgehogs seem particularly prone to neoplasia.[3,5,66] The incidence has been documented to be 30% or higher in two separate reports.[45,67] Over 80% of tumors in one survey were classified as malignant.[68] Reported tumor types are diverse, and any body system may be affected.[3] Clinical signs vary by the body system affected and may include the presence of a mass, chronic weight loss, anorexia, lethargy, diarrhea, dyspnea, and ascites.[3] Oral neoplasms (oral

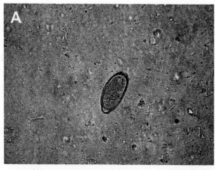
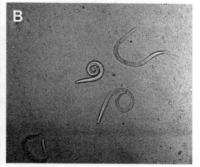

Fig. 6. Bipolar eggs typical of *Capillaria aerophila* (A) and larvae typical of *Crenosoma striatum* (B) may be found in feces, sputum, or nasal discharge of hedgehogs with lungworm infection. (*Images courtesy of* Bálint Márkus, DVM.)

fibrosarcoma or squamous cell carcinoma) are relatively common, representing 15% of tumors in one study.[68] Squamous cell carcinoma of the oral cavity is the third most common tumor type in the African pygmy hedgehog (**Fig. 7**).[66] Signs include decreased appetite, ptyalism, halitosis, and pawing at the mouth. Differential diagnosis includes foreign bodies and dental disease.[3] Squamous cell carcinoma may spread from the oral cavity to the nasal cavity, and pulmonary metastasis may occur.[5,66,69] Other reports of metastatic respiratory disease include adrenocortical carcinoma with metastasis to the lung, hepatocellular carcinoma with metastasis to the lung, lymphosarcoma with metastasis to the lung, and multicentric lymphosarcoma affecting the lung.[68,70] Primary neoplasia associated with the respiratory system seems to be less common, but includes bronchoalveolar carcinoma of the lung and osteosarcoma of a rib.[5,66,68] Dyspnea associated with pulmonary neoplasia can mimic pneumonia or heart disease.[3,5]

As in other species, neoplasia is confirmed via cytologic or histologic examination. Radiography may provide evidence of neoplastic invasion or metastasis. Hematology, blood chemistry, and ultrasonography may help to identify concurrent problems and location and extent of neoplasia. Treatment is usually limited to surgical excision and supportive care, although other treatment modalities may be possible in certain cases.[3] The high incidence of neoplasia encountered in hedgehogs can lead to the false conclusion that therapy for infection or other disease has failed, when neoplasia is actually the underlying etiology. Often a necropsy is not performed, and the neoplasia goes undetected.[71]

Heart disease
Cardiomyopathy can cause respiratory illness in pet hedgehogs.[72] Dilated cardiomyopathy is common, with an incidence of 38% according to one published report.[3,5,72] Affected hedgehogs are more likely to be male and 3 years of age or older, although the disease may occur in animals as young as 1 year of age.[3,5,19] The etiology remains unknown, although diet, toxins, stress, obesity, and genetics are possible contributing factors.[3,5,19] Nutritional imbalances, such as vitamin E, selenium, taurine, choline, and tryptophan deficiencies, have been considered.[72] Clinical signs are referable to cardiopulmonary dysfunction and include dyspnea, moist rhales, lethargy, anorexia,

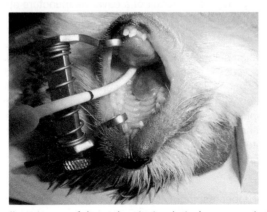

Fig. 7. Squamous cell carcinoma of the oral cavity is relatively common in the African pygmy hedgehog. It may spread from the oral cavity to the nasal cavity, and pulmonary metastasis may occur.

weight loss, dehydration, heart murmur, ascites, and acute death.[3,5,72] Death may occur without clinical signs, but overt disease is observed in most cases.[5,15]

Consider heart disease if heart murmur, irregular rhythm, or weak femoral pulse are detected.[3,5] Dyspnea, tachypnea, pallor or cyanosis of the lips, ears, feet and tail, and extremities that feel cool to the touch are common with heart disease. Clinical signs may improve with oxygen administration.[19] Affected hedgehogs tend to crouch while keeping the ventrum in contact with the table surface, whereas healthy hedgehogs walk with the ventrum raised clear off the table.[3] Diagnosis of heart disease involves radiography, echocardiography, and electrocardiogram.[3,5,19] Although normal radiographic cardiac size has not yet been reported in the hedgehog, radiographs typically demonstrate varying degrees of cardiac enlargement, aerophagia, tracheal elevation, pulmonary edema, pleural effusion, hepatic congestion, and abdominal fluid.[3,19] Normal echocardiographic measurements for hedgehogs have not been published, but a subjective evaluation of wall motion and chamber size is often sufficient to confirm a diagnosis of cardiomyopathy.[3,19] In one author's experience with a small number of healthy hedgehogs, fractional shortening should be at least 25% and wall thickness should be at least 1.5 mm.[3] Complete blood count and blood chemistry profile may be indicated to screen for concurrent problems and to serve as a reference for monitoring the effects of therapeutic agents.[3] Necropsy findings associated with cardiovascular disease in the hedgehog include cardiomyopathy, hepatomegaly, pulmonary edema, pulmonary congestion, hydrothorax, ascites, and pulmonary or renal infarcts.[3,5,72] Among the common findings on histology are acute and chronic passive congestion of the lungs, and renal tubular necrosis and vascular infarct.[5,72] Therapy with digoxin, furosemide, and enalapril may be helpful initially, but the long-term prognosis for hedgehogs with congestive heart failure is poor.[3,19]

Trauma

Respiratory injury can result from a fall, crushing injury, predator attack, or road trauma. Although hedgehogs are excellent swimmers, they may drown if trapped in a smooth-sided enclosure (eg, tub, toilet, or swimming pool) and unable to escape.[1] Nuts, seeds, and large items, such as carrots, can become lodged in the roof of a hedgehog's mouth and should be avoided.[3] Hemothorax and cardiac puncture are possible risks associated with vena cava blood collection because of the relatively cranial position of the hedgehog heart (**Fig. 8**).[3,32,35] The author has observed fatal hemothorax in a hedgehog as the result of a caval venipuncture attempt.

Sugar Glider

As for other companion animals, respiratory disease in the sugar glider may occur as a result of bacteria, viruses, parasites, fungi, yeast, neoplasia, and trauma. Primary respiratory disease is considered rare in marsupials. Instead, respiratory conditions are usually associated with another disease process or an opportunistic pathogen.[21] Clinical signs of respiratory disease in marsupials are similar to those seen in placental mammals: bilateral nasal discharge, sneezing, anorexia, and coughing are the more commonly encountered clinical signs. Diagnosis and treatment follows standard protocols for respiratory disease in other small mammals.[21]

Bacterial

In general, bacterial upper respiratory infection is rare in sugar gliders, whereas bacterial pneumonia is more common.[15,21,33,42] Clinical signs vary by location and severity of infection and include sneezing; bilateral, clear, or mucopurulent nasal discharge; pharyngitis; regional lymph node enlargement; coughing; audible respiratory noises;

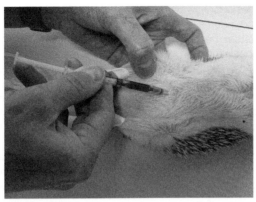

Fig. 8. While the cranial vena cava may be utilized for venipuncture in hedgehogs, there exists a potential for cardiac puncture due to the cranial position of the heart.

and anorexia.[21] Chilling and malnutrition may predispose sugar gliders to secondary infections including bacterial pneumonia.[18,22,73] Because of suboptimal body temperature, slow swallowing reflex, and high flow rate of artificial milk formula, hand-reared infant joeys are prone to aspiration with resulting aspiration pneumonia.[21,33] Respiratory infections in sugar gliders may be attributed to common bacteria including *Pasteurella, Escherichia coli, Klebsiella* spp, *Pseudomonas* spp, staphylococci, and streptococci.[20,21,33,73] When kept in the same area, rabbits may serve as a source of *P multocida* infection for sugar gliders.[23] *Mycobacterium* species are the causative agent of tuberculosis in other possum species and may affect sugar gliders.[20,23,74] Treatment for bacterial infection in sugar gliders should include bacteriocidal antibiotics with good coverage against gram-negative bacteria.[21] Although sugar gliders possess a well-developed cecum, antibiotic therapy is well tolerated.[20] Additional treatments include nebulization, bronchodilators, mucolytics, supportive care, and oxygen as needed. Husbandry problems should be corrected. For aspiration pneumonia in joeys, corticosteroids are indicated in the early stages to limit inflammation associated with the aspirated material; nonsteroidal antiinflammatory drugs may be used as an alternative.[21,33]

Viral

There are no known naturally occurring clinically relevant viral diseases in sugar gliders.[57] Viruses associated with respiratory disease that are seen in other marsupials (poxvirus, orbivirus, and herpesvirus) are not reported in sugar gliders.[21]

Fungal and yeast

Histoplasmosis has been documented in sugar gliders.[75] Most affected animals died without exhibiting clinical signs. Two of five sugar gliders necropsied were found to have systemic disease including lung involvement. The remaining sugar gliders were treated with oral itraconazole.[75] *Cryptococcus neoformans* is a significant pathogen in related glider species.[18,74]

Parasitic

Parasites are rare in the sugar glider and usually found in wild animals or in captive animals that are maintained outdoors.[18] Sugar gliders are highly susceptible to toxoplasmosis.[32,76] Clinical signs are nonspecific and similar to those seen in other animals including depression, loss of appetite, and weight loss.[20] Commonly, there are no visible gross lesions; however, microscopically, interstitial pneumonitis, pulmonary congestion and edema, myocardial, skeletal, and smooth muscle necrosis, central nervous system necrosis, and adrenal, pancreatic, and liver lesions are observed.[76,77] Diagnosis may be confirmed by immunostaining, enzyme-linked immunosorbent assay, immunoflorescent assay, latex agglutination, or polymerase chain reaction testing.[32,76,78,79] Although clindamycin is the drug of choice for toxoplasmosis because it has good tissue distribution and can cross the blood–brain barrier, complete elimination of the organism is considered unlikely.[76,80] Animals that survive the initial infection develop tissue cysts, and recrudescence may be triggered by chilling, shipping, overcrowding, or other stress.[76,81]

A new pentastome, *Rileyella petauri*, was identified from the lungs and nasal sinus of the sugar glider. Evidence suggests the parasite has a direct life cycle, making *R petauri* the only pentastome known to inhabit mammal lung through all instars.[82]

Neoplastic

Primary neoplasia is considered rare in sugar gliders and other marsupials.[33] Bronchogenic carcinoma and chondrosarcoma involving the jaw have been reported in other members of the superfamily Phalageroidea.[74]

Heart disease

Cardiac disease and myonecrosis have been reported in sugar gliders in association with malnutrition.[22] Obesity in sugar gliders may also lead to cardiac disease.[18] Ultrasound may be useful in the diagnosis of cardiac dysfunction in the sugar glider, although normal ultrasonographic parameters for this species have not been determined.[19]

Trauma

Trauma, particularly cat predation, is one of the most common presentations of wild sugar gliders in Australia.[33,74] Pneumothorax, hemothorax, and other injuries are typical, and the prognosis is guarded.[74] Cat attacks on sugar gliders often lead to pyothorax and infection with *P multocida*, to which marsupials seem to be particularly susceptible.[18,33] Clinical signs vary by the extent and location of damage and may include dyspnea, anorexia, and depression. Diagnosis is by history, clinical presentation, physical examination, and radiography. Injuries to the respiratory tract of sugar gliders can be treated in essentially the same manner as for other mammals.[33] Gliders that have been injured by a cat or other pet should be treated with amoxicillin–clavulanate or injectable penicillin procaine–benzathine combination.[33] Although the cranial vena cava may be the most accessible site for blood draw in sugar gliders, care must be used so as not to damage the vein, heart, or other thoracic structures. Possible risks include pneumothorax, hemothorax, and cardiac puncture.[35] Gliders may exhibit tachypnea or dyspnea secondary to abdominal distention from various causes.[18]

Sugar gliders become hyperthermic and begin to pant when ambient temperature rises above 87.8°F (31°C). They sprawl with their limbs extended and their patagium exposed, and they spread saliva on their forelimbs, but they do not sweat.[26] If grass hay or straw is used as bedding, particulates may inadvertently be inhaled and lodge in the nasal passage. Nasal foreign bodies usually result in unilateral purulent discharge, sneezing, and persistent pawing at the nares. These may be removed with the aid of anesthesia.[33] Pine or cedar shavings should be avoided as bedding because the aromatic oils in these products are considered toxic.[8,21] Sugar gliders are poor swimmers and may drown if they become trapped in a tub, toilet, or similar hazard.[18]

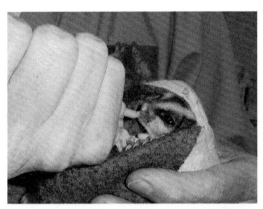

Fig. 9. Sugar gliders and hedgehogs may present in an unresponsive state of semihibernation. However, supportive care measures such as fluid therapy, supplemental heat, and assisted feeding often yield dramatic results, even in severely ill patients that appear beyond hope of recovery.

TREATMENT

Treatments for hedgehogs and sugar gliders are essentially no different than for other small mammals encountered in practice. The hedgehog's shy nature and tendency to roll when threatened make oral medications less attractive than injections and nebulization therapy. For vascular access, the intraosseous route is recommended.[42] Severely diseased hedgehogs and sugar gliders both may present in a moribund, unresponsive state of semihibernation. Although these patients may appear beyond hope of recovery, fluids, supplemental heat, and assisted feeding often yield dramatic results (**Fig. 9**). Therefore, a patient may require 24 to 48 hours of supportive care before it can be accurately assessed.

PREVENTION

Prevention of respiratory disease in hedgehogs and sugar gliders depends on good husbandry, frequent examination, and early intervention. Predisposing factors for respiratory tract infection include suboptimal environmental temperature, unsanitary conditions, obesity, malnutrition, concurrent disease, stress, and other causes of immunocompromise.[3,7,21] Dusty, unclean, or inappropriate substrates (ie, corncob, pine, or cedar) should also be avoided.[3,21] Because exotic companion mammals often hide signs of illness, annual or semiannual examinations are recommended.[3]

SUMMARY

Sugar gliders and hedgehogs are susceptible to many of the same respiratory conditions as other mammals. What sets hedgehogs and sugar gliders apart from other exotic companion mammals is their ability to slow respiration to save energy, and their need for supplemental heat in captivity to prevent disease. Diagnosis and treatment of respiratory disease in these animals is similar to that for other animals, the primary differences relating the small size of sugar gliders and hedgehogs, and the need for anesthesia to do many procedures. When compared with many other companion animals, there has been relatively little research on these species, few case reports, and the normal parameters for many diagnostic tests (eg, radiology, ultrasound, and electrocardiography) are either absent or poorly established. Thus, when presented with respiratory disease in a sugar glider or hedgehog, practitioners often have to apply diagnostic and treatment skills for which there is little published support.

REFERENCES

1. Reeve N. Hedgehogs. London: T&AD Poyser Ltd. 1994. p. 6–25, 43–51, 139–72, 214–64.
2. Mori M, O'Brien SE. Husbandry and medical management of African hedgehogs. Iowa State Univ Vet 1997;59(2):64–71.
3. Ivey E, Carpenter JW. African hedgehogs. In: Quesenberry KE, Carpenter JW, editors. Ferrets, rabbits and rodents, clinical medicine and surgery. 2nd edition. Philadelphia: Saunders; 2004. p. 339–53.
4. Nowak RM. 6th edition. Walker's mammals of the world, vol. 1. Baltimore (MD): Johns Hopkins University Press; 1999. p. 140, 170–7.
5. Heatley JJ. Hedgehogs. In: Mitchell MA, Tully TN, editors. Manual of exotic pet practice. St Louis (MO): Saunders; 2009. p. 433–55.
6. Gregory M. Observations on vocalization in the central African hedgehog, *Erinaceous albiventris*, including a courtship call. Mammalia 1975;39:1–7.
7. Smith AJ. Husbandry and medicine of African hedgehogs (*Atelerix albiventris*). J Small Exotic Anim Med 1992;2:21–8.
8. Larsen RS, Carpenter JW. Husbandry and medical management of African hedgehogs. Vet Med 1999;94(10):877–88.
9. Bartels H, Schmelzle R, Ulrich S. Comparative studies of the respiratory function of mammalian blood. V. Insectivora: shrew, mole and nonhibernating and hibernating hedgehog. Respir Physiol 1969;7(3):278–86.
10. Wallach JD, Boever WJ. Insectivora. In: Wallach JD, editor. Diseases of exotic animals: medical and surgical management. Philadelphia: Saunders; 1983. p. 653–63.
11. Isenbugel E, Baumgartner RA. Diseases of the hedgehog. In: Fowler ML, editor. Zoo and wild animal medicine: current therapy III. Philadelphia: Saunders; 1993. p. 294–301.
12. Kramm C, Sattrup G, Baumann R, et al. Respiratory function of blood in hibernating and non hibernating hedgehogs. Respir Physiol 1975;25(3):311–8.
13. Clausen G, Ersland A. The respiratory properties of the blood of the hibernating hedgehog *Erinaceus europaeus* L. Respir Physiol 1968;5(2):221–33.
14. Tähti H, Soivio A. Comparison of induced and spontaneous arousals in hibernating hedgehogs. Experientia Suppl 1978;32:321–5.
15. Johnson-Delaney CA. Hedgehogs. In: Johnson-Delaney CA, editor. Exotic companion medicine handbook for veterinarians. Lake Worth (FL): Zoological Education Network; 2000. p. 1–14.
16. Holloway JC, Geiser F. Seasonal changes in the thermoenergetics of the marsupial sugar glider, *Petaurus breviceps*. J Comp Physiol B 2001;171:643–50.
17. Bergin TJ. Physiology. In: Fowler ME, editor. Monotremes and marsupials (Monotremata and Marsupialia). Zoo and wild animal medicine. 2nd edition. Philadelphia: Saunders; 1986. p. 560–2.
18. Ness RD, Booth R. Sugar gliders. In: Quesenberry KE, Carpenter JW, editors. Ferrets, rabbits and rodents: clinical medicine and surgery. 2nd edition. Philadelphia: Saunders; 2004. p. 330–8.
19. Heatley JJ. Cardiovascular anatomy, physiology, and disease of rodents and small exotic mammals. Vet Clin North Am Exot Anim Pract 2009;12(1):99–113.
20. Available at: http://www.merckvetmanual.com/mvm/index.jsp?cfile=htm/bc/171600. htm. Accessed October 30, 2010.

21. Carboni D, Tully TN. Marsupials. In: Mitchell MA, Tully TN, editors. Manual of exotic pet practice. St Louis (MO): Saunders; 2009. p. 299–325.
22. Johnson-Delaney C. Practical marsupial medicine. Proc Assoc Avian Vet Assoc Exot Mammal Vet 2006;51–60. Available at: http://www.aemv.org/Documents/2006_AEMV_proceedings_6.pdf. Accessed March 21, 2011.
23. Pye GW, Carpenter JW. A guide to medicine and surgery in sugar gliders. Vet Med 1999;94:891–905.
24. Fleming MR. Thermoregulation and torpor in the sugar glider, Petaurus breviceps (Marsupialia: Petauridae). Aust J Zool 1980;28:521–34.
25. Körtner G, Geiser F. Torpor and activity patterns in free-ranging sugar gliders Petaurus breviceps (Marsupialia). Oecologia 2000;123:350–7.
26. Henry SR, Suckling GC. A review of the ecology of the sugar glider. In: Smith A, Hume I, editors. Possums and gliders. Chipping Norton (NSW): Surrey Beatty & Sons Pty Limited/Australian Mammal Society; 1996. p. 355–8.
27. Christian N, Geiser F. To use or not to use torpor? Activity and body temperature as predictors. Naturwissenschaften 2007;94(6):483–7.
28. Geiser F, Holloway JC, Körtner G. Thermal biology, torpor and behaviour in sugar gliders: a laboratory-field comparison. J Comp Physiol B 2007;177(5): 495–501.
29. Nagy KA, Suckling GC. Field energetics and water balance of sugar gliders, Petaurus breviceps (Marsupiala: petauridae). Aust J Zool 1985;33:683–91.
30. Tell L, Wisner E. Diagnostic techniques for evaluating the respiratory system of birds, reptiles and small exotic mammals. Exotic DVM 2003;5(2):38–48.
31. Lightfoot TL. Clinical examination of chinchillas, hedgehogs, prairie dogs, and sugar gliders. Vet Clin North Am Exot Anim Pract 1999;2(2):447–69.
32. Evans EE, Souza MJ. Advanced diagnostic approaches and current management of internal disorders of select species (rodents, sugar gliders, hedgehogs). Vet Clin North Am Exot Anim Pract 2010;13(3):453–69.
33. Blyde DJ. Respiratory diseases, diagnostics, and treatment of marsupials. Vet Clin North Am Exot Anim Pract 2000;3(2):497–512.
34. Capello V, Lennox AM. Clinical radiology of exotic companion mammals. Ames (IA): Wiley-Blackwell; 2008. p. 430–2, 482–5.
35. Dyer SM, Cervasio EL. An overview of restraint and blood collection techniques in exotic pet practice. Vet Clin North Am Exot Anim Pract 2008;11(3):423–43.
36. Carpenter JW, editor. Exotic animal formulary. 3rd edition. St Louis (MO): Saunders; 2005. p. 347–58, 359–73.
37. Majeed SK, Morris PA, Cooper JE. Occurrence of the lungworms Capillaria and Crenosoma spp. in British hedgehogs (Erinaceus europaeus). J Comp Pathol 1989;100(1):27–36.
38. Johnson D. Endoscopic tracheal wash in two guinea pigs. Exotic DVM 2005;7(3): 11–5.
39. Kohno S, Watanabe K, Hamamoto A, et al. Transthoracic needle aspiration of the lung in respiratory infections. Tohoku J Exp Med 1989;158(3):227–35.
40. Clifton-Hadley RS, Sauter-Louis CM, Lugton IW, et al. Mycobacterial diseases. In: Williams ES, Barker IK, editors. Infectious diseases of wild mammals. 3rd edition. Ames (IA): Iowa State Press; 2001. p. 340–61.
41. Johnson D. Endoscopic intubation of exotic companion mammals. Vet Clin North Am Exot Anim Pract 2010;13(2):273–89.
42. Lennox AM. Emergency and critical care procedures in sugar gliders (Petaurus breviceps), African hedgehogs (Atelerix albiventris), and prairie dogs (Cynomys spp). Vet Clin North Am Exot Anim Pract 2007;10(2):533–55.

43. Kraft SL, Dailey D, Kovach M. Magnetic resonance imaging of pulmonary lesions in guinea pigs infected with mycobacterium tuberculosis. Infect Immun 2004; 72(10):5963–71.

44. Beurgelt CD. Histopathologic findings in pet hedgehogs with nonneoplastic conditions. Vet Med 2002;97:660–5.

45. Raymond JT, White MR. Necropsy and histopathologic findings in 14 African hedgehogs (*Atelerix albiventris*): a retrospective study. J Zoo Wildl Med 1999; 30(2):273–7.

46. Hoefer HL. Hedgehogs. Vet Clin North Am Small Anim Pract 1994;24(1): 113–20.

47. Smith AJ. General husbandry and medical care of hedgehogs. In: Bonagura JD, editor. Kirk's current veterinary therapy XIII: small animal practice. Philadelphia: Saunders; 2000. p. 28–1133.

48. Robinson I, Routh A. Veterinary care of the hedgehog. In Practice 1999;21(3): 128–37.

49. Keymer IF, Gibson EA, Reynolds DJ. Zoonoses and other findings in hedgehogs (*Erinaceaus europaeus*): a survey of mortality and review of the literature. Vet Rec 1991;128(11):245–9.

50. Raymond JT, Williams C, Wu CC. Corynebacterial pneumonia in an African hedgehog. J Wildl Dis 1998;34(2):397–9.

51. Smith JM. Diseases of hedgehogs. Vet Bull 1968;38:425–30.

52. Lugton IW, Johnstone AC, Morris RS. *Mycobacterium bovis* infection in New Zealand hedgehogs (*Erinaceus europaeus*). N Z Vet J 1995;43(7):342–5.

53. Matthews PRJ, McDiarmid A. *Mycobacterium avium* infection in freeliving hedgehogs (*Erinaceus europaeus* L). Res Vet Sci 1977;22(3):388.

54. Ragg JR, Mackintosh CG, Moller H. The scavenging behaviour of ferrets (*Mustela furo*), feral cats (*Felis domesticus*), possums (*Trichosurus vulpecula*), hedgehogs (*Erinaceus europaeus*) and harrier hawks (*Circus approximans*) on pastoral farmland in New Zealand: implications for bovine tuberculosis transmission. N Z Vet J 2000;48(6):166–75.

55. Coleman JD, Cooke MM. *Mycobacterium bovis* infection in wildlife in New Zealand. Tuberculosis 2001;81(3):191–202.

56. Tappe JP, Weitzman I, Liu S. Systemic *Mycobacterium marinum* infection in a European hedgehog. J Am Vet Med Assoc 1983;183(11):1280–1.

57. Kashuba C, Hsu C, Krogstad A, et al. Small mammal virology. Vet Clin North Am Exot Anim Pract 2005;8(1):107–22.

58. Brooksby JB. Wild animals and the epizootiology of foot and mouth disease. Symp Zool Soc Lond 1968;24:1–11.

59. Vizoso AD, Thomas WE. Paramyxoviruses of the morbilli group in the wild hedgehog *Erinaceus europeus*. Br J Exp Pathol 1981;62:79–86.

60. Karstad L. Cytomegalic inclusion disease in the East African hedgehog. J Wildl Dis 1975;11(2):187–8.

61. Brunnert SR, Hensley GT, Citino SB, et al. Salivary gland oncocytes in African hedgehogs (*Atelerix albiventris*) mimicking cytomegalic inclusion disease. J Comp Pathol 1991;105(1):83–91.

62. Snider TA, Joyner PH, Clinkenbeard KD. Disseminated histoplasmosis in an African pygmy hedgehog. J Am Vet Med Assoc 2008;232(1):74–6.

63. Soulsby EJL. Helminths, arthropods and protozoa of domesticated animals. 7th edition. London: Bailliere Tyndall; 1982. p. 282–3, 339–40.

64. Urquhart GM, Armour J, Duncan JL, et al. Veterinary parasitology. England. Harlow (Essex): Longman Scientific & Technical; 1987. p. 94.

65. Sweatman GK. Mites and pentastomes. In: Davis JW, Anderson RC, editors. Parasitic diseases of wild mammals. Ames (IA): The Iowa State University Press; 1971. p. 3–64.
66. Greenacre CB. Spontaneous tumors of small mammals. Vet Clin North Am Exot Anim Pract 2004;7(3):627–51.
67. Done LB, Dietze M, Cranfield M, et al. Necropsy lesions by body systems in African hedgehogs: clues to clinical diagnosis. Proc Am Assoc Zoo Vet 1992;110–2.
68. Raymond JT, Garner MM. Spontaneous tumours in captive African hedgehogs (*Atelerix albiventris*): a retrospective study. J Comp Pathol 2001;124:128–33.
69. Rivera RY, Janovitz EB. Oronasal squamous cell carcinoma in an African hedgehog (*Erinaceidae albiventris*). J Wildl Dis 1992;28(1):148–50.
70. Juan-Sallés C, Raymond JT, Garner MM, et al. Adrenocortical carcinoma in three captive African hedgehogs (*Atelerix albiventris*). J Exotic Pet Med 2006;15(4): 278–80.
71. Lightfoot TL. Therapeutics of African pygmy hedgehogs and prairie dogs. Vet Clin North Am Exot Anim Pract 2000;3(1):155–72.
72. Raymond JT, Garner MM. Cardiomyopathy in captive African hedgehogs (*Atelerix albiventris*). J Vet Diagn Invest 2000;12(5):468–72.
73. Butler R. Bacterial diseases. In: Fowler ME, editor. Monotremes and marsupials (Monotremata and Marsupialia). Zoo and wild animal medicine. 2nd edition. Philadelphia: Saunders; 1986. p. 572–6.
74. Booth RJ. General husbandry and medical care of sugar gliders. In: Bonagura JD, editor. Kirk's current veterinary therapy XIII: small animal practice. Philadelphia: Saunders; 2000. p. 1157–63.
75. Tocidlowski M. Histoplasmosis outbreak at the Houston zoo. Proc Am Assoc Zoo Vet 2003;141–8.
76. Barrows M. Toxoplasmosis in a colony of sugar gliders (*Petaurus breviceps*). Vet Clin North Am Exot Anim Pract 2006;9(3):617–23.
77. Canfield PJ, Hartley WJ, Dubey JP. Lesions of toxoplasmosis in Australian marsupials. J Comp Pathol 1990;103:159–67.
78. Garell DM. Toxoplasmosis in zoo animals. In: Fowler ME, Miller RE, editors. Zoo and wild animal medicine current therapy IV. Philadelphia: Saunders; 1999. p. 131–5.
79. Hafid J, Flori P, Raberin H, et al. Comparison of PCR, capture ELISA and immunoblotting for detection of *Toxoplasma gondii* in infected mice. J Med Microbiol 2001;50:1100–4.
80. Wolfe BA. Toxoplasmosis. In: Fowler ME, Miller RE, editors. Zoo and wild animal medicine. 5th edition. St Louis (MO): Saunders; 2003. p. 745–9.
81. Juan-Salles C, Lopez S, Borras D, et al. Disseminated toxoplasmosis in susceptible zoo species: a sporadic disease? Proc Am Assoc Zoo Vet 1997;227–30.
82. Spratt DM. *Rileyella petauri* gen. nov., sp. nov. (Pentastomida: Cephalobaenida) from the lungs and nasal sinus of *Petaurus breviceps* (Marsupialia: Petauridae) in Australia. Parasite 2003;10(3):235–41.

A Review of Respiratory System Anatomy, Physiology, and Disease in the Mouse, Rat, Hamster, and Gerbil

Melissa A. Kling, DVM

KEYWORDS

• Rodent • Chronic • Respiratory • Disease • Mycoplasmosis
• Sendai virus • Cilia-associated respiratory bacillus

The purpose of this article is to provide for practitioners a comprehensive overview of respiratory diseases[1,2] in the mouse, rat, hamster, and gerbil, whether they treat family-owned pets, classroom pets, animals housed in nature/wildlife centers, pet stores, zoos, commercial breeding operations, or laboratory animal facilities. The information presented will also be useful for veterinarians pursuing board certification. Anatomy and physiology are briefly addressed, as those two facets alone could encompass an entire article for these species.

Print and electronic resources have vastly increased in recent years, and our knowledge of exotic animal medicine continues to develop. Therefore, practitioners must stay on the cutting edge of this information.

Basic principles of a sound workup should be followed when dealing with respiratory disease in these species, including anamnesis, husbandry evaluation, physical examination, differential diagnoses, diagnostics, treatments, disease control (prevention and quarantine), research complication assessment, and zoonotic potential. Multiple animal outbreaks should employ the same systematic approach as individual animal situations. Standard criteria are discussed here, and specifics as they apply to individual diseases are addressed in later sections.

Genetically engineered mice (GEMs), immunodeficient (ID), and immunosuppressed animals are at increased risk for disease expression than their immunocompetent (IC)

The author has nothing to disclose.
Division of Basic Medical Sciences and Laboratory Animal Resources, Mercer University School of Medicine, 1550 College Avenue, Box 165, Macon, GA 31207, USA
E-mail address: kling_m@mercer.edu

counterparts. Lack of genetic diversity within a commercial breeding operation also predisposes animals to infection because of their weakened immune systems.

When an individual or group of animals is presented for respiratory disease, it is crucial to obtain a thorough and accurate history. Significant information includes:

- Date of birth or approximate age
- Sex, breed, and/or strain of the animal
- Time of acquisition
- Acquisition source (if acquired from a store/vendor, where did the store/vendor obtain the animal)
- Husbandry practices including cage size/construction, substrate material(s), room temperature, humidity levels, lighting (intensity and cycle), ventilation, and sanitation/disinfection protocols (intervals, chemicals)
- Diet, water supply, nutritional supplementation in the form of treats, vitamins, and/or minerals. How is the food stored/has it expired/is fresh food free of contamination
- Are there other species of animals housed in the same room/facility and are any of these animals sick/recently deceased?
- Have any new animals recently been added to the household/facility?
- Has the animal been exposed to other animals recently such as a show/boarding/and so forth?
- How long has the animal been ill?
- What symptom(s) is the animal exhibiting?
- Has the animal received treatment for a previous illness(es), when was it treated, and what treatment was provided?
- Are any caretakers ill?
- The country in which the animal resides can be another diagnostic clue with regard to disease syndromes known to occur in specific geographic locations.

Husbandry procedures and perceived stress cannot be overemphasized as to their role in respiratory disease in these rodent species.

These animals are normally comfortable in warm ambient temperatures ranging from 26° to 28°C (79°–82°F) with a relative humidity of 30% to 70%. The animals should be protected from drafts and because they do not have efficient cooling mechanisms, and should never be placed in direct sunlight. Temperature and humidity must be monitored closely, as extremes and variations can cause stress and significantly contribute to disease susceptibility. Ventilation is another important factor, taking into consideration the size of the room, strain and sex of the animals, number of animals present, number of animals per cage, and sanitization interval. Ten to 15 complete air changes per hour should occur in facilities housing large numbers of animals in high-density situations, with fewer air exchanges being adequate for small numbers of pet rodents in private homes. If recycled air is used within a housing system, it should be HEPA (high-efficiency particulate air) filtered. Closed systems should be avoided, as they result in poor air circulation and a buildup of potentially toxic levels of ammonia and carbon dioxide. Ammonia gas reduces the disease-resistance capabilities of the respiratory system. The metaplastic and ciliary inhibiting effects of ammonia can extend an innocuous upper respiratory infection into a bronchopneumonia. If an ammonia smell is detected with one's nose down at the level of the animal(s) in the cage, the level is too high for the occupants (Angela M. Lennox, DVM, Indianapolis, IN, personal communication, January 2010). Controversy remains on the minimal concentration of ammonia that is deleterious, but levels as low as 25 ppm increase the severity of *Mycoplasma*-induced lesions.[3] Other considerations of air quality might include factors such as dusts, fungal spores, disinfectant vapors, and environmental pollutants.

Strict sanitation and disinfection procedures should be followed on a regular basis. Dishwashers reaching temperatures of 82°C (180°F) can be used to disinfect food and water vessels once organic matter has been removed. Dishcloths or other utensils that could inadvertently be shared between humans and animals should never be used for cleaning. Knowledge of the biology and behavior of infectious organisms is necessary to select appropriate disinfectants that will be active against a particular agent in the environment.

Appropriate pest control must be implemented, as feral mice and rats are often a source of disease.

Other known stressors that affect these animals include transport to and from the veterinary hospital, long-distance shipping from vendors, concurrent disease(s), handling for a physical examination and/or diagnostic procedures, disruption of normal biorhythms, incorrect light intensity and cycles, overall room activity, overcrowding, excessive noise, and experimental manipulations. Stress can exacerbate symptoms, making a subclinical infection become apparent or worsening already existing signs.

Clinical signs are dependent on the aspect of the respiratory system that is affected and the severity of disease expression. However, many respiratory infections are subclinical, and signs may be absent altogether or animals may be found dead without premonitory symptoms. Symptoms are not always diagnostic, but coupled with an accurate history they can provide important clues. General signs associated with respiratory disease include:

- Nasal discharge
- Ocular discharge/chromodacyorrhea
- Sneezing
- Audible clicking, "chattering," or "snuffling" when breathing
- Dyspnea
- Open-mouth breathing
- Cyanosis
- Head tilt or other vestibular involvement.

Signs of overall ill health such as decreased appetite, anorexia, lethargy, hunched posture, dehydration, and wasting commonly accompany respiratory disease. Respiratory signs can also occur as secondary manifestations of cardiac or other systemic illness.

Obtaining a correct diagnosis is essential, especially when dealing with multiple animal outbreaks; rare and costly research animals; and the pet that is a treasured member of the family. Many respiratory infections are multifactorial, necessitating a thorough investigation. Fundamental diagnostic procedures and methodology employed for traditional species are readily adaptable to rodents. Early and accurate diagnosis can lead to more successful treatment strategies and formulation of a prognosis. All options should be presented because owners can form very strong bonds with these animals, especially rats. The practitioner must be cognizant that performing an examination or stressful diagnostic procedures could be detrimental; therefore in some cases supportive care must be instituted without the aid of diagnostics. Preemptive sedation to relieve anxiety and distress when appropriate can be beneficial to some animals. Procedures requiring anesthesia in the severely compromised animal must be carefully considered, especially when using inhalant anesthetics. Clinical pathology, microbiology, serology, parasitology, environmental screening, and surveillance testing can furnish pieces of the diagnostic puzzle. Necropsy and histopathology should be considered standard elements of the diagnostic plan, especially when epizootics occur. Cases submitted to one diagnostic laboratory typically fall into two general categories: (1) young, recently shipped animals for the pet trade and (2) older animals kept as pets (Drury Reavill, DVM, West Sacramento, CA, personal communication, August 2010). It is important to use a diagnostic laboratory familiar with the specific testing needs of these species and their pathogens. Several independent, commercial, and university-based diagnostic laboratories now offer an array of testing services as outlined in **Table 1**. Imaging studies using plain radiography, contrast computed tomography, and magnetic resonance imaging comprise yet another diagnostic and, in some cases, prognostic tool.

Treatment requires an intimate knowledge of adverse side effects of drugs used in rodents. Very few drugs used in these species are approved by the United States Food and Drug Administration, which presents not only legal but therapeutic considerations, and similar restrictions may exist in other countries. It must be conveyed to the owner that treatment is not always curative and is ameliorative at best for some diseases. The use of particular antimicrobials administered orally, parenterally, or via nebulization can result in dysbiosis with subsequent fatal enterotoxemia. This side effect is seen most commonly in hamsters and gerbils and infrequently in mice and rats. Drugs that fall into this category are β-lactams, macrolides, and lincosamides. Aminoglycosides can cause an ascending flaccid paralysis with respiratory arrest, coma, and death in addition to its ototoxic and nephrotoxic potential. Neuropathological lesions in rats have been associated with nitrofurantoin. Examples of "safe" antibiotics are enrofloxacin, ciprofloxacin, marbofloxacin, trimethoprim/sulfonamide combinations, tetracycline, doxycycline, azithromycin, erythromycin, clarithromycin, and chloramphenicol. However, even antibiotics considered safe can cause problems. Nebulization can be an adjunctive modality to administer with antimicrobials, bronchodilators (aminophylline), mucolytics (acetylcysteine), or mucokinetics (saline, F10) (**Fig. 1**). The nebulizer must be capable of producing particle sizes smaller than 3 μm to reach the alveolar space.[4] Nonsteroidal anti-inflammatory drugs and analgesics can be administered if the animal seems to be in pain or discomfort. Corticosteroids are typically reserved for refractory cases. Numerous exotic animal formulary resources are available for specific drug dosages and contraindications.[5–13] Chloramphenicol has been associated with aplastic anemia in humans; therefore, appropriate client education with documentation must occur when prescribing this drug.

For animals presenting with decreased appetite, anorexia, and/or dehydration, nutritional support is an important component of the therapeutic plan. Some animals may require oxygen supplementation and/or thermal support.

The situation must be evaluated as regards the risk to other rodents in the environment when dealing with diseases that are infectious and contagious. For commercial breeding or research situations, this often means depopulation or rederivation procedures by embryo transfer or cesarean section. Strict sanitation and decontamination procedures must be followed and appropriate quarantine measures implemented. Nonessential materials should be discarded and essential items cleaned with an appropriate disinfectant and/or autoclaved before new animals are introduced.

Consideration must be given to organisms carried by human caretakers and research investigators. Organisms such as Streptococcus spp and Klebsiella spp commonly colonize humans. Humans can also transmit viruses that may result in serologic cross-reactions, if not outright infection. In addition, veterinarians must be knowledgable regarding organisms transmissible from rodents to humans.

ANATOMY AND PHYSIOLOGY

It is beyond the scope of this article to provide in-depth anatomy and physiology of these species; however, there are unique features, discussed here. **Table 2** summarizes basic physiologic functions and lung lobation. **Fig. 2** illustrates the anatomy of the lung in the rat.

Rodents are obligate nasal breathers; therefore, disease processes affecting the nasal cavity interfere with humidification and filtering of inspired air, respiration, and olfaction. Cartilage envelopes are present only in extrapulmonary airways in mice, rats, and hamsters. In rabbits and rodents, the lung volume increases with age, and the ratio of residual volume to vital capacity does not change. Mice, rats, guinea pigs, and rabbits have very high chest wall compliances and low functional residual capacities. Smaller rodents have proportionately wider airways than do larger animals. Rodents posses Clara cells in the bronchial epithelium, which are thought to provide the major component of the distal mucociliary escalator.

Of particular interest are the cardiac muscle fibers surrounding major branches of pulmonary veins that extend into the lung tissue in most rodents, making the pulmonary vein thicker. This route could allow infectious agents to spread from the heart, through the pulmonary veins, and into the lungs.

Mouse

In the mouse,[14–19] the nostrils open laterally at the tip of the snout and are guarded externally by folds of thickened skin. A vertical groove just below them forms a cleft in the upper lip, exposing the incisors. The nostrils communicate internally via vestibules with the anterior nasal cavities, which are separated by a median septum. The sinuses are also divided by the median septum, and are highly developed olfactory organs containing 7 rows of turbinal bones. The nasopharynx forms the posterior part of the pharyngeal duct, lying dorsal to the soft palate and communicating with both the oropharynx and the Eustachian tubes. The intermediate section of the respiratory tract consists of the larynx, trachea, and bronchi, all of which have cartilaginous support. The larynx is formed by 3 single (epiglottis, thyroid, and cricoid) and 3 paired (arytenoids, corniculate, and cuneiform) cartilages. Incomplete cartilaginous rings support the walls of the trachea by branching and fusing with one another dorsally. The trachea branches into the left and right bronchi dorsal to the aortic arch. Extrapulmonary bronchi have complete cartilaginous rings, whereas intrapulmonary bronchi have no cartilaginous rings. There are no muscle swellings in the pulmonary artery of the mouse as there are in the rabbit, guinea pig, and opossum. There are no bronchial artery-pulmonary artery precapillary anastomoses in the mouse as there are in humans. Nerve density in the lung is greater in the mouse than in the dog, cat, rabbit, or guinea pig. Respiratory bronchioles are short or nonexistent. Bronchus-associated lymphoid tissue is normally present only at the hilus of the lung. Lymphoid accumulations are present on the visceral pleura of mice, within interlobar clefts.

A mouse at rest can use up to 3.5 mL of oxygen per gram of body weight per hour, which is approximately 22 times that used by an elephant. To accommodate for this high metabolic rate, the mouse has a rapid respiratory rate, short air passage, high alveolar Po_2, moderately high erythrocyte concentration, high red blood cell hemoglobin and carbonic anhydrase concentrations, high capillary density, and high blood sugar concentration. The hemoglobin affinity for oxygen with changes in pH is more pronounced (Bohr effect). Mice also exhibit a slight shift in the oxygen-dissociation curve, enabling oxygen to be unloaded in the tissue capillaries at a high Po_2.

Table 1
Diagnostic laboratories performing rodent health testing

Diagnostic Laboratory	Mailing Address	Phone Number/ Fax Number	Web Site Address	Email Address	Services Provided
Bioreliance Laboratory Animal Diagnostic Services (LADS)	14920 Broschart Road, Rockville, MD 20850-3349	(p) 800-804-3586 (f) 301-610-2587	www.bioreliance.com	lads@bioreliance.com	Clinical pathology, microbiology, parasitology, serology (ELISA, IFA, HAI, WIB), PCR, cell line testing, molecular antigen PCR identification test (MAP-IT), reagents for in-house testing, health assessment panels, necropsy, histopathology, environmental monitoring, custom profiles, consultations
Charles River	251 Ballardvale Street, Wilmington, VA 01887	(p) 800-338-9680	www.crvier.com	comments@crl.com askcharlesriver@crl.com	Clinical pathology, microbiology, serology (MFIA, ELISA, IFA, WIB, HAI), PCR, prevalent rodent infectious agent (PRIA) panel (alternative to mouse and rat antibody production), necropsy, histopathology, environmental screening, custom testing, technical services/consultations
Comparative Pathology Laboratory, University of California, Davis	UCD Comparative Pathology Laboratory, 1000 Old Davis Road, Building R-1, Davis, CA 95616-8520	(p) 530-752-2832	www.vetmed.ucdavis.edu	cpl@ucdavis.edu	Clinical pathology, microbiology, parasitology, serology (MFIA, ELISA, IFA), PCR, necropsy, histopathology, environmental testing, custom testing, consultation
Molecular Diagnostic Services, Inc	204 Sorrento Valley Blvd., Suite G, San Diego, CA 92121	(p) 858-450-9990 (f) 858-450-0619	www.mds-usa.com	services@mds-usa.com	Clinical pathology, microbiology, serology (ELISA), necropsy, histopathology, environmental monitoring

Laboratory	Address	Phone/Fax	Website	Email	Services
Northwest Zoo Path	654 W. Main Street, Monroe, WA 98272	(p) 360-794-0630 (f) 360-794-4312	www.zoopath.com	zoopath@aol.com	Histopathology
Research Animal Diagnostic Laboratory	Discovery Ridge, Research Park, 4011 Discovery Drive, Columbia, MO 65201	(p) 800-669-0825 (f) 573-882-5983	www.radil.missouri.edu	RADIL@missouri.edu	Clinical pathology, microbiology, parasitology, serology (MFI, IFA, WIB), PCR, necropsy, histopathology
Research Associates Laboratory	14556 Midway Road, Dallas, TX 75244	(p) 972-960-2221 (f) 972-960-1997	www.vetdna.com	Not available	DNA-based testing, microbiology
University of Georgia, Veterinary Diagnostic Laboratory, Georgia Animal Diagnostic Services	AVDL, College of Veterinary Medicine, University of Georgia, Athens, GA 30602	(p) 706-542-5568 (f) 706-542-5977	www.vet.uga.edu/dlab	Not available	Clinical pathology, microbiology, parasitology, serology (ELISA, confirmatory testing using MFIA and IFA), PCR, necropsy, histopathology, custom testing, consultation
University of Miami, Leonard M. Miller School of Medicine, Department of Pathology	1611 NW 12th Avenue, Miami, FL 33136	(p) 305-585-6303 (f) 305-326-9363	www.cpl.med.miami.edu	compathlab@med.miami.edu	Clinical pathology, microbiology, parasitology, serology (ELISA), histopathology, custom testing
Veterinary Molecular Diagnostics, Inc	5989 Meijer Drive, Suite 5, Milford, OH 45150	(p) 513-576-1080 (f) 513-576-6177	www.VMDLABS.com	Not available	DNA-based testing
Zoo/Exotic Pathology Service	2825 KOVR Drive, West Sacramento, CA 95605	(p) 916-725-5100 (f) 916-725-6155	www.zooexotic.com	mail@zooexotic.com	Nucleic acid-based diagnostics, toxicology, necropsy, histopathology, consultations
Zoologix	9811 Owensmouth Avenue, Suite 4, Chatsworth, CA 91311-3800	(p) 818-717-8880 (f) 818-717-8881	www.zoologix.com	info@zoologix.com	PCR

This is not a complete listing of all laboratories providing diagnostic testing to rodents but laboratories with which the author has experience.
Abbreviations: ELISA, enzyme-linked-immunosorbent serologic assay; HAI, hemagglutination inhibition; IFA, immunofluorescent assay; MFIA, multiplexed fluorimetric immunoassay; PCR, polymerase chain reaction; WIB, Western immunoblot.

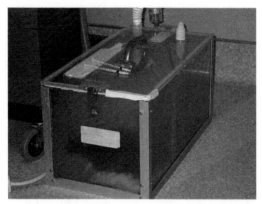

Fig. 1. Use of nebulization for treatment of rats with severe respiratory disease. Nebulizing formulas usually contain acetylcysteine, a bronchodilator, and an antibiotic with normal saline. (*Courtesy of* Cathy A. Johnson-Delaney, DVM, Dipl ABVP (Avian), Edmonds, WA.)

Rat

In the rat,[20–24] the external nares are shaped like inverted commas, open on the lateral aspect of the nose, and can be closed under water. The rat has several well-developed nasal glands but the largest is the Steno's gland (*glandula nasalis lateralis*), which lies in the rostral maxillary sinus and its duct empties at the vestibule. This gland is homologous with the salt gland of marine birds. It produces a watery, nonviscous secretion at the nasal airway entrance where it may help to humidify inspired air and regulate mucus viscosity. Because of the large number of autonomic nerves that are found in close contact with its acinar cells, it is believed that this gland is regulated by the nervous system in such a way that rapid adjustment of the secretory activity to changes in the humidity of the inspired air or to airborne irritants is possible. Tracheal diameter is approximately 1.6 to 1.7 mm in the adult rat, and the shape is maintained

Table 2
Basic physiologic respiratory functions and lung lobation of the mouse, rat, hamster, and gerbil

Parameter	Mouse	Rat	Hamster	Gerbil
Respiratory rate (breaths/min)	60–230	70–115	100–250	90–160
Tidal volume (mL)	0.09–0.38	0.60–1.5	0.91–1.4	NA[a]
Minute volume (mL/min)	11–36	75–130	64	NA[a]
Oxygen use per hour (mL O_2/g body weight/h)	1.63–3.5	0.68–1.10	0.6–1.4	1.4
Left lung lobation	Single lobe	Single lobe	Single lobe	Single lobe
Right lung lobation	4 lobes (cranial, middle, caudal, accessory)	4 lobes (cranial, middle, caudal, accessory)	5 lobes (cranial, middle, caudal, intermediate, accessory)	4 lobes (cranial, middle, caudal, accessory)

[a] Data not available.

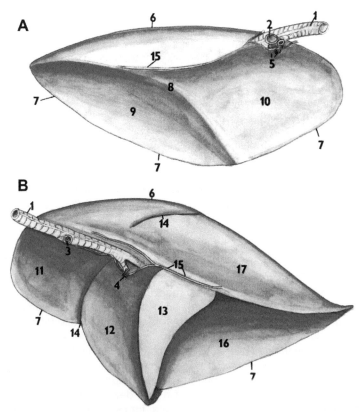

Fig. 2. View of the mediastinal surfaces of left (*A*) and right (*B*) rat lungs. Key features include cranial (11), medial (12), accessory (13), and caudal (16, 17) lobes of the right lung. The left lung has only a single lobe. (*Reprinted from* Popesko P, Rajtova V, Horak J. A colour atlas of anatomy of small laboratory animals, vol. 2: rabbit, guinea pig. Elsevier; 1992; with permission from Elsevier.)

by 18 to 24 rigid C-shaped cartilage structures that form the framework of the trachea. Tracheal length from the first cartilage to bifurcation is 33 mm and because of the cartilaginous rings, extension of the head of the rat can result in lengthening of the trachea by 50% with no decrease in lumen diameter. The lung in the newborn rat is immature and contains no alveoli or alveolar ducts; instead, gas exchange occurs in smooth walled channels and saccules, and the prospective alveolar structures. Once the rat reaches 4 days old, a rapid restructuring of lung parenchyma occurs so that by day 7, the lung is morphologically more mature. Respiratory bronchioles are also absent at birth but by day 10 are easily identified. Rats have the thinnest pulmonary artery and the thickest pulmonary vein of all rodent species. In the conscious resting rat, blood flow preferentially distributes to the central and hilar regions of the lung lobes, with less blood flow to the peripheral regions. Precapillary anastomoses between the bronchial and pulmonary arteries have been demonstrated in the rat, as they have been in man and guinea pig, and are limited to the hilar region in the rat. Innervation of the lung is complex, with high neuronal density similar to the calf, mouse, and guinea pig. The rat and rabbit do not have an adrenergic nerve supply to the bronchial musculature, and bronchoconstriction is controlled by vagal tone. At least 10 morphologically distinct cell types have been identified in the intrapulmonary airways. Rats possess serous cells in respiratory epithelium, which are unique to this species. These cells secrete a product that has less viscosity than the mucous cell, and is thought to be responsible for the low-viscosity pericilliary liquid layer found at all levels of the rat's respiratory tract.

Total lung capacity of the rat is 11.3 ± 1.4 mL and vital capacity 8.4 ± 1.7 mL. Although surfactant is composed of mostly monounsaturated phospholipids in many mammals, rat surfactant has a high content of polyunsaturated phospholipids. Carotid bodies located in the bifurcation of the common carotid artery function as chemoreceptors and respond when the tissue partial pressure of oxygen decreases to below 100 mm of mercury. Similar chemoreceptors located in the aorta are called aortic bodies, whose afferents travel via the vagi to the brain. Regulation of respiration occurs through tissue CO_2 exchange in the medullary respiratory center, with the carotid bodies playing a role. Rats have high serotonin activity and low histamine activity in the lungs.

Hamster

Hamsters[25–28] have several nasal serous glands that open into the internal ostium of the external nares. These glands include 1 infraseptal, 2 nasoturbinate, 5 maxilloturbinate, 1 ventromedial nasal, 4 or 5 dorsal medial nasal, and the lateral nasal gland (Steno's gland). There are 4 endoturbinates and 3 ectoturbinates, unlike the rat which has 4 endoturbinates and 2 ectoturbinates. These very intricately folded turbinates project into the lumen of the nasal cavity and thus provide for an increased nasal mucosal surface. The trachea bifurcates at the height of the fourth rib pair into thicker right and thinner left main bronchi. Reisseisen's membrane, a layer of smooth muscle and elastic tissue, lines the lobar bronchi. The diaphragm originates dorsally on the first lumbar vertebrae and is composed of a well-developed *pars muscularis* and a transparent *centrum tendineum*. The pleura forms a large right and left sac surrounding the lungs. There are no respiratory bronchioles as in the rat and guinea pig, although the guinea pig and hamster have a transition to alveolar airways within a single generation that could be classified as producing one order of respiratory bronchioles. The conductive airways contain a limited number of glandular structures, primarily in the proximal trachea. The histologic appearance of the hamster trachea closely resembles the human bronchus. The pulmonary vascular bed is similar to that of humans in many ways, and hamsters develop pulmonary lesions that resemble human centrilobular emphysema. This similarity makes the Syrian hamster a potential model for studies of chronic bronchitis. Bronchus-associated lymphoid tissue, normally present only at the hilus of the lung in rodents, is absent in hamsters. Spontaneous bronchiogenic and pulmonary cancers are rare; hence, the Syrian hamster is a good model in which to study chemical carcinogenesis in the respiratory tract.

Resting respiration rate is inversely proportional to the body weight, whereas tidal volume and mean minute volume are directly related. Arterial blood pH is 7.4 and P_{CO_2} is 45.3 mm Hg. Blood pH increases slightly during hibernation and P_{CO_2} decreases, indicating that hibernating animals are slightly acidotic. Hamsters are fairly resistant to pulmonary infection and are able to decompose nicotine, and therefore make good subjects for the study of effects of long-term smoke inhalation.

Gerbil

The gerbil[29,30] has not been studied as extensively as the mouse, rat, and hamster, but its respiratory anatomy and physiology are similar to those of other small rodent species.

INFECTIOUS DISEASES
Bacterial Agents

Bordetella bronchiseptica

Bordetella bronchiseptica[31–34] is a gram-negative bacillus or coccobacillus belonging to the family Alcaligenaceae. Infection is more likely in pet rodents and rabbits, especially those exposed to other species such as cats and dogs. Because of the frequency of *Bordetella* in the laboratory guinea pig and rabbit, contact with these species should be avoided. Frequently there is an identifiable concurrent infection, such as coronavirus.

Transmission is by direct contact with clinically affected animals, carrier hosts, contaminated fomites, and respiratory aerosols. Although many surviving animals develop immunity and eliminate the infection, subclinical and carrier animals are common. The bacteria can form biofilms in vitro that may serve to protect it from host defenses.

Diagnosis is best achieved by isolation of the organism in large numbers from affected tissues. Enzyme-linked immunosorbent serologic assay (ELISA) is commercially available and the polymerase chain reaction (PCR) is possible. Treatment is usually not practical with the exception of small numbers of pets, and even then treatment of chronic infections is palliative at best. The organism is normally sensitive to trimethoprim-sulfonamide products, chloramphenicol, enrofloxacin, and marbofloxacin. If the animal is anorexic, nutritional support should also be provided.

The importance of infection of humans in minimal, although the organism is recovered occasionally from the human nasopharynx and could serve as a source of infection to animals. The organism could cause a whooping-cough syndrome and bronchopneumonia in young, elderly, or immunocompromised humans.

Mouse Although no naturally occurring disease has been reported, mice are susceptible to experimental infection. Strains such as C3H/HeJ show increased susceptibility to clinical disease.

Rat Infection is typically opportunistic, but aerosol exposure in laboratory rats has resulted in lesions characterized by suppurative rhinitis. The organism tends to colonize on the apices of the ciliated respiratory epithelial cells, resulting in impaired clearance. In spontaneous cases, there has been a suppurative bronchopneumonia with consolidation of affected anteroventral areas of the lung. Multifocal bronchopneumonia with polymorphonuclear cell and lymphocytic infiltration, and peribronchial lymphoid hyperplasia are seen microscopically.

In experimental trials, *B bronchiseptica* caused pneumonia and was more pathogenic for the respiratory system of weanling rats than *Pasteurella pneumotropica*.[35]

Hamster The hamster appears to be uniquely resistant to intranasal inoculation with this organism.

Gerbil This organism is a potential problem for gerbils, but has not been reported as a natural disease. Young gerbils inoculated intranasally with *B bronchiseptica* developed a severe disease with high mortality, whereas older gerbils appeared to be more resistant. Both the *Meriones unguiculatus* and *Meriones shawi* species appear to be susceptible.

Chlamydophila spp

Chlamydophila spp[36,37] belong to the family Chlamydiaeceae, and are gram-negative obligate intracellular bacteria whose name remains in a state of constant flux. Mice are susceptible to natural infections with *Chlamydophila muridarum*, the mouse pneumonitis (MoPn) agent. Clara Nigg discovered the agent, so it has also been referred to as the "Nigg Agent." Mice are experimentally susceptible to both *Chlamydophila trachomatis* and *Chlamydophila psittaci* of human origin. IC animals develop transient infections that are typically silent in natural infections. Natural infection of laboratory mice is rare, but infection with other chylamidiae, such as *C psittaci* or *Chlamydophila pneumoniae*, does occur, with increased incidence in ID animals. Experimental lung infections are more severe in BALB mice than in B6 mice. In addition, *C psittaci* can experimentally cause respiratory and septicemic disease in mice. These infections are more severe in C3H, BALB/c, or A/J strains than in resistant B6 mice. Immunity to the MoPn agent is dependent on functional CD4 T cells. B-cell–deficient mice (Igh6 null) recover from infection, but T-cell–deficient RAG, SCID, and MHC class II (CD4 null) (but not β2-microglobulin [CD8] null mice) develop severe disease. Mice of the C3H/HeN strain develop infections of longer duration than those of BALB/c or B6 strains.

Based on experimental infection, transmission is presumed to occur via respiratory aerosols and/or venereal transmission. Contact exposure rarely results in transmission. Both mouse and human agents are used in laboratory mice as models for respiratory and genital chlamydiosis, therefore serving as potential iatrogenic sources of infection for mouse colonies. Severe acute infections are characterized by ruffled fur, hunched posture, and labored respiration due to interstitial pneumonitis, followed by death within 24 hours. Mice dying more slowly may develop progressive emaciation and cyanosis of the ears and tail.

Intranasal inoculation results in nonsuppurative interstitial pneumonia with atelectasis and pulmonary perivascular/peribronchiolar lymphocytic infiltration. Lesions are manifested grossly as pinpoint, elevated gray foci on the pleural surfaces. Organisms grow within bronchiolar epithelium, type I alveolar cells, and macrophages, which can possess intracytoplasmic vesicles containing inclusions. The agent readily disseminates hematogenously and by lymphatics to multiple organs regardless of route of inoculation, due to its affinity for macrophages.

Diagnosis can be made with impression smears, growth in cell culture, or embryonated chicken eggs. Accurate speciation can be made via DNA sequencing.

Cilia-associated respiratory bacillus

The cilia-associated respiratory bacillus (CARB)[38–47] organism is an unclassified, gram-negative, motile, non–spore-forming bacterium. It is closely related genetically to *Flexibacter* spp and the *Flavobacterium* group of bacteria known as "gliding bacteria," based on the fact they are motile but without visible means for such motility. These bacteria are widespread and noteworthy respiratory pathogens in rats, commonly infect rabbits, and probably infect mice at a higher rate than is currently recognized. Disease has also been reported in wild rats, hamsters, guinea pigs, dogs, cats, goats, swine, and cattle. No data exist for pet populations but infections are likely to be common. CARB can act as a primary pathogen or can exacerbate infections caused by other agents. Colonization with the organism leads to interference with the mucociliary apparatus, and secondary infections with other opportunistic invaders in chronic cases may occur.

CARB is transmitted via direct contact, and there is no evidence for transmission by fomites, vectors, or aerosols. With an infected population, CARB tends to spread slowly. Serology can be used to monitor healthy populations using multiplexed fluorimetric immunoassay (MFIA), ELISA, or immunofluorescent assay (IFA) along with PCR and/or histopathology to detect the organism in diseased animals. However, CARB serology has a higher rate of false positives because the reagents used are often bacterial lysates containing numerous antigens. PCR is the preferred confirmatory method for follow-up to positive serology, and is best performed on nasopharyngeal or tracheal swabs or lavages. Because transmission is by direct contact, screening of sentinel rats exposed to bedding may miss infections.

Culture and sensitivity testing have demonstrated that CARB is sensitive to sulfonamides, procaine penicillin G, ampicillin, chloramphenicol, neomycin, gentamicin, and streptomycin. The efficacy of antimicrobial therapy in eliminating CARB from enzootically infected colonies or in chronically infected pets remains unknown.

The primary consideration for exclusion of this agent from a facility or colony should be the avoidance of direct contact between infected and uninfected animals. Colony animals should be screened regularly for CARB, and incoming animals should be quarantined and screened. The appearance of this organism in an established facility, previously free of it, would indicate the entry of infected rodents, most likely feral or wild. Repopulation or rederivation are generally recommended. It is unlikely that survival of the organism in the environment should play a significant role in the transmission of CARB. Typical animal room sanitation and disinfection should serve to remove any CARB from the environment.

Mouse In breeding populations, CARB is transmitted from infected dams to pups shortly after birth, and infection can be transmitted among adult mice by direct contact. Natural outbreaks of disease in mice seem to be associated with concurrent viral infections, including Sendai virus (SeV) and pneumonia virus of mice (PVM). Experimental, and probable natural, infections may be inapparent with no discernible lesions. Chronic disease and seroconversion have been produced in BALB/c mice inoculated intranasally with the CARB, but B6 mice developed less severe lesions and lower antibody responses. The organism has been associated with chronic respiratory disease in conventional B6 and B6 obese mutant mice dying of the disease. Microscopic changes include chronic suppurative cranioventral bronchopneumonia with marked peribronchiolar infiltration with lymphocytes and plasma cells, and luminal neutrophilic exudation.

Rat CARB was first reported in association with respiratory disease in rats in 1980; however, the organisms have been found in archived tissues collected in the 1950s, and are seen on electron microscopy photographs published in the 1960s.[48]

Naturally occurring, uncomplicated disease has been observed in rats, and signs are similar to those seen with *Mycoplasma pulmonis* infection. Although infected rats are often asymptomatic, signs generally associated with respiratory disease can occur. Rats appear to have a more significant clinical presentation than mice. Lesions similar to those seen in confirmed cases of mycoplasmosis have been produced in *Mycoplasma*-free rats inoculated intranasally with CARB. Its pathogenic potential as a potentiator of *M pulmonis* respiratory disease has been demonstrated most clearly in the rat. Intranasal inoculation of young Wistar rats resulted in colonization of the upper respiratory tract and airways by 14 days. Necropsy signs are variable, and depend on the pathogenicity of the bacterial strain involved and the chronicity of the infection. CARB can be present anywhere there is ciliated respiratory epithelium, including the Eustachian tubes and middle ears. A multifocal to coalescing pyogranulomatous bronchopneumonia with bronchiectasis, enlarged mediastinal and bronchial lymph nodes, and dilated bronchi are seen microscopically. Chronic suppurative bronchitis and bronchiolitis, with peribronchiolar cuffing with lymphocytes and plasma cells, are typical microscopic findings.

Hamster A multifocal to coalescing pyogranulomatous bronchopneumonia with bronchiectasis, enlarged mediastinal and bronchial lymph nodes, and dilated bronchi are seen in experimentally infected hamsters.

Gerbil Gerbils are susceptible to experimentally induced CARB infections. Young gerbils inoculated intranasally with a rat isolate remained asymptomatic during the study. At necropsy, there was colonization of the apices of epithelial cells lining the trachea and airways, with marked peritracheal and peribronchial lymphocytic infiltration.[49]

Corynebacterium kutscheri

Corynebacterium kutscheri[50–59] is a gram-positive bacillus belonging to the family Corynebacteriaceae. It causes corynebacteriosis or pseudotuberculosis, and is considered an opportunistic pathogen in IC animals (**Fig. 3**). This infectious disease syndrome was one of the first to be recognized in mice and rats by Kutscher in 1894. It remains a significant pathogen that occasionally infects colonies of rats and mice, and infection is usually latent and subclinical. Infections only become overt after immunosuppression or other stressors such as nutritional deficiencies. Natural transmission is via the oral-fecal route, with prenatal transmission occurring experimentally. Infected animals may shed the bacterium into the environment for extended periods of time, as it has been detected in the feces of mice up to 5 months post infection. Pet rodents, and rats in particular, can transmit the bacterium to their human handlers.

The acute clinical disease has high morbidity and low mortality, and infected animals exhibit signs associated with respiratory disease in addition to abnormal gait, with septic and swollen joints. Death usually occurs in 1 week. A chronic infection, with low morbidity and mortality, may be inapparent or produce nonspecific signs.

Hematogenous extension of the organism from the oral cavity via small abrasions or from regional lymph nodes results in focal embolic abscessation in a variety of organs, including the lungs. Histologically, lesions are chronic and consist of a pyogranulomatous infiltrate around the central necrotic core, surrounded by a mantle of infiltrating lymphocytes, plasma cells, and fibroblasts. Lung lesions eventually become granulomatous, giving rise to the name pseudotuberculosis.

Diagnosis is by examination of impression smears from affected tissues or tissues sections. Definitive diagnosis requires characterization of the cultured bacteria or serology. Positive ELISA should always be confirmed by culture. The isolation rate of this organism is most successful from specimens collected from the oral cavity and submaxillary lymph nodes. This agent is difficult to recover from animals latently infected in enzootically affected colonies, although oral swabs of the gingiva may be helpful. PCR is not widely available.

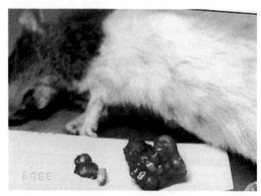

Fig. 3. Gross necropsy of rat lung with abscesses due to *Corynebacterium kutcheri*. (*Courtesy of* Cathy A. Johnson-Delaney, DVM, Dipl ABVP (Avian), Edmonds, WA.)

The bacterium is sensitive to a variety of antimicrobials, including ampicillin, chloramphenicol, and tetracyclines. Treatment of animals with antimicrobials may serve to treat illness, but would probably not resolve the carrier state nor eliminate the bacteria from the bedding or cage surfaces. Thus, treatment is only recommended to ameliorate clinical signs or for rederivation, if necessary.

Mouse The usual sites of colonization in mice are the oral cavity, cecum, and colon. Clinical manifestations usually occur in conjunction with predisposing factors that compromise the immune system.

Susceptibility to this organism among various strains of mice is attributed to the effectiveness of the mononuclear phagocyte system. BALB/c-nude, A/J, CBA/N, MPS, and BALB/cCr mice are most susceptible, C3H/He mice intermediate, and C57BL/6Cr, B10.BR/SgSn, ddY, and ICR resistant to colonization and disease induction. Male mice harbor higher numbers of bacteria and a higher carrier rate. Strains of mice sensitive to *C kutscheri* infections tend to be resistant to *Salmonella* spp infections and vice versa.

Raised gray nodules may be present in the lungs along with other organ involvement. Lesions may contain material that varies from friable caseous exudate to liquefied pus. Microscopically, lesions feature coagulation to caseation necrosis, with peripheral aggregations of leukocytes composed primarily of neutrophils. Suppurative thrombosis and embolization involving the pulmonary or mesenteric and portal vessels may be evident.

Rat Rats are more resistant to acute spontaneous disease than mice. Rats infected with sialodacryoadenitis virus (SDAV), SeV, or parvovirus do not transform preexisting subclinical *C kutscheri* into clinically apparent disease. Clinical symptoms are those typically seen with respiratory disease. Gross lesions include raised pale foci of suppuration of variable size with a characteristic hyperemic peripheral zone in the lung. Affected areas frequently coalesce with adjacent lesions. Fibrinous exudate may be present on the pleura and/or pericardial sac. Histologically, lesions occur most frequently in the lung. There are foci of coagulation to caseation necrosis, with leukocytic infiltration as in the mouse. Neutrophils are the predominant cellular infiltrates in the early stages. Subsequently there are mononuclear cells composed of macrophages, lymphocytes, and plasma cells. Lesions are usually not associated with airways and are interpreted to be hematogenous in origin. There is an associated pneumonia, with hypercellularity of alveolar septa, perivascular cuffing, and pulmonary edema. Some airways adjacent to affected areas may contain purulent exudate.

The presence of bacterial colonies is pathognomonic. Lymphoid hyperplasia is a frequent finding in chronic cases, and residual scars may be present in target tissues of recovered animals.

There is one report of a human *C kutscheri* infection in an infant after a bite from an infected rat.[60]

Hamster Both *C kutscheri* and *Corynebacterium paulometabulum* have been isolated from the respiratory tracts of hamsters. Although the hamster can serve as a host, it appears to be relatively resistant to systemic infection.

Haemophilus *spp*
During routine quality control of a laboratory rodent colony, 16.8% of the rats were found to be infected with this organism, which was characterized as a member of the family Pasteurellaceae.[61] The organism was cultured from the nasal cavity, trachea, lung, and the female genital tract. Investigation of rats immediately on receipt

from the breeder showed that they were culturally and serologically positive for *Haemophilus* spp. Histologic examination of the lungs in rats infected with *Haemophilus* spp demonstrated a mild inflammatory cell infiltration and diffuse hyperemia. The prevalence of this organism is unknown. In view of the sites of colonization and the presence of lesions in the respiratory tract, this represents a possible complicating factor in the laboratory rat under experiment.

Klebsiella pneumoniae

Klebsiella pneumoniae[62–65] is a gram-negative anaerobic rod belonging to the family Enterobacteriaceae that can be a normal component of the intestinal flora in mice and rats. The bacterium may be also common in the environment. It is considered an opportunistic pathogen in these species, but is not a significant cause of naturally occurring disease.

K pneumoniae can be readily transmitted from one species to another, including humans to animals and vice versa. Transmission is probably fecal-oral or via direct contact. Colonization of animals may be from human caretakers or from exposure to infected soil.

Clinical signs and lesions are very rare in IC animals. These organisms are low-level opportunists; therefore, ID animals are more susceptible to disease. Infection may also be seen after antibiotic treatment. There is no pattern of infection or characteristic lesions, but it has been associated with mild suppurative rhinitis in otherwise pathogen-free rats. It has been associated with bacteremic disease in mice with cervical lymphadenopathy, liver and kidney abscesses, emphysema, pneumonia, ventricular endocarditis and myocarditis, and thrombosis.

Diagnosis is by culture and biochemical identification to differentiate the species. Treatment with antimicrobials may serve to treat illness, but rarely, if ever, resolves the carrier state; nor will therapy eliminate bacteria from the bedding or cage surfaces. This organism is an important cause of human nosocomial infection, and human isolates of are often multidrug resistant.

Mycobacterium avium-intracellulare

Mycobacterium avium-intracellulare[66,67] is a gram-positive, acid-fast, obligate intracellular bacterium belonging to the family Mycobacteriaceae that can be found in soil, water, and bedding materials. Naturally occurring infections are rare but mice are susceptible to experimental infections. A naturally occurring outbreak of infection in C57BL/6N mice within a B6C3F1 hybrid production colony has been documented. B6C3F1 hybrid mice did not develop lesions of mycobacterial infection when intratracheally inoculated. Adult mice were more susceptible to infection than 8-week-old animals. Grossly, subpleural 1- to 5-mm diameter tan-colored masses were present in the lungs. Microscopic findings consisted of focal accumulations of epithelioid cells, foamy macrophages, and lymphocytes in alveolar spaces and septa, with variable amounts of necrosis and neutrophilic leukocyte infiltration.

Mycoplasma *spp*

Mycoplasma pulmonis[68–77] is a gram-negative, small bacterium devoid of cell walls and is a member of the family Mycoplasmataceae. Infection and disease are common in pets, nonbarrier-housed rats and mice, and wild rodents. The organism can be carried in the in the upper respiratory passages in the absence of disease.

Mycoplasmosis is exacerbated by viral infections, particularly SeV; by other bacteria including *P pneumotropica*, *Actinobacillus* spp, *Streptococcus pneumoniae*, *B bronchiseptica*, CARB, and *C kutscheri*; and by environmental ammonia levels. These cofactors play a significant role in causing subclinical infections to manifest into outright disease. The most important aspect for clinicians is that respiratory mycoplasmosis varies greatly in disease expression because of environmental, host, and pathogen factors that influence the host-pathogen relationship. *M pulmonis* colonizes the apical cell membranes of respiratory epithelium, interferes with mucociliary clearance, and is mitogenic for B cells, which contributes to the pathology observed in the lungs. The acquired immune response is important in limiting hematogenous dissemination but does little to eliminate infection or resolution of disease.

Diagnosis is based on history, clinical findings, gross and microscopic lesions, and isolation of the organism from tissues. PCR offers a rapid way to screen cell lines, biologic agents, and other tissues. Colony surveillance can employ serology (MFIA, ELISA, or IFA), as the organisms persist despite the presence of antibodies. However, animals may be infected for months before antibodies develop against these surface-dwelling organisms, yielding false-negative results in early stages of the disease. Therefore, culture and PCR are recommended to detect early infections. CARB is frequently a copathogen with *M pulmonis*, and diagnostic investigations should also include screening for this organism.

Despite developing high antibody titers to *Mycoplasma* and high antibiotic tissue levels, affected animals typically have persistent *M pulmonis* infection; therefore, antimicrobial therapy may alleviate clinical signs but does not eliminate the infection. For many years the standard of treatment for laboratory rats was to add tetracycline to sweetened drinking water; however, this treatment is ineffective because blood antibiotic concentrations are below minimum inhibitory concentration (MIC) and pulmonary tissue concentration of tetracycline is not inhibitory. Tetracyclines in water can cause a reduction in water consumption, and those at high concentrations in tap water form a scale that can block sipper tubes. Although scientific studies of effectiveness have not been conducted, tylosin administered in drinking water has been shown to reach concentrations in serum and lung well above MIC concentrations. Enrofloxacin (10 mg/kg) in combination with doxycycline (5 mg/kg) administered per os every12 hours for 7 to 10 days appears to be an effective regimen to control symptomatic animals. Sulfamethazine at 0.02% in the drinking water or 1 mg/4 g feed, tylosin at 66 mg/L (2.5 g/gallon) for 21 days, and chloramphenicol at 30 mg/kg for 5 days are other treatment protocols used in colony situations. Nebulization, anti-inflammatory and analgesic medication, and nutritional support are indicated in chronic cases of infection. Environmental factors contributing to the severity of the disease must also be corrected.

Effective control and prevention depend primarily on maintenance of *Mycoplasma*-free colonies under barrier conditions supported by careful surveillance for infection. Progress has been made in developing DNA-based vaccines against *M pulmonis*, but these have not achieved clinical application. Prevention of this organism in a facility should focus on the entry of animals and biologic materials. Animals should be obtained from reputable vendors or quarantined and screened before entry. Vigorous pest control should be in place. Pet rats and mice commonly harbor this organism, and caretakers in laboratory facilities should not keep pet rodents or have secondary employment that may expose them to pets or wild rodents. *Mycoplasma* spp are common contaminants of animal and human tumor cell lines, but *M pulmonis* is rarely confirmed in these materials. Nonetheless, these materials should be screened via PCR or antibody production.

Elimination of *M pulmonis* from large populations of rats and mice, for all practical purposes, is impossible without rederivation or depopulation. The organism can be found in both male and female reproductive tissues, so the pretreatment of donor animals with antibiotics may be helpful in decreasing the chance of vertical transmission.

In general, these organisms are not considered to be viable for long periods of time outside of a host. Some mycoplasmas are able to form biofilms, which may afford them better resistance to heat and desiccation than previously thought. Decontamination appropriate for more robust non–spore-forming bacteria should be sufficient for decontamination after an outbreak.

Research protocols involving inhalation toxicology and pulmonary carcinogenesis can be compromised by chronic, progressive infection. One of the most important complications is contamination of cell lines and transplantable tumors. There is evidence that *M pulmonis* may depress humoral and cellular mediated responses. Animals with *M pulmonis* infection have decreased delayed hypersensitivity responses, T-cell subset changes, and increased total lymphocyte and neutrophil counts.

Although the organism can be carried in the nasal passage, it does not normally affect humans. *M pulmonis* has been detected, isolated, and sequenced in animal facility workers exposed to infected rats. The mode of transmission is unknown.[78]

Mouse *M pulmonis, Mycoplasma arthritidis*, and *Mycoplasma neurolyticum* inhabit the upper respiratory tract of mice. *M arthritidis* may cause respiratory disease following intranasal inoculation, but under natural conditions it is generally nonpathogenic. However, it is problematic because it can cause seroconversion to *M pulmonis*.

The organism referred to as the gray lung agent (GLA) has been characterized as a *Mycoplasma* spp. It appears to be closely related to *Mycoplasma hominis* and distantly related to *M pulmonis*. The name *Candidatus Mycoplasma ravipulmonis* has been proposed.[79]

Compared with rats, mice are relatively resistant to the disease caused by *M pulmonis*, and there has been a marked decrease in incidence of clinical disease in laboratory mice. Asymptomatic infection is more common. Exposure occurs by aerosol transmission, but venereal transmission may also occur. Although not documented, transplacental transmission is likely in ID mice with disseminated infections. Disease severity in experimental infection is closely linked to inoculum dose, and disease susceptibility depends on the strain or isolate of *M pulmonis* and the strain of mouse. Genetic resistance is complex and does not appear to be *H-2* linked. Mice of the C57BR, B6, and B10 strains are resistant, whereas C57L, SJL, BALB, A/J, C3H/HeJ, C3H/HeN, C3HeB, SWR, AKR, CBA/N, C58, and DBA/2 have varying susceptibility. Experimental studies compared infections between susceptible C3H and resistant B6 mice, and found that female mice develop more severe disease. Athymic nude, thymectomized, CBA/N (X-linked ID), and SCID mice inoculated intranasally with *M pulmonis* develop significantly less severe respiratory disease than IC mice, but have disseminated infection with severe polyarthritis.

When clinical signs occur they reflect a suppurative rhinitis, otitis media, and chronic pneumonia. Affected mice may display inactivity, weight loss, and ruffled hair coat, but the most prominent signs are "chattering" and dyspnea, due to rhinitis and purulent exudate in the nasal passages. Otitis media may cause head tilt, circling, and other vestibular signs. Suppurative inflammation in the brain and spinal cord, although rare, can cause flaccid paralysis. Survivors develop chronic bronchopneumonia, bronchiectasis, and occasionally pulmonary abscesses.

Rat *M pulmonis* infection is common in rats and should be considered essentially ubiquitous in rats other than specific pathogen-free laboratory rats. It is by far the most common cause of clinical respiratory disease in pet rats. Chronic respiratory disease (CRD) in rats has experienced an interesting evolution, as it was initially believed to be multifactorial, but later it became apparent that *M pulmonis* was the primary pathogen of the disease. Hence, the term murine respiratory mycoplasmosis

(MRM) became the preferred nomenclature over CRD. Although other pathogens of the respiratory tract can play a role in the development of the disease, *M pulmonis* remains the major pathogen in cases of CRD in rats. Some seropositive animals may be cross-reacting because of exposure to *M arthritidis*. Reports of naturally occurring infections with clinical disease due to *M arthritidis* are rare, but this organism has been isolated from the respiratory tract and middle ear.

Transmission of *M pulmonis* among cage-mates and to adjacent cages occurs primarily through aerosols. It may require several months to establish an infection in contact animals, and clinical disease may not occur for up to 6 months. Intrauterine transmission also occurs, although newborn pups appear to be frequently infected by exposure to the dam during the postnatal period. Placentitis and fetal broncho-pneumonia have been produced in pregnant rats inoculated intravaginally with *M pulmonis* prior to breeding.

As with mice, the incidence and intensity of the disease are influenced by a variety of factors, such as strain of rat, concurrent infection, and environmental conditions. LEW rats develop a more severe disease than do F344 rats. Concurrent infections with organisms such as SeV, rat coronavirus, CARB, or *P pneumotropica* have an additive effect on the disease.

Clinical signs include mild to severe respiratory distress, sniffling, torticollis, and infertility (**Fig. 4**). Dyspnea, ruffled hair coat, and weight loss may occur. Porphyrin-containing dark red encrustations may be present around the eyes and nares. Infections frequently extend from the Eustachian tube to the middle ear and then to the inner ear, causing labyrinthitis. Rats with labyrinthitis will spin, rotating their bodies rapidly when they are held in a vertical position by the tail. Unless the respiratory infections are complicated by bacterial infections, the terminal clinical stages of MRM may last weeks or months, which is common in the geriatric pet rat.

The organism has an affinity for the epithelial cells of the respiratory tract, middle ear, and endometrium. Invasion of the middle ear occurs via the Eustachian tube and usually results in a chronic infection because the Eustachian tube opens into the tympanic bulla on the dorsal aspect, affording poor drainage to the nasopharynx. Rats have cartilaginous rings only around primary bronchi. Damage to respiratory epithelium with ciliostasis and resultant accumulation of lysozyme-rich inflammatory exudate in the airways frequently results in weakening of bronchiolar walls and ensuing bronchiolectasis. *Mycoplasma*-associated host cell damage may occur by a variety of means, including uptake of essential cell metabolites and release of cytotoxic substances. Both the intact organisms and the cell membranes are

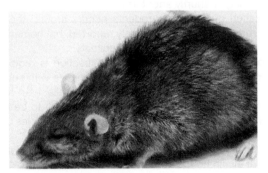

Fig. 4. Rat with chronic murine respiratory disease and typical hunched postural presentation. (*Courtesy of* Cathy A. Johnson-Delaney, DVM, Dipl ABVP (Avian), Edmonds, WA.)

nonspecifically mitogenic for lymphocytes. Thus, the marked lymphocytic infiltration seen in response to mycoplasmal infections does not appear to be due only to a response to a specific antigenic stimulus. The extensive lesions seen in some rat strains after exposure to *M pulmonis* may be attributable to an exaggerated and misdirected cellular immune response. The organism usually persists in infected rats, even in the presence of relatively high antibody titers. Microscopic changes in the affected tympanic bullae, turbinates, and major airways are characterized by a leukocytic infiltrate in the submucosa consisting of neutrophils, lymphocytes, and plasma cells. Peribronchial, peribronchiolar, and perivascular infiltration with lymphocytes and plasma cells is a prominent feature in all stages of the disease. Chronic bronchitis and bronchiolitis frequently progress to bronchiectasis and bronchiolectasis, which are characterized by dilation of airways and peribronchiolar cuffing with lymphocytes, with varying degrees of hyperplasia and metaplasia of respiratory epithelium.

At necropsy, serous to catarrhal exudate may be present in nasal passages, trachea, and major airways. In animals with copious viscous exudate in the airways, there may be patchy vesicular to bullous emphysema in the lungs. In affected lobes, lesions are unilateral or bilateral, and usually cranioventral in distribution. In advanced cases there are scattered areas of abscessation involving one or both lungs and in some animals the normal architecture may completely obliterated by the chronic suppurative process. One or both tympanic bullae may contain serous to inspissated purulent material, with thickening of the tympanic membrane.

Hamster *M pulmonis* has been isolated from hamsters, but its pathogenic potential in these animals is not known.

Gerbil *M pulmonis* has been isolated from gerbils, but disease due to natural infection or experimental inoculation is rare.

Pasteurella pneumotropica

P pneumotropica[80-89] is a very common commensal gram-negative coccobacillus belonging to the family Pasteurellaceae. Rats and mice are the main carriers although guinea pigs, hamsters, and gerbils may also be infected. *P pneumotropica* represents an important secondary bacterial invader and opportunistic infection in primary *M pulmonis* or SeV infections.

P pneumotropica is shed from upper respiratory secretions and feces, and is transmitted through direct contact. The organism has been found to be associated with conjunctivitis, rhinitis, otitis, and cervical lymphadenitis in rats and mice. The uterus and vagina are often colonized without disease, and thus transmission can occur from dam to pups during or shortly after birth. In enzootically infected colonies, nasopharyngeal colonization of laboratory rodents occurs around the time of weaning. Transmission from rodents to humans is rarely reported, but humans may be inadvertent sources of infection for barrier-sustained animals.

Culture of the organism with subsequent identification is required for diagnosis. Screening with serology is not recommended, as animals with subclinical infections are often negative and animals with other Pasteurellaceae may show cross-reactivity. In live animals, oral swabs or fecal culture appear to be the sites of choice for collection. PCR assay and DNA extraction are other techniques used to identify the organism.

Therapy with enrofloxacin may be beneficial in controlling clinical manifestations of infection, but will not eliminate the carrier state.

Prevention is best achieved by exclusion of carriers from the facility. Embryo transfer, rather than hysterectomy rederivation, may be the best choice for an infected colony. Fetuses may also be infected in utero, which may explain why this organism is the most frequent agent in failure of cesarean rederivation. Exclusion of wild or feral animals from facilities is also important. Sentinel monitoring programs for this organism are unreliable. Once a colony is free of the agent, there is relatively little risk of reinfection except through the introduction of infected animals.

Because of its fragility in the environment, stringent environmental decontamination is not necessary, and regular cleaning and use of a high-level disinfectant should suffice to rid the environment of the organism.

Mouse *P pneumotropica* is ubiquitous in almost all wild mice and is common among laboratory mouse populations. Most infections in mice are asymptomatic; however, because of growing use of GEMs and ID mice, the incidence of clinical disease is also increasing. As an opportunistic invader it is associated with several lesions, but its true nature as a primary pathogen is questionable. Elimination of this organism from a mouse population allows other gram-negative bacteria, such as *Klebsiella*, to fill its opportunistic niche. Seroconversion normally occurs only in mice with overt disease.

Clinical signs are varied and include conjunctivitis, panophthalmitis, dacryoadenitis, periorbital abscessation, rhinitis, otitis (externa, media, interna), and cervical lymphadenitis. Lesions are also seen in the dermatologic, urinary, and reproductive organs. Severe suppurative bronchopneumonia has been documented in B-cell–deficient mice coinfected with *Pneumocystis murina*.

Prophylactic administration of trimethoprim/sulfamethoxazole (50–60 mg/kg) in the drinking water has been shown to prevent infection in immunodeficient mice. Enrofloxacin (25.5–85 mL/kg) in the drinking water for 2 weeks may be effective in eliminating infection in mice.[90]

Rat In rats *P pneumotropica* readily colonizes in the intestine, where it may be carried for long periods of time. It can also be carried as an inapparent infection in the nasopharynx, conjunctiva, lower respiratory tract, and uterus. Transmission is most likely primarily by direct contact or fecal contamination in the rat, rather than by aerosols. Lesions associated with pasteurellosis include rhinitis, sinusitis, conjunctivitis, otitis media, suppurative bronchopneumonia, and interstitial pneumonia with polymorphonuclear cell infiltration has been observed. *Pasteurella* may cause a severe, multifocal to coalescing, acute to subacute, necrotizing to fibrinous bronchopneumonia, which must be differentiated from *Streptococcus* and *Corynebacterium*. Subcutaneous abscessation, suppurative or chronic necrotizing mastitis, and pyometra have been reported. The organism can be recovered from various tissues in the absence of lesions.

Hamster In hamsters *P pneumotropica* can cause acute or chronic respiratory infections or be present in the carrier state. Lesions seen are associated with upper respiratory disease, otitis, and bronchopneumonia.

Gerbil *P pneumotropica* has been isolated from gerbils, but disease due to natural infection or experimental inoculation is rare.

Proteus mirabilis

Proteus mirabilis[91–93] is a gram-negative facultative anaerobe and a member of the family Enterobacteriaceae. Ubiquitous in the environment, it can be isolated from the upper respiratory tract and feces of normal mice. Opportunistic infections have been observed in both IC and ID laboratory mice.

Disease is often septicemic, with suppurative lesions in various organs, including pneumonia, hepatitis, splenitis, pyelonephritis, and peritonitis. Pulmonary lesions, when present, are typified by serous flooding of alveoli and mobilization of alveolar macrophages. Lung infection has also been found in reduced nicotinamide adenine dinucleotide phosphate (NADPH) oxidase-deficient B6.129S6-Cybb^{tm1Din}/J mice.

Streptobacillus moniliformis

Streptobacillus moniliformis[94–96] is a gram-negative pleomorphic bacillus. This zoonotic agent is virtually nonexistent in modern laboratory animals but can lead to infection in humans, with potentially serious consequences. In humans it is the cause of rat bite fever. A similar syndrome, called Haverhill fever, has been associated with ingestion of rat-contaminated foodstuffs, particularly milk. Rats may act as zoonotic reservoirs for mice.

The organism inhabits the nasopharynx, middle ear, and respiratory tract. It is present in the blood and urine of infected rats and is transmitted to humans by bite wounds, aerosols, and fomites. Clinical signs in humans follow a 3- to 10-day incubation period and include fever, vomiting, arthralgia, and rash.

S moniliformis can be associated with opportunistic respiratory infections in rats, and can cause wound infections and abscesses. It has been found in bronchiectatic abscesses or rats with CRD, in concert with *Mycoplasma* and CARB.

Colonies of laboratory rats should be monitored by culture of blood and nasopharyngeal swabs, and any animals with a positive diagnosis should be euthanized immediately. Because wild rats are the reservoir for *S moniliformis*, its detection in a laboratory rat colony would indicate exposure to wild rats.

Streptococcus pneumoniae

S pneumoniae[97–106] is a gram-positive α-hemolytic aerobic diplococcus belonging to the family Streptococcaceae. Numerous serotypes exist, and disease is predominantly associated with infection by the more pathogenic serotypes 2, 3, 8, 16, and 19. In rats serotypes 2, 3, and 19 are most common, but they may also have serotypes 8, 16, and 35.

Inapparent infections and carrier states are very common. Despite its periodic detection in large breeding colonies, no outbreaks have been reported in laboratory colonies for almost 35 years, raising the possibility that previous outbreaks were the result of *S pneumoniae* and other concurrent agents. When it occurs, disease is usually seen in young animals, especially after disruption of host defense mechanisms, such as concurrent infection, experimental manipulation, or a change in environment. Mortality is greater in the winter, after shipment, and in animals on marginal diets.

S pneumoniae can cause respiratory and meningeal disease in man, especially in immunocompromised individuals. Humans are a natural host of *S pneumoniae*, with both adults and children frequently colonized.

Depending on the season, 40% to 70% of human populations carry it in their respiratory passages and may be a source of animal infections. Human caretakers with pneumococcal pneumonia, otitis media, conjunctivitis, or other diagnosed or possible streptococcal infections should not work with animals until a course of antibiotics has been completed. Zoonotic transmission from rats or mice to humans has never been reported, but should be considered.

Transmission occurs primarily via aerosol or contact with nasal or lacrimal secretions of an infected animal. Carriers may have upper respiratory infection without clinical signs. Acute episodes or prolonged epizootics with variable morbidity and mortality may occur. Affected animals have signs apparent with generalized respiratory disease in addition to hematuria. Gross lesions include pleuritis, otitis media and interna, and bronchopneumonia.

Diagnosis is established by observation of the bacteria in inflammatory exudate. Samples for culture can be collected from the nasopharynx, tympanic bullae, and nasal passages by swab or lavage. Unlike for many bacterial diseases, large numbers of this organism can be seen in smears and tissue sections via histopathology. Serology using ELISA is also available.

Treatment of animals with antimicrobials may serve to abate clinical signs but does not resolve the carrier state, nor will antibiotic treatment eliminate bacteria from the bedding or cage surface. These organisms are generally sensitive to benzathine-based penicillins, methicillin, ampicillin, chloramphenicol, erythromycin, and linco-mycin, Treatment must be aggressive, and the use of β-lactamase–resistant penicillins such as cloxacillin, oxacillin, and dicloxacillin is generally recommended.

Monitoring is conducted by nasopharyngeal culture onto blood agar. However, because of the occurrence of nonpathogenic isolates, isolation of *S pneumoniae* from rats, even if a respiratory problem is present in the colony, does not necessarily provide a diagnosis, nor does isolation of the organism from asymptomatic rats necessarily indicate a health threat to the colony. Action to eliminate is indicated in the presence of characteristic lesions or detection of known pathogenic serotypes.

Mouse Bacterial pneumonia in mice is nearly always caused by this organism, but seldom develops in the absence of some combination involving *M pulmonis*, SeV, or CARB.

Rat In clinically normal rats *S pneumoniae* is carried primarily in the nasoturbinates and tympanic bullae. Infection is rarely present in commercially obtained rats and is now considered to be a pathogen of low significance in laboratory animals. *S pneumoniae* in rats may cause acute primary disease with mortality, but more often it represents an important secondary invader, particularly in respiratory infections. Young rats are more severely affected than are older ones, and often the only sign they exhibit is sudden death.

Clinical signs can include serosanguinous to mucopurulent nasal discharge, rhinitis, sinusitis, conjunctivitis, vestibular signs consistent with middle ear infection, dyspnea, snuffling, and abdominal breathing. Infection in rats resembles that in both human and nonhuman primates, characterized by suppurative inflammation in the upper respiratory tract, which spreads to the lung to cause bronchopneumonia.

In the acute systemic form there are variable patterns of characteristic fibrinopuru-lent polyserositis, including pleuritis. Grossly, there is serous to mucopurulent exudate in the nasal passages, with variable involvement of the tympanic bullae. There may be consolidation of one or more lobes of the lung, and affected areas are dark red to dull tan and relatively firm and nonresilient. Pulmonary changes vary from localized suppu-rative bronchopneumonia to acute fibrinopurulent bronchopneumonia, with oblitera-tion of the normal architecture in affected lobes. Suppurative rhinitis and otitis media may also occur. There is pericarditis in some cases. Fibrinopurulent peritonitis and pleuritis with minimal involvement of the lung parenchyma are not uncommon.

Hamster *S pneumoniae* in hamsters is relatively uncommon and frequently associated with stress. Signs include depression, anorexia, nasal and ocular discharge, dehydra-tion, and weight loss. The course of the disease is about 3 days.

Gerbil *S pneumoniae* has been isolated from gerbils, but disease due to natural infec-tion or experimental inoculation is rare.

Mycotic Agents

Pneumocystosis

The pneumocystosis organism[107–113] was originally classified as a protozoan, but study of its nucleic acids and proteins places it among the fungi. The genus *Pneumocystis* has undergone sequence analysis of its genes, including the 18S rRNA gene, bringing about identification of distinct species that were once all classified as *Pneumocystis carinii*. These species include *P murina* in mice, *P carinii* and *Pneumocystis wakefieldiae* in rats, and *Pneumocystis jirovecii* in humans. *Pneumocystis* is an important respiratory pathogen in ID mice, rats, and guinea pigs but does not cause overt disease in IC animals. The organism is widespread, naturally acquired by airborne transmission of the respiratory tract, and establishes a persistent, quiescent infection in the lungs. Infection may also be transmitted through the atypical colonized and shedding IC animals. This shedding may occur after infection of an IC animal, but before the infection is eliminated by the immune system. Subclinical infections that resolve in 5 to 6 weeks are relatively common in IC mice and rats, whereas ID animals are unable to clear the organism from their respiratory tract and develop a chronic infection. Treatment with trimethoprim (40 mg/mL)/sulfamethoxazole (200 mg/mL) suspension at a rate of 15.6 mL per 500 mL water will control disease symptoms but will not extinguish the infection. Daily treatment or pulse therapy following a 3 days on/4 days off pattern are recommended protocols. The water bottle must be shaken at least daily to resuspend the agent. Antibiotic resistance due to mutations in the gene targeted by sulfa drugs has been reported in human isolates, so care should be taken with long-term administration of these drugs.

The organism's widespread distribution strongly suggests that susceptible animals should be protected by microbarrier combined with macrobarrier housing. It does not cross the placenta, so cesarean section or embryo transfer rederivation will eliminate the organism. The strains of this organism appear to be species specific; therefore, interspecies transmission is unlikely and, although pneumocystosis occurs in humans, there has not been any confirmation of transmission between rodents and humans.

Mouse Spontaneous enzootics pose a serious threat in colonies of ID mice, with high morbidity and mortality. Mice are typically infected as 3- to 4-week-old juveniles and because of the ubiquitous nature of the organism, virtually all mice in the 4- to 12-week-old age groups should be considered to be infected and shedding. Immunity to the organism develops rapidly, with young animals being protected initially by colostral antibodies. Infection in susceptible mice proceeds slowly, leading to clinical signs of suppurative bronchopneumonia within several months. Primary signs include dyspnea and a hunched posture, which may be accompanied by wasting and scaly skin. Severe cases, such as those that occur with advanced disease, may be fatal. At necropsy, lesions are especially severe in SCID or athymic nude mice. Nonfilamentous trophic forms attach to type I pneumocytes with clusters of developmental stages spreading into the alveolar lumen. The lungs collapse poorly and have a rubbery consistency, with pale, patchy areas of consolidation. The type of pneumonia can be variable depending on the host's type of immune deficiency. Some ID mice may have very few visible cysts or alveolar exudation, with principally interstitial pneumonia. Histologic changes are characterized by interstitial alveolitis, with thickening of alveolar septa from proteinaceous exudate and infiltration with mononuclear cells. Immunocompromised mice subclinically infected with *P murina* that are inoculated with PVM develop severe respiratory tract lesions attributed to the dual infection. Superimposed viral infection and/or bacterial infections such as *P pneumotropica* can exacerbate pneumocystosis. Respiratory distress in ID mice should elicit suspicion of pneumocystosis. Pathologic examination of the lung with special staining is essential to confirm the presumptive diagnosis. Past infections may be detected through ELISA, and PCR is used to detect active infection.

Rat The immunocompromised rat is a common animal model for *P carinii* pneumonitis that occurs in human AIDS patients. *P carinii* and *P wakefieldiae* can exist as coinfections in the same animal. Signs commonly seen in rats are weight loss, cyanosis, and dyspnea. There is diffuse to focal consolidation; lungs collapse poorly, and routinely have an opaque pale pink color. In athymic rats, pulmonary lesions vary from mild to severe interstitial pneumonia. Pulmonary lesions associated with this infection have been created in young laboratory rats from naturally infected colonies that were treated with immunosuppressants, such as cortisone, and fed a diet deficient in protein for several weeks. Diagnosis of infection in IC rats usually requires at least 6 weeks of treatment with corticosterioids or cyclophosphamide to elicit a histologically detectable level of infection. Special stains demonstrate the fungal cysts within the alveoli. PCR has been used to detect infection in rat lungs consistently after only 1 week of treatment. PCR can also be performed on oral swabs and bronchoalveolar lavage samples. Routine screening of asymptomatic animals, such as IC sentinels in colonies of ID animals, is best accomplished by PCR.

Miscellaneous mycotic agents
B6-*p47* (*phox*) null mice, which are defective in NADPH oxidase, have been reported to develop pyogranulomatous lesions in the lung, liver, lymph nodes, salivary gland, and skin, from which *Trichosporon beigelii* was cultured. Another colony of B6-*p47(phox)* null mice with a concomitant γ-interferon mutation was found to develop granulomatous pneumonia in association with *Aspergillus terreus*. Mice that lack NADPH oxidase function through null mutation of *gp91 (phox)* developed pulmonary infections with *Paecilomyces variotii*. Chronic granulomatous disease in mice, especially in the lungs, was associated with *Paecilomyces* sp, *Aspergillus fumigatus*, *Rhizopus* sp, and *Candida guilliermondii*.[114]

One report described almost one-fifth of Wistar rats in a 2-year carcinogenesis study as having chronic rhinitis associated with *A fumigatus*. The predisposing factor in these animals was thought to be subclinical SeV infection. Clinical signs included sniffling and nasal exudation. Yellowish, friable material was present either unilaterally or bilaterally in the nasal cavities, and in severe cases the nasal cavities were completely occluded. Lesions were, in most cases, limited to the nasoturbinates and maxilloturbinates. A bronchial abscess containing hyphae and multiple fruiting heads occurred in one rat.[115]

Tracheobronchial aspergillosis was reported in an aged F-344 rat with concurrent large granular cell leukemia. Immunodeficiency due to the leukemia was thought to be associated with the multifocal, transmural necrotic lesions of the trachea and bronchi.[116]

Two cases of *Aspergillus* spp rhinitis in rats that had no known immunosuppression were reported. Corncob and hardwood bedding from 2 sources were analyzed to determine if the source of the fungus was the substrate material. Six genera of fungi were isolated from corncob samples, whereas only negligible counts were isolated from hardwood samples. The investigators recommended that the use of either autoclaved or γ-irradiated corncob bedding should be considered as a method to eliminate fungal contamination of bedding.[117]

Parasitic Diseases

Primary respiratory tract parasitism in mice, rats, hamsters, or gerbils has not been confirmed in the United States; however, cases have been documented in other countries.

There is a report of *Spleorodens clethrionomys* observed in epizootic proportions in the nasal cavities of Syrian hamsters in Stockholm, Sweden. Mites were detected in the nasal cavities of the animals during preparations for an inhalation experiment. More than 90% of the adult animals and all offspring were infested within the colony. Examination of animals from the vendor revealed a pervasive infection. Surveillance of hamsters at 2 other research institutes in Stockholm, which obtained animals from the same source, revealed similar infection rates. The origin of nasal mites at the breeding facility was not determined. Affected animals did not show any clinical signs. This species of mite was originally reported from field voles in Holland, and has not been reported in other species of laboratory rodents.[118]

Trichosomoides sp, possibly *Trichosomoides nasalis*, was reported in England in parasagittal sections through the nose and in adjacent tissues in 5-week-old hamsters. Some animals had a distinctive pug-faced deformity, believed to be associated with the inoculation of sarcoma material as neonates. The parasitic ova were seen in the feces of 37 of 185 stock hamsters in the facility. The ova were infective for rats when given orally. *T nasalis* was later reported in the nasal cavities of hamsters in Switzerland. This nematode was originally described by Biocca and Azrizi in 1961 in the nasal cavities of *Rattus norvegicus* in Rome, Italy.[119]

Trichosomoides crassicauda, a nematode that affects the urinary tract of rats, has a migratory phase in its life cycle, which may produce lesions in the lung and other organs.[120]

Viral Agents

Hantavirus

Hantavirus (HV)[121–123] is discussed from a zoonotic aspect, as it remains an agent of severe disease in humans, although humans are inadvertent hosts.

Hantaviruses are members of the family Bunyaviridae. Rodents are the primary reservoir hosts of the hantaviruses worldwide, with each virus in the genus being associated with a specific rodent species. Hantaviruses infect the majority of wild mouse and rat populations in the United States, with an antibody prevalence rate of up to 8%. In the laboratory animal facility, the rat is the primary animal responsible with the spread of these viruses. Rabbits, guinea pigs, cats, and dogs housed in the same room as infected rats can become seropositive.

Infected rodents shed the virus in saliva, urine, and feces for many weeks with lifetime persistence. Transmission occurs via contaminated fomites; by direct introduction into broken skin, mucous membranes, or conjunctiva; by ingestion of contaminated food/water; or by aerosols. Biting may be an important mode of transmission during conspecific aggression. Hantavirus infections in rodents are characterized by being chronic and subclinical, and although clinical signs and lesions have not been reported in laboratory mice or rats, they develop high antibody titers.

Transmission to humans occurs in a similar way as for rodents, and transmission between humans is unlikely. Two major lineages of hantaviruses are of zoonotic importance. One represents those associated with hemorrhagic fever and renal syndrome (HFRS) in humans, and the other represents viruses of the New World that are associated with hantavirus pulmonary syndrome (HPS). Hantaviruses that can cause HFRS include Hantann virus, Puumala virus, Dobrava virus, and Seoul virus. The deer mouse, *Peromyscus maniculatus*, is the reservoir for Sin Nombre virus (SNV), which is responsible for the great majority of human HPS cases in North America. However, HPS can be caused by infection from at least 11 other hantaviruses.

Mouse cytomegalovirus infection

Mouse The official name for the agent responsible for mouse cytomegalovirus (MCMV) infection is murid herpesvirus 1 (MuHV-1), which is a member of the family Herpesviridae, genus *Muromegalovirus*.[124,125] The virus can be isolated from saliva or salivary glands in the majority of wild mice, and there are multiple MCMV strains within wild mouse populations. Outbreaks in laboratory mice are rare or nonexistent in most colonies. Lesions are primarily found in the salivary glands, but lung pathology can occur as well. Latency of MCMV has been documented to occur in the lung tissue and can persist for the life of the mouse.

The virus is transmitted oronasally by direct contact and is excreted through saliva, tears, urine, and semen. Although MCMV does not readily cross the placenta and in utero transmission does not appear to take place, latently infected dams have been documented to transmit low-level or latent infection to fetuses in utero. Experimental transmission by artificial insemination has been reported, making sexual transmission likely.

Experimental infection is greatly influenced by viral strain, host factors, dose, and route of inoculation. Neonates of all mouse strains are susceptible to disease, and severity of disease expression is significantly influenced by host strain genotype. Resistance begins to develop after weaning and increases until about 8 weeks of age. Resistant strains include B6, B10, CBA, and C3H mice. Susceptible strains include BALB/c and A strain mice. Resistance is associated with *H-2k* haplotype, but non-*H2* associated factors exist, including one that is linked to loci on chromosome 6 within the natural killer (NK) cell complex.

Within 1 week of experimental infection, viremia with multisystemic dissemination occurs, including the lung and a variety of reproductive tissues. Monocytes are important for the viremic phase of infection, and macrophages are also targeted. Following dissemination, the virus is rapidly cleared from the host with exception of the salivary glands. Virus clearance is significantly prevented in beige mice or mice depleted of NK cells. Athymic or SCID mice fail to control active infection whereas B-cell deficient mice can recover. Of interest, MCMV can actively persist and replicate in the salivary glands of fully IC mice, due to genes of the virus that function to control immune response, determine cell tropism, and inhibit apoptosis. MCMV can persist in a nonreplicative state as a latent infection, but can be reactivated by stress or immunosuppression.

Overt clinical disease with disseminated lesions usually does not occur in naturally infected mice. Experimentally induced disease produces focal necrosis, cytomegaly, inclusions, and inflammation in many tissues, including the lung, during the acute phase. Diffuse interstitial pneumonitis has been described in BALB/c mice that were immunosuppressed by a variety of methods, and athymic nude mice develop progressive multifocal nodular pulmonary inflammation. A single case of naturally occurring MCMV disseminated infection has been reported in an aged laboratory mouse.[126]

Diagnosis of MCMV can be made via serology using MFIA, ELISA, IFA, PCR, and virus isolation.

Hamster Inclusions have been identified in hamsters but overt clinical disease has not been reported.

Mouse hepatitis virus

The official name for the mouse hepatic virus is murine hepatitis virus (MHV),[127–129] which is a member of the family Coronaviridae, genus *Coronavirus*. MHV encompasses several genetically and antigenically related strains that vary tremendously in their virulence and organotropism. MHV is generally separated into two biologically distinct groups, respiratory strains and enterotropic strains. Respiratory strains exhibit primary affinity for upper respiratory mucosa. As with all RNA viruses, MHV is capable of extreme mutation rates with resultant antigenic drift.

MHV continues to plague conventionally housed laboratory mouse populations in the United States and Europe as a major infectious agent. It is pervasive in wild mouse populations throughout the world.

Strains with respiratory affinity initially replicate in the nasal mucosa followed by dissemination to a variety of other organs, due to their polytropic nature. This disseminated pattern of infection is exhibited by highly virulent strains of the virus in mice younger than 2 weeks, in genetically susceptible strains, or in immunocompromised mice. Dissemination occurs from the nasal mucosa to the pulmonary vascular endothelium and then to draining lymph nodes. Secondary viremia further spreads the virus to multiple organs. Immune-mediated clearance of the virus begins after 5 to 7 days, with no persistence or carrier state detectable beyond 3 to 4 weeks. The majority of natural respiratory/polytropic MHV infections are subclinical, with mild or no gross lesions. The obvious exception is ID mice, which cannot clear the virus and develop progressively severe disease with chronic wasting, or die acutely. Fetal infection with MHV is fatal, as is infection in naïve nursing pups. In general, BALB/c mice are fairly susceptible whereas SJL mice are quite resistant. However, experimental infections clearly demonstrate that the biologic behavior of the wild-type MHV is unpredictable. Host immunity is decidedly virus strain dependent, which has given rise to the misconception that the virus has a latent phase. Recovery from one strain provides solid resistance to reexposure with the homotypic strain, but only partial to no resistance to infection with an antigenically heterotypic strain. Maternally derived passive immunity is also important in MHV epizootiology.

MHV is highly contagious, and is spread via respiratory aerosol and feces. Vertical transmission from infected dams to fetuses has been documented experimentally, but is highly unlikely in naturally occurring infections.

Pulmonary vascular endothelium syncytia are common in ID mice. Animals can also develop nasoencephalitis due to localized infection of olfactory mucosa, nerves, bulbs, and tracts of the brain. This pattern of infection occurs regularly after intranasal inoculation of many MHV strains, but is uncommon with natural exposure.

Active infection is confirmed by immunohistochemistry or virus isolation. During the acute phase, histologic diagnosis can be made by finding characteristic syncytial lesions in target tissues. Recovered mice may have perivascular lymphocytic infiltrates in the lung. Serology is the most useful means for detection of retrospective infection in a colony. Female mice usually have higher titers than do males, as they ingest the infected feces of nursing pups. C57BL/6 mice produce a high antibody titer and are commonly used in sentinel testing. PCR can detect the virus in feces or tissues of infected mice.

Research complications are attributable to the viruses' polytropic, contagious, and persistent nature, making it the most probable virus to interfere with biologic responses in mice and to contaminate transplantable tumors and cell lines. MHV can also infect embryonic stem cells without cytopathic effects.

Elimination of MHV from a colony requires complete cessation of breeding of seropositive animals and no introduction of new animals for an 8-week period in conjunction with meticulous environmental decontamination. This action allows for "burn-out" of the infection within the colony. For extensive outbreaks, it may be necessary to rederive the populations by embryo transfer or cesarean section of pups to clean foster dams.

Maintenance of disease-free populations depends on the exclusion of infected animals, domestic or wild.

Murine norovirus

Murine norovirus (MNV-1) is a member of the family Caliciviridae, genus *Norovirus*, and mice are the only known host for this virus. MNV-1 is present in a relatively high percentage (≥30%) of laboratory animal facilities where viral monitoring has been initiated.[130–132] Its prevalence in wild and pet populations is unknown.

The virus was first reported in 2003, in a study[133] that described isolation of a calicivirus from a colony of ID mice experiencing unexpected mortality. The investigators later classified the virus as a norovirus, thus naming it murine norovirus 1 (MNV-1). In the outbreak, mice lacking both interferon-αβ receptors and interferon-γ receptors were very susceptible to lethal infection, demonstrating that interferons are necessary for resistance to MNV-1. STAT1-dependent innate immunity is also needed for resistance to MNV. Therefore, unlike human noroviruses, MNV-1 is remarkably nonpathogenic except under highly specific circumstances. There is no evidence for zoonotic transmission to date.

The virus is transmitted by the fecal-oral route. Fecal shedding following infection in both IC and ID mice can persist for months. STAT1 null mice with intact B and T cells, STAT1 null mice lacking B and T cells (RAG null), and STAT1 null mice lacking RNA-dependent protein kinase (PKR null) exhibit high mortality with encephalitis, pneumonia, and hepatitis. Other strains showed low mortality but became persistently infected. Infection of 129, B6, RAG1, RAG2, interferon-αβ receptor null, interferon-γ receptor null, inducible nitric oxide synthase null, or PKR null mice with functional STAT1 resulted in no clinical disease. IC mice appear to seroconvert and are only transiently infected, with no clinical signs. Most ID mice are asymptomatic and only those with severe deficiencies in innate immunity as described can have an infection leading to wasting and death.

Microscopic lesions in STAT1 null mice inoculated per os or intranasally include alveolitis, pulmonary edema, pneumonia, and multifocal areas of coagulation necrosis in the liver, with minimal or no inflammatory cell response. In another study, microscopic and gross lesions encountered were strain dependent.

MNV-1 can be diagnosed using serology via MFIA, ELISA, and IFA. Antibody titers may be slow to increase; therefore, 8 weeks of exposure is recommended for sentinel mice housed on soiled bedding. There are many field strains of MNV having antibodies that only faintly cross from strain to strain, so it is important that the diagnostic laboratory uses assays validated for the full spectrum of MNV strains. At least 6 strains of MNV have been identified to date. PCR can detect strains 2, 3, and 4 from tissues 8 weeks post infection, with jejunal and mesenteric lymph nodes being the preferred sites for sampling.

Caliciviruses are notoriously difficult to eradicate from the environment. Aggressive chemical decontamination with the help of detergents and disinfectants is recommended, with bleach being the only disinfectant known to kill this virus.

Murine pneumotropic virus or Kilham polyomavirus

Murine pneumotropic virus (MPTV) or Kilham polyomavirus (KPYV)[134] is a member of the family Polyomaviridae, genus *Polyomavirus*, which is different from murine polyoma virus (MPyV). It is sometimes referred to as K-virus and should not be confused with Kilham rat virus.

This disease is of interest from a historical aspect, and rarely occurs in modern mouse colonies although it is found in wild mouse populations. It was discovered by Lawrence Kilham while performing investigations with the mammary tumor virus.

Adult nude mice are susceptible to experimental infection with resultant pathologic lesions. Other highly susceptible strains are AKR and CB, with C57BL/6 being resistant to disease. Transmission is via the oronasal route. Oral inoculation of neonatal mice causes initial replication in the intestinal capillary endothelium followed by dissemination to other organs, including the lung, where it replicates in the vascular endothelium. There is a rapid onset of dyspnea due to pulmonary vascular edema and hemorrhage, resulting in death 6 to 15 days post infection. MPTV may be suspected if 6- to 15-day-old mice or ID mice present with an interstitial pneumonia. Mice that are inoculated between 12 and 18 days of age do not develop pulmonary disease because of passive immunity from the dam, allowing them to mount an early and effective immune response and thereby preventing the viremic phase of infection. Regardless of age, mice remain persistently infected, and the site for virus persistence is renal tubular epithelium.

Gross lesions are restricted to lungs of neonatal or immunodeficient mice. Pulmonary lesions consist of hemorrhage, congestion, edema, atelectasis, and septal thickening with prominent basophilic nuclear inclusions in affected endothelial cells. Interstitial pneumonia with lymphocytic infiltrates develops in recovering mice.

Antibodies may be detected via MFIA, ELISA, or IFA. Because of the extreme rarity of this virus, positive serology results have a very low predictive value and are likely to be false positives. PCR can also detect the virus.

Pneumonia virus of mice

The PVM[133–143] is a member of the family Paramyxoviridae, subfamily Pneumovirinae, and genus *Pneumovirus*. The official name of this virus is murine pneumovirus (MPV), which should not be confused with the other official MPV, mouse parvovirus, not to mention murine pneumotropic virus. PVM can cause natural infections in mice, rats, hamsters, gerbils, guinea pigs, and probably other rodents, and may be infectious for rabbits. Serologic data indicate that PVM is prevalent in mice, is infrequently reported in rats, and has a worldwide distribution. The possibility of interspecies transmission to other animals within the facility should be considered when dealing with this disease.

Mouse PVM is relatively benign in IC mice, causing an acute and self-limiting infection, but causes significant disease in GEMs. As with many other viral infections, susceptibility is strain dependent and can be increased by a variety of local and systemic stressors. DBA/2, C3H/HeN, and 129Sv are very susceptible when inoculated with a pathogenic strain, followed by BALB/cBy and B6 exhibiting intermediate susceptibility, while SJL strains are highly resistant. Infection appears to persist in ID mice. MPV is transmitted via aerosol and contact exposure to the respiratory tract. Because the virus has a low degree of contagion and environmental inactivation occurs rapidly, close contact between mice is required for transmission.

Clinical signs of disease and gross lesions are typically absent in natural infections of IC mice. ID mice exhibit listlessness, cyanosis, and dyspnea with chronic wasting.

Experimental infection of immunocompetent BALB/c mice with an intranasal pathogenic PVM strain produced pulmonary lesions peaking within 2 weeks and commencing resolution within 3 weeks. Virus replication occurs in alveolar lining cells, alveolar macrophages and, to a lesser extent, bronchiolar epithelium. Natural isolates of PVM are nonpathogenic, with replication occurring primarily in the nasal mucosal epithelium with few pathologic lesions. The low pathogenicity of PVM allows ID mice to develop a progressive severe interstitial pneumonia with the wasting syndrome instead of acute death. In these mice, PVM antigen is confined to alveolar type II cells and occasionally bronchiolar epithelial cells. SCID mice naturally infected with *P murina*, then inoculated with a nonpathogenic isolate of PMV, developed more severe *Pneumocystis* pneumonia. PVM-associated pneumonia in ID mice is often complicated by pneumocystosis and vice versa, as both are common agents in mouse colonies.

Microscopic lesions of experimentally infected mice consist of mild necrotizing rhinitis, necrotizing bronchiolitis, and nonsuppurative interstitial pneumonia. Lungs are pale, firm, and do not collapse. Alveolar septa are thickened as a result of edema and infiltrating macrophages and leukocytes. Alveolar spaces are collapsed and filled with fibrin, blood, macrophages, and large mononuclear cells, representing desquamated alveolar type II cells. Although MPV lesions are similar to Sendai viral lesions microscopically, MPV tends not to cause proliferative bronchiolar lesions as does SeV.

Serologic diagnosis can be achieved via MFIA, ELISA, and IFA. Seroconversion confirmation is the most practical method to make a diagnosis; however, because PVM is not highly contagious, the number of seropositive animals within a colony can be small. Nude mice do not seroconvert to PVM. During active infections, PVM can be identified by virus isolation, PCR, or mouse antibody production testing of suspect tissues. Immunohistochemistry staining can demonstrate viral antigen within infected pneumocytes in tissue sections.

Rat Based on serologic surveys, enzootics do occur in laboratory rats. Intranasal inoculation of F344 rats resulted in gross and microscopic lesions by the sixth day, although animals showed no overt disease. In experimental infections, complement-fixing antibodies to PVM peaked at 14 days and declined markedly by 19 days. Multifocal, nonsuppurative vasculitis and interstitial alveolitis with necrosis are typical lesions seen during the acute stages of the disease. There are prominent perivascular infiltrates, with hyperplasia of bronchus-associated lymphoid tissue, perivasculitis, and multifocal interstitial pneumonitis. These lesions tend to persist for weeks in the rat. The presence of microscopic lesions attributed to PVM requires confirmation by serologic conversion, as in mice. PVM may also be a copathogen in other respiratory diseases, such as mycoplasmal infections.

Hamster PVM infection in this species normally goes undetected as a subclinical event. Animals inoculated with PVM exhibit sneezing, dyspnea, and weakness, with death ensuing 6 to 15 days post infection. Gross lesions include patchy, plum-colored lung consolidation involving 50% to 75% of the lung. Multifocal, nonsuppurative vasculitis and interstitial pneumonitis with necrosis are prominent lesions seen during the acute phase of the disease. Alveolar walls are thickened and contain a predominantly mononuclear cell infiltrate.

Poxvirus
This poxvirus is also known as Turkmenian rodent poxvirus, and infections have been reported to occur in laboratory rats from Europe and the former Soviet Union.[144] The virus is closely related to cowpox virus, but distinctly different from ectromelia virus (ECTV), which causes mousepox. Clinical signs in affected rats resemble those seen in ectromelial infections in mice, with both dermal and respiratory lesions occurring. Microscopically, rats with respiratory signs have severe interstitial pneumonia with edema, hemorrhage, and pleural effusion. Focal inflammatory lesions occur in the upper respiratory tract.

Serologic surveys of wild rodents have identified animals that are seropositive for cowpox virus, and the reservoir hosts were usually asymptomatic. There have been documented reports of the transmission of cowpox from rats to humans, felids, and nonhuman primates. Whether the Turkmenian rodent poxvirus in previous reports was actually cowpox virus is not known.

Rat polyoma virus

The rat polyoma virus[145] is serologically distinct from the MPTV/Kilham polyomavirus of mice, and its incidence is unknown. The virus was discovered in a colony of 32 athymic nude (rnu) rats. Clinically, affected animals developed a wasting disease with interstitial pneumonia and parotid sialoadenitis. The rats had bronchitis, bronchiolitis, and secondary bacterial pneumonia. Less commonly, rhinitis and Harderian gland adenitis were seen. Intranuclear inclusion bodies were seen in the ductal and acinar epithelial cells of the parotid salivary gland. Euthymic rats did not develop disease. Because this virus has not been isolated, serologic screening of populations is not performed.

Rat respiratory virus

Based on initial characterization studies, the rat respiratory virus (RRV)[146] was classified as a member of the *Hantavirus* genus. Further investigations revealed that the reactions seen on IFA were nonspecific and false positive. Attempts to demonstrate a relationship with other hantaviruses using hantavirus-specific PCR primer sets have been consistently negative. Therefore, more studies are needed to classify the virus. Investigators at the Research Animal Diagnostic Laboratory in Columbia, Missouri have data strongly supporting *P carinii* as the agent responsible for lung lesions previously attributed to RRV in rats. This information was presented at the annual American Association for Laboratory Animal Science National Meeting in October 2010.

Sendai virus

The official name for this pathogen is Sendai virus (SeV), a member of the family Paramyxoviridae, genus *Paramyxovirus*.[147–154] It was first isolated in Sendai, Japan; hence, the name. SeV is antigenically related to parainfluenza virus (HPIV) serotype 1 of humans, and there has long been a debate as to the human or mouse origin, or if humans are naturally susceptible to SeV infection. Studies have demonstrated that both SeV and HPIV serotype 1 replicate equally well in the upper and lower respiratory tracts of African green monkeys and chimpanzees, suggesting that SeV lacks a significant host range restriction and could very well be an anthropozoonotic agent.

From a historical perspective, SeV infections have caused some of the most significant disease outbreaks among laboratory rodents. Mice, rats, hamsters, guinea pigs, and swine are natural hosts for infection whereas gerbils seem resistant to infection. As with many diseases, improvements in housing systems, production standards, and health monitoring have led to a drastic decline in the incidence of SeV over recent years. Although SeV was once very pervasive in commercial sources of mice and rats, it now rarely occurs in barrier-maintained commercial sources. However, conventionally maintained commercial and institutional colonies may still be sources for introduction of the virus to naïve populations.

The disease is highly contagious, with morbidity in infected colonies commonly reaching 100%, with mortality rates of 0% to 100%. Transmission occurs through aerosol exposure, direct contact, contaminated tissues, and fomites. In utero infections do not occur.

Introduction of SeV into a susceptible population can result in epizootic disease, the severity of which depends on age, genetic factors, and presence of other potential pathogens. This virus is one of the few that may cause overt disease in IC animals. SeV can predispose animals to secondary bacterial infections, affect the immune response, and delay wound healing. Although vertical transmission does not occur, SeV infections of dams is associated with fetal resorption, prolonged gestation, fetal death, and poor growth in surviving pups.

Humans commonly serve as a source of non-Sendai parainfluenza infections in laboratory rodents. Mouse and rat antibody production or PCR testing should be done on all transplantable tumors, cell lines, and other biologic materials to prevent transmission of SeV from infected materials to recipient animals.

In the past, a killed vaccine of duck embryo origin was available commercially. The vaccine was administered intraperitoneally and afforded approximately 7 months of protection. Rats were resistant to intranasal virus challenge after receiving 2 doses of the vaccine. The vaccine was equally effective when administered by intravenous, intramuscular, or subcutaneous routes, but not the intranasal route. Animals receiving intraperitoneal SeV vaccine were also protected from contact infection. Nursing pups born to immunized dams were resistant to challenge infection at 3 weeks of age, but the resistance was not demonstrated after weaning at 4 weeks of age.[155]

A temperature-sensitive mutant of the original vaccine was also used with some success. Experimental infections of mice with a SeV temperature-sensitive (ts) mutant (HVJ-pB) were studied. Infection with the mutant induced the priming effect of interferon production and both humoral and cellular immune responses, although the mutant virus neither propagated satisfactorily in the respiratory tracts of mice nor caused appreciable microscopic lesions. Inoculation with the mutant protected mice from subsequent challenge with a parental wild-type virus. The efficacy of this protection began as little as 1 day after vaccination and continued for a minimum of 12 weeks. The report also suggested that serum antibodies were efficacious in the nasal turbinates, whereas specific immune cells acted more protectively in the lungs.[156]

Mouse SeV is the most likely pathogen to cause clinical respiratory disease in adult IC mice. Nursing and weanling mice are most commonly and most seriously affected. Neonatal mice, aged mice; strains 129/Re, DBA/2, C3H, and male BALB/c mice are highly susceptible to lethal disease. C57BL/6, SJL, female BALB/c, and random bred mice are moderately resistant whereas B6, AKR, SJL, and outbred Swiss mice are highly resistant. Susceptibility also is increased in protein-deprived mice.

Enzootic infection is commonly detected in post-weaned mice that seroconvert within 7 to 14 days, at which time the infection is terminated. Therefore, entrenched infection is perpetuated by the introduction of susceptible animals. There is no evidence of persistent infection in IC mice, but prolonged infection is common in ID mice. Maternally acquired immunity protects young mice from infection, and actively acquired immunity is thought to be long lived. Adults usually have mild respiratory signs including a characteristic "chattering," and recover fully in a few days; whereas nursing, weanling, and aged mice can have more severe disease with respiratory distress. Acute outbreaks in breeding colonies can cause production to decrease, then return to normal in a few weeks, although enzootic subclinical infection can persist. Athymic and immunosuppressed animals develop illness later than their IC counterparts.

Gross lesions are often absent but when present, the lungs are plum-colored with sharply demarcated foci and consolidation of the anteroventral lung or entire lobes.

These areas may turn gray in surviving mice. Mice develop a descending infection of respiratory epithelium, which is eliminated by a cell-mediated immune response that clears the infection but also provokes tissue pathology. The location to which the infection extends into the respiratory tract is determined by mouse strain, differences in mucociliary clearance, virus burden, and kinetics of the immune response. SeV infects nasal, tracheal, bronchial, bronchiolar, and middle ear epithelium, and spreads to type II alveolar cells. T-cell–immunodeficient mice develop progressive pulmonary consolidation with wasting. These mice develop severe, diffuse alveolitis, similar to PVM pneumonia. SeV and PVM lesions in nude and SCID mice are similar, although in SCID mice, bronchial and bronchiolar lesions are more extensive with PVM than with SeV infection. Proliferation with or without destruction of bronchiolar epithelium, increased cellularity of alveolar septa, proteinaceous exudation, and the presence of alveolar macrophages and neutrophils in bronchioles and alveoli are frequent findings during the acute phase of infection. Necrotizing bronchiolitis is a classic lesion. The sloughing of virus-infected bronchiolar epithelial cells corresponds with the appearance of measurable antibody. During the regenerative phase, there is hyperplasia of type II pneumocytes lining airways, with fibrosis, thickening, and mononuclear cell infiltration in alveolar septa. The squamous metaplasia found in recovering lungs has been misconstrued as neoplasia. Lesions are more pronounced in ID animals, and the terminal bronchioles can be severely damaged, with scarring, distortion, or polypoid outgrowths of the mucosa in survivors.

Clinical signs of respiratory distress along with gross and microscopic lesions are highly suggestive of SeV infection, especially among infant mice or adults of genetically susceptible strains. Antibody titers increase rapidly, and serologic diagnosis may be made 8 to 12 days after infection using MFIA, ELISA, or IFA. PCR is recommended on symptomatic animals. Sentinel animals can be added to seropositive colonies to detect active infection. Histopathology, immunohistochemistry and, where possible, virus isolation should be used to confirm infection. In rats, guinea pigs, and rodents other than mice, positive serology using SeV antigen can be due to exposure to PI-2 or PI-3 virus. Positive MFIA, ELISA, or IFA should be confirmed by strain-specific hemagglutination inhibition (HAI), which will discriminate between PI-1, PI-2, and PI-3.

In enzootically infected colonies there is a danger of transmission to other susceptible species. Control and eradication measures must eliminate exposure of susceptible animals, so that infection can "burn out" as previously described for MHV. Control is also aided by the fact that SV is highly labile; therefore, no special measures are required for disinfection. Barrier housing is preferred for prevention and control of transmission.

This virus may alter the incidence of pulmonary neoplasia in experimental carcinogenesis studies. This effect has been attributed to virus-induced modification of tumor cell surface membranes. Pulmonary changes during SeV pneumonia can compromise interpretation of experimentally induced lesions.

Rat As in mice, susceptibility varies with age, genotype, and immune status. An asymptomatic self-limiting disease is usually induced in rats, unlike for SeV-induced disease in mice. Clinical respiratory signs infrequently occur. Based on experimental infection, lesion severity is more pronounced in Brown Norway and LEW rats than in F-344 rats. Reduced production and litter sizes, as well as delayed growth of young within breeding colonies, may be seen in rats as in mice. SeV in the rat is recognized to have an additive effect on respiratory infections with *M pulmonis*. Concurrent bacterial and other viral infections increase the severity of clinical disease and pulmonary lesions. In Lewis rats inoculated intranasally with SeV, the draining lymph nodes of the upper respiratory tract are the initial and major site of antibody production. Development of serum immunoglobulin G (IgG) antibodies coincides with clearance of respiratory tract infection and recovery from viral infection.

Following exposure, the virus replicates in the upper respiratory tract, then spreads down the trachea and smaller airways. Pathogenesis of SeV infection in the rat parallels SeV in genetically resistant strains of mice. Acute bronchitis and bronchiolitis are features of the disease. Multifocal, nonsuppurative vasculitis and interstitial alveolitis with necrosis are typical lesions seen during the acute phase of the disease. There are prominent perivascular infiltrates, with hyperplasia of bronchus-associated lymphoid tissue, perivasculitis, and multifocal interstitial pneumonia. These lesions tend to persist for several weeks to months in the rat.

MFIA or ELISA are the best serologic choices for diagnosis of Sendai in rats, due to their sensitivity in detecting early antibody and detecting small amounts of antibody, as compared with complement fixation and HAI. PCR testing is also very sensitive.

If the virus is introduced into a colony of IC animals, neutralizing antibody in infected rats renders the infection self-limiting. Allowing "burn-out" of the virus as in mice is an effective means to eliminate the virus from a colony. In addition to research complications associated with the respiratory tract affinities of the virus, it may modulate some immunologic responses, for example, reducing the severity of adjuvant arthritis and depressing T-cell and thymocytotoxic autoantibody.

Hamster Infection is often clinically silent with low mortality, and there are very few reports of confirmed clinical disease due to SeV infections in this species. Seronegative animals introduced into a facility housing infected rodents may seroconvert, but it is unlikely that any clinical signs will be observed, although there are reports of mortality in newborn Syrian and Chinese hamsters. One colony of enzootically infected animals experienced occasional deaths in nursing pups as the only clinical sign.

Young adult Syrian hamsters inoculated intranasally with SeV remained asymptomatic during one study, and the animals seroconverted by day 7 post infection. There was a focal to segmental rhinitis progressing to necrotizing tracheitis and multifocal bronchoalveolitis. Immunohistochemistry can demonstrate viral antigen in respiratory epithelial cells during the acute phase of the disease. In animals examined at 3 to 9 days post inoculation, lesions were very similar to those present in mice. In the reparative stages of the disease, hyperplasia of epithelial cells lining affected airways and peribronchial lymphocytic infiltration were seen. Overall, most lesions had resolved by 12 days post infection.

Sialodacryoadenitis virus and Parker's rat coronavirus

Sialodacryoadenitis virus (SDAV) and Parker's rat coronavirus (PRC) belong to the family Coronaviridae, genus *Coronavirus*.[157–164] SDAV is a morphologic classification and represents all coronavirus isolates that produce sialodacryoadenitis. These viruses should be considered as part of a single biologic grouping (rat coronaviruses) but because of historical precedent, the separation and nomenclature continues. PRC was initially isolated from the lungs of rats after intranasal inoculation of newborn and weanling rats produced rhinitis, tracheitis, and interstitial pneumonia, with focal atelectasis and high mortality in infants. PRC also induced salivary and lacrimal gland lesions in early studies, but these were omitted in the original descriptions. SDAV produces lacrimal and salivary gland lesions in addition to pulmonary disease in young rats. Like MHV, the rat coronavirus groups likely contain many constantly changing strains that shift in virulence. Although the two viruses were once thought to cause distinctly different diseases, clinical signs or pathology cannot differentiate infection with either virus.

Rat coronavirus and mouse coronavirus share antigenic similarities, and antisera against SDAV cross-react with MHV strains. IFA and enzyme immunoassay were not able to differentiate antibodies to MHV or SDAV. Thus at present no diagnostic method is available to differentiate between the two. The hypervariable region identified in the SDAV S sequence may be used as a genetic marker to develop a reliable diagnostic PCR.[165]

Mouse Mice may develop a transient interstitial pneumonia with seroconversion. Athymic nude mice are particularly susceptible to coronavirus infections, and develop chronic persistent disease and wasting.

Rat SDAV is a highly infectious enzootic or epizootic disease of rats, and probably is the single most common viral infection in these animals. Mortality is usually low, but morbidity and subclinical infection commonly reach 100%. These viruses are common in both pets and conventionally housed rat populations. Natural infection can be epizootic, if newly introduced into a susceptible colony, or enzootic within a breeding colony. Age and genetic factors affect susceptibility. Pneumotropic strains of rat coronaviruses may cause an interstitial pneumonia in young rats, especially of the F-344 strain.

Immunity is not lifelong, and it has been shown that rats are susceptible to reinfection as early as 6 months after initial infection and that such rats are able to transfer infection to naïve rats by cage contact. However, the severity of lesions in reinfected rats is minimal compared with initial infection. Neutralizing antibodies to one virus prototype will not offer significant cross-protection from the other virus strain, thus allowing viral shedding and recurrence of clinical signs and lesions, although diminished.

The respiratory tract is the primary portal of entry with transmission occurring via aerosol or direct contact exposure with respiratory secretions. Passage among exposed rats is exceptionally rapid, with infected animals shedding the virus for about 7 days. The disease can become endemic but like MHV, SDAV does not exist in a latent carrier state in IC animals. Extension of the infection from the respiratory epithelium occurs via ducts of the salivary, lacrimal, and Harderian glands. The virus has not been detected in feces.

Clinical signs are seen in a colony for several weeks during epizootics, with individuals exhibiting signs for up to 1 week. Chromodacryorrhea, squinting, photophobia, blepharospasm, and eye rubbing are followed by sneezing and cervical swelling within 5 to 7 days. Keratoconjunctivitis may be the only clinical sign of infection in some outbreaks. Acute keratoconjunctivitis can resolve or progress to keratitis with opacities, ulceration, scarring, and even perforation, in which case there can be secondary bacterial anterior uveitis or panophthalmitis. Swelling under the neck is caused by cervical edema, enlarged cervical lymph nodes, and necrotic and inflamed salivary glands. In general, the swelling subsides in 10 to 14 days and the rat returns to normal. Unilateral or bilateral suborbital or periorbital swelling, prominent or bulging eyes, and keratitis sicca can develop secondary to decreased lacrimation. Self-mutilation may occur as a result of scratching at the eyes and other affected areas, and very young animals may enucleate the globe. During the infection rats usually remain active and continue to eat, although certain behavioral activities may be suppressed; for example, pain may reduce food intake and complicate feeding studies. Glaucoma or persistent megaglobus may be permanent side effects in recovered animals. Infection may be exacerbated by concurrent SeV infection or mycoplasmosis, resulting in death. There may be high mortality associated with general anesthesia during the pneumonic form of the disease. Behavioral changes and reproductive disorders, including irregularities of the estrous cycle and neonatal mortality, have also been associated with epizootics of the disease. Athymic rats develop chronic, active lesions that persist in target organs for months, with accompanying wasting.

The infection progresses rapidly from the respiratory epithelium to the lacrimal and serous or serous-mucous mixed salivary glands, regional lymph nodes, and adjacent tissues. Affected glands are enlarged, edematous, pale, and often reddened. The thymus becomes atrophic; however, this lesion and the chromodacryorrhea may be stress responses. The salivary, Harderian, and exorbital lacrimal glands may all be affected as a group or individually. Lesions are frequently unilateral, and paired salivary and lacrimal glands should be harvested for histopathologic examination. The glands will return to normal or become permanently scarred, depending on the severity of the infection and the degree of tissue damage, within 2 to 4 weeks of infection. Epithelial cells of the respiratory tract and ducts and acini of the glands undergo severe necrosis and inflammation. As the virus is eliminated from the lesion in about 1 week, the restoration process ensues. Harderian glands often have blotchy brown pigmentation with focal residual inflammatory lesions persisting for several weeks, resulting in prominent squamous metaplasia. During the reparative stages, cellular infiltrates of the affected glands are primarily lymphocytes, plasma cells, mast cells, and macrophages. In salivary glands, regeneration of acinar and ductal epithelial cells is usually completed within 3 to 4 weeks post exposure. In the respiratory tract, necrotizing rhinitis with mononuclear and polymorphonuclear cell infiltration occurs in the initial stages of the disease. Both respiratory and olfactory epithelium are affected, and although major repair is complete by 14 days post exposure, residual lesions may persist longer in specialized areas such as the vomeronasal organ. In the lower respiratory tract there is transient tracheitis, focal bronchitis and bronchiolitis with leukocytic infiltration, hyperplasia of respiratory epithelial cells, and flattening and loss of ciliated cells. Focal alveolitis, when present, is characterized by hypercellularity of alveolar walls and mobilization of alveolar macrophages. Lesions in the distal tract are transient, and usually dissipate by 8 to 10 days post exposure.

The presence of typical lesions in the salivary and lacrimal glands confirmed on histopathologic examination is sufficient to make the diagnosis. Viral antigen may be demonstrated in the respiratory tract and affected tissues (including the urinary bladder) by 4 to 6 days post exposure. In general, virus isolation is not a practical procedure in most circumstances. Serology (MFIA, ELISA, IFA) can detect enzootic infections. The combination of pathognomonic clinical signs and histopathology in animals will confirm the diagnosis in the first week of infection, and serology should be employed after 7 to 10 days of infection. PCR is also available for salivary or lacrimal tissue.

Treatment is not indicated unless ophthalmic lesions are present for which topical preparations are indicated. This disease process warrants supportive care in the form of a warm environment, comfortable quarters, and tasty food treats, especially for pet rats. Treatment with antibiotics during the rapid phase of the disease can alleviate the effects of secondary ophthalmic trauma and bacterial opportunistic invaders. Anti-inflammatory medications and analgesics are indicated for any animals exhibiting signs of pain and/or distress.

Preventing transfer of this highly contagious coronavirus to naïve colonies is predicated on preventing entry of infected rats into a facility through knowledge of the pathogen status of vendor colonies and an effective quarantine program. Control of an infection within a colony or facility is based on the fact that rats only shed the virus for about 1 week, after which they are immune and not latently infected. The virus is not transmitted vertically. Strict control of movement of animals, materials, and people into the animal house is useful in preventing contamination with SDAV. Elimination of the virus can be accomplished by the typical "burn-out" method previously described. Strict isolation and microbarrier caging are usually required to prevent an outbreak from infecting an entire facility.

As an enveloped virus, SDAV probably does not remain infectious in the environment for more than a few days and is susceptible to detergents, disinfectants, drying, and ethanol.

There may be significant effects on particular types of research in view of the confirmed effect of epidermal growth factor (EGF) on functions such as reproduction and carcinogenesis. There is a significant depletion of EGF in affected submandibular salivary glands during the convalescent stages of the disease. Active infection has been reported to precipitate graft-versus-host disease in the salivary and lacrimal glands of rats with allogenic bone marrow grafts.

NONINFECTIOUS DISEASES
Neoplasia

Neoplastic diseases have been studied in a variety of laboratory animals, including mice, rats, and hamsters.[166–170]

Mouse

The National Cancer Institute's Mouse Models of Human Cancer Consortium (MMHCC) consensus has endeavored to classify murine pulmonary tumors with those that occur in humans. Therefore, the terms "bronchiolo-alveolar" or "alveolar/bronchiolar" are no longer used. Spontaneous or carcinogen-induced tumors are now simply classified as pulmonary adenomas or carcinomas with approximate qualifications (solid, papillary, or mixed). Other types of tumors included in the new designations are papilloma, squamous cell carcinoma (SCC), and adenosquamous carcinoma.

Primary pulmonary respiratory tumors of mice occur at a relatively high frequency. It has been estimated that more than 95% of these tumors are pulmonary adenomas that arise from either type II pneumocytes and/or Clara cells lining terminal bronchioles. The onset and prevalence of pulmonary tumors can be enhanced with chemical carcinogens or viral infections, such as SeV. The tumors invade pulmonary parenchyma and are prone to metastasize. The prevalence of spontaneous respiratory tumors is mouse strain–dependent and the number of tumors per lung is also higher in susceptible mice. "A" strain mice are uniquely susceptible because of their K-ras allele, with activation of K-ras in the tumors. Tumors can arise by 3 to 4 months of age and can reach 100% prevalence by 18 to 24 months. Less susceptible strains are outbred Swiss, inbred FVB, BALB/c, 129, B6, and C57BL.

Pulmonary tumors are often encountered as incidental findings on necropsy, but those that grow expansively can result in clinical signs. There may be evidence of pleural invasion, with seeding of the visceral and parietal pleura, and there may be occasional extension into the intercostal muscles. Malignant alveologenic tumors are infrequent and consist of adenocarcinomas and SCC. Neoplasms must be differentiated from focal alveolar hyperplasia of mucin-containing epithelial cells (pulmonary adenomatosis) and from multifocal inflammatory lesions. Mammary carcinoma and hepatocellular carcinoma should be considered in the differential diagnosis, as these commonly metastasize to the lungs.

Rat

Nasal cavity tumors, including SCC and rhabdomyosarcoma, occur in rats. SCC is reported to have a relationship with malocclusion syndrome in aging rats.

Primary lung tumors are uncommon, but when they do occur they are usually of alveolar type II pneumocyte and/or Clara cell origin, as in mice. An unusual component of pulmonary oncogenesis in the rat is the predilection of this species to develop primary pulmonary neoplasm when exposed to low-toxicity, insoluble particulates at extremely high concentrations. This process overwhelms the ability to maintain alveolar macrophage-mediated lung clearance, and is known as "pulmonary overload" tumorigenesis. Other reported pulmonary tumors include adenoma, hemangioma, SCC, carcinoma, and adenocarcinoma.

Hamster

Neoplasia is rare but when it does occur, benign tumors (nasal polyps) of the nasal cavity and proximal trachea are most common, with carcinoma of the nasoturbinates occurring infrequently. Clear-cell carcinomas of the larynx have been seen in several colonies without gross lesions, and are of unknown cellular origin. Malignant epithelial tumors of the lower bronchial tree, such as polyps of the trachea covered with mucus-producing tracheal epithelium, bronchogenic adenomas with mucus production, and rare bronchial carcinomas, are extremely uncommon. Because spontaneous bronchogenic and pulmonary cancers are rare, the hamster serves as a good animal model in which to study chemical carcinogenesis in the respiratory tract. Many pulmonary tumors have arisen elsewhere including carcinomas of the adrenal cortex, melanomas of the skin, lymphomas, and sarcomas from a variety of sites. Intratracheal instillation of polynuclear hydrocarbons results in benign and malignant squamous cell lesions of the tracheobronchial lumen and bronchioalveolar tumors, which are usually benign. The squamous lesions are accompanied by anaplastic carcinomas and adenocarcinomas of the bronchi.

Miscellaneous Conditions

A range of miscellaneous noninfectious conditions also cause respiratory illness in the mouse, rat, hamster, or gerbil.[171–179]

Acidophilic macrophage pneumonia/epithelial hyalinosis

Acidophilic macrophage pneumonia (AMP), or epithelial hyalinosis, is characterized by focal to diffuse aggregation of acidophilic crystals within macrophages, alveolar spaces, and airways, and is prevalent among many strains of mice. Strains such as B6, 129 (particularly 129S4/SvJae), and Swiss mice tend to have an increased incidence and earlier onset of this lesion. AMP can cause mortality in various types of GEMs on the B6 or 129 background, and is particularly severe in B6 (*ptpn6^{me}*) moth-eaten mice. AMP tends to be most evident in older animals and can occur in wild mice as well. Any disease that impairs normal clearance (pulmonary tumors, pneumocystosis, or other chronic pneumonias) can predispose to AMP and will lead to dyspnea if very extensive. Grossly there is lobar to diffuse tan to red discoloration of the lungs, which do not collapse. Microscopically, macrophages have abundant cytoplasm filled with large numbers of needle-shaped to rhomboid-shaped eosinophilic crystals, present in alveolar spaces, alveolar ducts, terminal airways, and bronchiolar glands. The crystalline material is a conglomerate of substances primarily composed of Ym1 chitinase, but also contains iron, α-1 antitrypsin, immunoglobulin, and granulocyte breakdown products. Based on ultrastructural studies, the crystals resemble Charcot-Leyden crystals, which are unique to nonhuman primates and humans in association with eosinophil-related diseases.

Although AMP is the most overt manifestation of this condition, hyalinosis of multiple organs can occur, including olfactory, nasal, middle ear, trachea, lung, stomach, gall bladder, bile duct, and pancreatic duct epithelium as part of the syndrome. Neonatal mice with lesions in the olfactory and vomeronasal areas fail to nurse.

Agent-induced pulmonary edema

A report in 1991 documented that xylazine administration in rats resulted in pleural effusion and alveolar edema. The optimal "edemagenic" dose was approximately 43 mg/kg, which has been used to study the progression of increased pulmonary vascular permeability. Other agents causing varying degrees of pulmonary edema in rats are pentobarbital and carbon dioxide.

Allergic disease/allergic rhinitis

Animals may be allergic to components of their food, dusty hay, bedding, cigarette smoke, and a variety of aerosols. Allergies in hamsters may be hereditary.

Alveolar hemorrhage

Regardless of the cause of death, focal intra-alveolar hemorrhage is a uniform agonal finding in lungs of mice, which must be differentiated from congestive heart failure and other causes.

Pulmonary histiocytosis/alveolar histiocytosis/alveolar proteinosis/alveolar lipoproteinosis

Mouse Focal accumulations of foamy lipid-laden macrophages are sporadically observed in the peripheral, particularly subpleural, regions of the lung in aging mice of all types. These lesions are rare in specific pathogen-free (SPF) mice. Some of the macrophages may contain cholesterol crystals. These changes can follow pulmonary hemorrhage, and hemoglobin crystals may also be present in the area. Alveolar lipoproteinosis is a more severe condition, in which there is hypertrophy and vacuolization of type II pneumocytes, mobilization of scattered macrophages, and progressive intra-alveolar accumulation of granular, pale, eosinophilic phospholipid. Experimental procedures (inhalation of toxic aerosols and so forth) are frequently used to produce this type of lesion. To add to the perplexity, there appears to be considerable overlap in the interpretation and nomenclature assigned to these changes, and they may overlap with AMP.

Rat Aggregates of alveolar macrophages and pulmonary foam cells (PFC) are seen occasionally in the lungs of older rats. The cause is unknown and does not appear to be infectious, although there is usually a minimal concurrent inflammatory cell response. Factors such as excess surfactant production over breakdown and clearance or impaired mucociliary clearance have been implicated to explain the excess recruitment of alveolar macrophages. Lesions are grossly visible on the pleural surface as white to pale tan foci, usually about 1 mm diameter. Foci may extend slightly above the pleural surface in the uninflated lung. Microscopically, clusters of alveoli, often in a subpleural location or adjacent to a terminal bronchiole, contain increased numbers of large, pale, foamy-appearing macrophages. Occasionally cholesterol clefts may be visible in denser accumulations of macrophages, and a slight infiltration of lymphocytes may be present around adjacent vessels, probably as a response to proinflammatory mediators released by the macrophages. This condition should not be mistaken for any of the viral pneumonias of rats, because affected animals are seronegative, and any lymphoid infiltrate is slight and localized to the area of macrophage accumulation.

Hamster Alveolar histiocytosis similar to that seen in rats also occurs in hamsters.

Amyloidosis
Mouse Amyloidosis is a common event in many aging laboratory and wild mice, and can be difficult to distinguish between primary and secondary in spontaneous cases There are two types of amyloid in the mouse, AapoAll and AA. The prevalence of spontaneous amyloidosis is significantly affected by stress; ectoparasitism; and chronic inflammatory conditions, such as ulcerative dermatitis, preputial adenitis, cervical lymphadenitis, conjunctivitis, pyometra, and others. There does not appear to be a clear sex-related predisposition, although it can be more common in males that are prone to fighting due to stress. Individually housed SPF mice have lower prevalence of amyloidosis compared with group-housed mice. Amyloidosis tends to occur at high prevalence and early onset in A, SJL, and outbred Swiss mice, at high prevalence but late onset in C57BL, B6, and B10 mice, and is extremely rare in BALB/c, C3H, and DBA mice.

AapoAll is known as "primary" or "senile amyloid." Although the precursor is produced by the liver, deposition of AapoAll tends to be less severe in spleen and liver (compared with AA), with more deposition in the lungs and other internal organs. Primary amyloidosis is common among aging mice but also may occur in young mice of highly susceptible strains. AA amyloid is associated with an increase in serum precursors apoSAA, which is induced in hepatocytes and elevated in response to cytokines produced during inflammatory and neoplastic disease. AA amyloidosis can be induced by repeated injections of casein and other inflammatory stimuli, thereby earning the name "secondary amyloidosis." Localized amyloidosis can also be found. Tumor-associated amyloid can be found in pulmonary adenomas of A and BALB mice. A common site for amyloid-like deposition is in the nasal submucosa, particularly above the vomeronasal organs.

Hamster Tracheal and lung amyloidosis has been reported in hamsters.

Aspiration pneumonia
Although rodents are obligate nasal breathers, aspiration pneumonia is a common sequela to accidental inhalation of foreign material, which occurs under several circumstances but especially when shipping containers using wood shavings are handled roughly during transportation. It can also occur secondary to megaesophagus or gastrointestinal impaction.

Eosinophilic granulomatous pneumonia in brown Norway rats
The brown Norway (BN) rat has been a model to study the pathogenesis of asthma because they readily develop increased bronchiolar responsiveness and elevated Immunoglobulin E (IgE) after exposure to allergens. However, they can develop a spontaneous eosinophil-rich granulomatous pneumonia in the absence of any experimental manipulations. The changes have been attributed to inadvertent exposure to the allergen, but because of the inflammatory nature of the lesions, they could be due to an unidentified infectious agent. Incidence can be up to 100% in both males and females at 3 to 4 months of age. BN rats from colonies worldwide are affected, including those maintained in isolators. Affected animals are seronegative for all known agents, and rats of other strains housed with affected animals do not develop lung lesions. The lesions are distributed throughout the parenchyma and are characterized by well-organized granulomas of Langerhans giant cells, macrophages, and eosinophils. No foreign material, fungi, or bacteria can be demonstrated microscopically. This syndrome remains an important complication for the researcher evaluating histopathological changes in the lung of the BN rat. Transient pulmonary eosinophilia and granulomatous vasculitis have been produced in laboratory rats following

intravenous administration of Sephadex. However, the pulmonary lesions are markedly different to those of the spontaneous disease.

Freund adjuvant pulmonary granuloma
Focal histiocytic granulomas can be found in the lungs of mice immunized with Freund adjuvant, regardless of the site of immunization.

Hyperplasia of alveolar or bronchial epithelium
This condition occurs in old mice and must be differentiated from pulmonary tumors.

Inflammation of nasal mucosa
Common nasal lesions of aging mice include squamous epithelial hyperplasia in the nasal vestibule, intracytoplasmic hyaline inclusions, inflammation of the nasal mucosa and nasolacrimal duct, and olfactory degeneration with atrophy.

Lymphohistiocytic lung lesions
An unidentified agent has been associated with this condition in rats. Lesions occur in 8- to 18-week-old animals, with rats 8 to 12 weeks of age the most severely affected. Grossly, lesions appear as multiple small gray to tan foci on the pleural surface of the lung. Microscopically, mild to moderate multifocal histiocytic alveolitis and perivascular cuffing are present. Microbiological culturing and PCR assays suggest that the lesions are not bacterial in origin. A viral etiology is suggested, because inoculation of lung tissue homogenates passed through bacteriologic filters induces cytopathic effects in tissue culture, and lesions have been reported in barrier-maintained commercial breeding colonies.

Miscellaneous lesions reported in hamsters
Other lesions reported in hamsters include tracheal mucosal gland adenitis, ossification of tracheal rings, tracheal gland degeneration, lung mineralization, and heterotopic bone in the lung.

Perivascular lymphoid infiltrates
Mild to severe infiltrates can be seen in the adventitia of pulmonary vessels, with extension into adjacent alveolar septa in mice. This condition is consistently found in response to antigenic stimuli, such as viral infection. Perivascular lymphoid infiltrates also frequently appear in older mice with perivascular mononuclear cell infiltrates in salivary glands, kidneys, and other organs. The condition seems to precede lymphoproliferative disorders.

Tracheal cartilage degeneration
F-344 rats seem particularly susceptible to developing age-related tracheal cartilage degeneration and seromucinous adenitis. The use of rigid, metal gavage tubes and the irritant properties of the gavaged material may play a role, although spontaneous lesions did occur in untreated animals and may be seen as early as 6 weeks of age. These inflammatory lesions are thought to lead to impaired salivation. Food and bedding may become lodged in the oropharyngeal cavity, resulting in asphyxia.

REFERENCES

1. Harkness JE, Turner PV, VandeWoude S, et al. Introduction, general husbandry, and disease prevention. In: Greenacre CB, editor. Harkness and Wagner's biology and medicine of rabbits and rodents. 5th edition. Ames: Wiley Blackwell; 2010. p. 11–7.
2. Jenkins JR. Rodent diagnostics. J Exot Pet Med 2008;17:16–25.

3. King WW, Russell SP. Metabolic, traumatic, and miscellaneous diseases. In: Suckow MA, Weisbroth SH, Franklin CL, editors. The laboratory rat. 2nd edition. Orlando: Academic Press; 2005. p. 521.
4. Mayer J. Annoying respiratory tract diseases in rats. In: Proceedings from the North American Veterinary Conference. Orlando: 2008. p. 1859.
5. Carpenter JW. Rodents. In: Exotic animal formulary. 3rd edition. St Louis: Elsevier Saunders; 2005. p. 377–97.
6. Johnson-Delaney CA. Small rodents. In: Exotic companion medicine handbook. Lake Worth: Zoological Education Network; 1996. p. 3–9.
7. Sayers I, Smith S. Mice, rats, hamsters, and gerbils. In: Meredith A, Johnson-Delaney CA, editors. BSAVA manual of exotic pets. 5th edition. Gloucester, England: BSAVA; 2010. p. 26–7.
8. deMatos R. Rodents: therapeutics. In: Keeble E, Meredith A, editors. BSAVA manual of rodents and ferrets. Gloucester, England: BSAVA; 2009. p. 52–62.
9. Hrapkiewicz K, Medina L. Mice. In: Clinical laboratory animal medicine. 3rd edition. Ames: Blackwell Publishing; 2007. p. 58–60.
10. Hrapkiewicz K, Medina L. Rats. In: Clinical laboratory animal medicine. 3rd edition. Ames: Blackwell Publishing; 2007. p. 95–6.
11. Hrapkiewicz K, Medina L. Gerbils. In: Clinical laboratory animal medicine. 3rd edition. Ames: Blackwell Publishing; 2007. p. 121–3.
12. Hrapkiewicz K, Medina L. Hamsters. In: Clinical laboratory animal medicine. 3rd edition. Ames: Blackwell Publishing; 2007. p. 140–3.
13. Harkness JE, Turner PV, VandeWoude S, et al. Clinical procedures. In: Harkness and Wagner's biology and medicine of rabbits and rodents. 5th edition. Ames: Wiley Blackwell; 2010. p. 141–6.
14. Feldman SH, Gograge SI, Kohn DF, et al. Biology. In: Laboratory mouse handbook. Memphis: AALAS; 2006. p. 14.
15. Hrapkiewicz K, Medina L. Mice. In: Clinical laboratory animal medicine. 3rd edition. Ames: Blackwell Publishing; 2007. p. 42–3.
16. Percy DH, Barthold SW. Mice. In: Pathology of laboratory rodents and rabbits. 3rd edition. Ames: Blackwell Publishing; 2007. p. 7–11.
17. Jacoby RO, Fox JG, Davisson M. Biology and diseases of mice. In: Fox JG, Anderson LC, Loew FM, et al, editors. Laboratory animal medicine. 2nd edition. San Diego: Academic Press; 2002. p. 43–5.
18. Cook MJ. Anatomy. In: Foster HL, Small JD, Fox JG, editors. The mouse in biomedical research, vol. 3. New York: Academic Press; 1983. p. 102–20.
19. Kaplan HM, Brewer NR, Blair WH. Physiology. In: Foster HL, Small JD, Fox JG, editors. The mouse in biomedical research, vol. 3. New York: Academic Press; 1983. p. 248–92.
20. Hofstetter J, Suckow MA, Hickman DL. Morphophysiology. In: Suckow MA, Weisbroth SH, Franklin DL, editors. The laboratory rat. 2nd edition. Orlando: Academic Press; 2002. p. 106–8.
21. Hrapkiewicz K, Medina L. Rats. In: Clinical laboratory animal medicine. 3rd edition. Ames: Blackwell Publishing; 2007. p. 81–2.
22. O'Malley B. Rats. In: Clinical anatomy and physiology of exotic species. St Louis: Elsevier Saunders; 2005. p. 13.
23. Percy DH, Barthold SW. Rats. In: Pathology of laboratory rodents and rabbits. 3rd edition. Ames: Blackwell Publishing; 2007. p. 125–6.
24. Kohn DF, Clifford CB. Biology and diseases of rats. In: Fox JG, Anderson LC, Loew FM, et al, editors. Laboratory animal medicine. 2nd edition. San Diego: Academic Press; 2002. p. 124–5.

25. Bivin WS, Olsen GH, Murray KA. Morphophysiology. In: vanHoosier GL Jr, McPherson CW, editors. Laboratory hamster. Orlando: Academic Press; 1987. p. 19–24.

26. Hrapkiewicz K, Medina L. Hamsters. In: Clinical laboratory animal medicine. 3rd edition. Ames: Blackwell Publishing; 2007. p. 131–3.

27. Hankensen CF, vanHoosier GL Jr. Biology and diseases of hamsters. In: Fox JG, Anderson LC, Loew FM, et al, editors. Laboratory animal medicine. 2nd edition. San Diego: Academic Press; 2002. p. 171–2.

28. Percy DH, Barthold SW. Hamsters. In: Pathology of laboratory rodents and rabbits. 3rd edition. Ames: Blackwell Publishing; 2007. p. 180.

29. Hrapkiewicz K, Medina L. Gerbils. In: Clinical laboratory animal medicine. 3rd edition. Ames: Blackwell Publishing; 2007. p. 113–4.

30. Percy DH, Barthold SW. Gerbils. In: Pathology of laboratory rodents and rabbits. 3rd edition. Ames: Blackwell Publishing; 2007. p. 207.

31. Winsser J. A study of Bordetella bronchiseptica. Proc Anim Care Panel 1960;10: 87–104.

32. Harkness JE, Turner PV, VandeWoude S, et al. Specific diseases and conditions. In: Harkness and Wagner's biology and medicine of rabbits and rodents. 5th edition. Ames: Wiley Blackwell; 2010. p. 262–5.

33. Percy DH, Barthold SW. Rat. In: Pathology of laboratory rodents and rabbits. 3rd edition. Ames: Blackwell Publishing; 2007. p. 141–2.

34. Weisbroth SH, Kohn DF, Boot R. Bacterial, mycoplasmal, and mycotic infections. In: Suckow MA, Weisbroth SH, Franklin DL, editors. The laboratory rat. 2nd edition. Orlando: Academic Press; 2002. p. 380–1.

35. Burek JD, Jersey CG, Whitehair CK, et al. The pathology and pathogenesis of Bordetella bronchiseptica and Pasteurella pneumotropica infection in conventional and germ-free rats. Lab Anim 1993;27:342–9.

36. Percy DH, Barthold SW. Mouse. In: Pathology of laboratory rodents and rabbits. 3rd edition. Ames: Blackwell Publishing; 2007. p. 63–4.

37. Jacoby RO, Fox JG, Davisson M. Biology and diseases of mice. In: Fox JG, Anderson LC, Loew FM, et al, editors. Laboratory animal medicine. 2nd edition. San Diego: Academic Press; 2002. p. 96.

38. Schoeb TR. Respiratory diseases of rodents. Vet Clin North Am Exot Anim Pract 2000;3(2):487–8.

39. Harkness JE, Turner PV, VandeWoude S, et al. Specific diseases and conditions. In: Harkness and Wagner's biology and medicine of rabbits and rodents. 5th edition. Ames: Wiley Blackwell; 2010. p. 269–72.

40. Percy DH, Barthold SW. Mouse. In: Pathology of laboratory rodents and rabbits. 3rd edition. Ames: Blackwell Publishing; 2007. p. 64.

41. Jacoby RO, Fox JG, Davisson M. Biology and diseases of mice. In: Fox JG, Anderson LC, Loew FM, et al, editors. Laboratory animal medicine. 2nd edition. San Diego: Academic Press; 2002. p. 83.

42. Hrapkiewicz K, Medina L. Mice. In: Clinical laboratory animal medicine. 3rd edition. Ames: Blackwell Publishing; 2007. p. 61.

43. Weisbroth SH, Kohn DF, Boot R. Bacterial, mycoplasmal, and mycotic infections. In: Suckow MA, Weisbroth SH, Franklin DL, editors. The laboratory rat. 2nd edition. Orlando: Academic Press; 2002. p. 366–9.

44. Hrapkiewicz K, Medina L. Rats. In: Clinical laboratory animal medicine. 3rd edition. Ames: Blackwell Publishing; 2007. p. 98.

45. Kohn DF, Clifford CB. Biology and diseases of rats. In: Fox JG, Anderson LC, Loew FM, et al, editors. Laboratory animal medicine. 2nd edition. San Diego: Academic Press; 2002. p. 140–2.
46. Percy DH, Barthold SW. Rat. In: Pathology of laboratory rodents and rabbits. 3rd edition. Ames: Blackwell Publishing; 2007. p. 142–3.
47. Percy DH, Barthold SW. Gerbil. In: Pathology of laboratory rodents and rabbits. 3rd edition. Ames: Blackwell Publishing; 2007. p. 211.
48. Schoeb TR, Lindsey JR. Cilia-associated respiratory bacillus infection, rat, mouse, and rabbit. In: Jones TC, Mohr U, Hunt RD, editors. International life sciences institute monographs on pathology of laboratory animals: respiratory system. Berlin: Springer-Verlag; 1996. p. 325.
49. St. Claire MB, Besch-Williford CL, Riley LK, et al. Experimentally induced infection of gerbils with cilia-associated respiratory bacillus. Lab Anim Sci 1999;49(4):421–3.
50. Harkness JE, Turner PV, VandeWoude S, et al. Specific diseases and conditions. In: Harkness and Wagner's biology and medicine of rabbits and rodents. 5th edition. Ames: Wiley Blackwell; 2010. p. 283–7.
51. Percy DH, Barthold SW. Mouse. In: Pathology of laboratory rodents and rabbits. 3rd edition. Ames: Blackwell Publishing; 2007. p. 72.
52. Percy DH, Barthold SW. Rat. In: Pathology of laboratory rodents and rabbits. 3rd edition. Ames: Blackwell Publishing; 2007. p. 130–2.
53. Kohn DF, Clifford CB. Biology and diseases of rats. In: Fox JG, Anderson LC, Loew FM, et al, editors. Laboratory animal medicine. 2nd edition. San Diego: Academic Press; 2002. p. 135.
54. Hrapkiewicz K, Medina L. Rats. In: Clinical laboratory animal medicine. 3rd edition. Ames: Blackwell Publishing; 2007. p. 99.
55. Weisbroth SH, Kohn DF, Boot R. Bacterial, mycoplasmal, and mycotic infections. In: Suckow MA, Weisbroth SH, Franklin DL, editors. The laboratory rat. 2nd edition. Orlando: Academic Press; 2002. p. 362–6.
56. Jacoby RO, Fox JG, Davisson M. Biology and diseases of mice. In: Fox JG, Anderson LC, Loew FM, et al, editors. Laboratory animal medicine. 2nd edition. San Diego: Academic Press; 2002. p. 92.
57. Hankensen CF, vanHoosier GL Jr. Biology and diseases of hamsters. In: Fox JG, Anderson LC, Loew FM, et al, editors. Laboratory animal medicine. 2nd edition. San Diego: Academic Press; 2002. p. 182.
58. Frisk CS. Bacterial and mycotic infections. In: vanHoosier GL Jr, McPherson CW, editors. Laboratory hamster. Orlando: Academic Press; 1987. p. 129.
59. Percy DH, Barthold SW. Hamster. In: Pathology of laboratory rodents and rabbits. 3rd edition. Ames: Blackwell Publishing; 2007. p. 192.
60. Holmes NE, Korman TM. Corynebacterium kutscheri infection of skin and soft tissue folloing rat bite. J Clin Microbiol 2007;45:3468–9.
61. Nicklas W. Haemophilus infection in a colony of laboratory rats. J Clin Microbiol 1989;27:1636–9.
62. Percy DH, Barthold SW. Mouse. In: Pathology of laboratory rodents and rabbits. 3rd edition. Ames: Blackwell Publishing; 2007. p. 64.
63. Jacoby RO, Fox JG, Davisson M. Biology and diseases of mice. In: Fox JG, Anderson LC, Loew FM, et al, editors. Laboratory animal medicine. 2nd edition. San Diego: Academic Press; 2002. p. 95.
64. Percy DH, Barthold SW. Rat. In: Pathology of laboratory rodents and rabbits. 3rd edition. Ames: Blackwell Publishing; 2007. p. 152.

65. Weisbroth SH, Kohn DF, Boot R. Bacterial, mycoplasmal, and mycotic infections. In: Suckow MA, Weisbroth SH, Franklin DL, editors. The laboratory rat. 2nd edition. Orlando: Academic Press; 2002. p. 380.

66. Waggie KS, Wagner JE, Lentsch RH. A naturally occurring outbreak of *Mycobacterium avium-intracellulare* infections in C57BL/6N mice. Lab Animal Sci 1983;33:249–53.

67. Waggie KS, Wagner JE, Lentsch RH. Experimental murine infections with a *Mycobacterium avium-intracellulare* complex organism isolated from mice. Lab Anim Sci 1983;33:254–7.

68. Harkness JE, Turner PV, VandeWoude S, et al. Specific diseases and conditions. In: Harkness and Wagner's biology and medicine of rabbits and rodents. 5th edition. Ames: Wiley Blackwell; 2010. p. 331–4.

69. Donnelly T. Small rodents: disease problems. In: Quesenberry KE, Carpenter JW, editors. Ferrets, rabbits, and rodents clinical medicine and surgery. 2nd edition. St Louis: Elsevier Publishing; 2004. p. 304–7.

70. Goodman G. Rodents: respiratory and cardiovascular disorders. In: Keeble E, Meredith A, editors. BSAVA manual of rodents and ferrets. Gloucester, England: BSAVA; 2009. p. 147.

71. Schoeb TR. Respiratory diseases of rodents. Vet Clin North Am Exot Anim Pract 2000;3(2):485–7.

72. Percy DH, Barthold SW. Mouse. In: Pathology of laboratory rodents and rabbits. 3rd edition. Ames: Blackwell Publishing; 2007. p. 65–8.

73. Jacoby RO, Fox JG, Davisson M. Biology and diseases of mice. In: Fox JG, Anderson LC, Loew FM, et al, editors. Laboratory animal medicine. 2nd edition. San Diego: Academic Press; 2002. p. 80–3.

74. Percy DH, Barthold SW. Rat. In: Pathology of laboratory rodents and rabbits. 3rd edition. Ames: Blackwell Publishing; 2007. p. 143–6.

75. Kohn DF, Clifford CB. Biology and diseases of rats. In: Fox JG, Anderson LC, Loew FM, et al, editors. Laboratory animal medicine. 2nd edition. San Diego: Academic Press; 2002. p. 142–3.

76. Hrapkiewicz K, Medina L. Rats. In: Clinical laboratory animal medicine. 3rd edition. Ames: Blackwell Publishing; 2007. p. 97–8.

77. Weisbroth SH, Kohn DF, Boot R. Bacterial, mycoplasmal, and mycotic infections. In: Suckow MA, Weisbroth SH, Franklin DL, editors. The laboratory rat. 2nd edition. Orlando: Academic Press; 2002. p. 389–93.

78. Ferreira JB, Yamaguti M, Marques LM, et al. Detection of *Mycoplasma pulmonis* in laboratory rats and technicians. Zoonoses Public Health 2008;55(5):229–34.

79. Neimark H, Mitchelmore D, Leach RH. An approach to characterizing uncultivated prokaryotes: The grey lung agent and proposal of a candidatus taxon for the organism, "*Candidatus Mycoplasma ravipulmonis*". Int J Syst Bacteriol 1998;48:389–94.

80. Schoeb TR. Respiratory diseases of rodents. Vet Clin North Am Exot Anim Pract 2000;3(2):491.

81. Harkness JE, Turner PV, VandeWoude S, et al. Specific diseases and conditions. In: Harkness and Wagner's biology and medicine of rabbits and rodents. 5th edition. Ames: Wiley Blackwell; 2010. p. 235–6, 281–2.

82. Percy DH, Barthold SW. Mouse. In: Pathology of laboratory rodents and rabbits. 3rd edition. Ames: Blackwell Publishing; 2007. p. 66–8.

83. Jacoby RO, Fox JG, Davisson M. Biology and diseases of mice. In: Fox JG, Anderson LC, Loew FM, et al, editors. Laboratory animal medicine. 2nd edition. San Diego: Academic Press; 2002. p. 87–8.

84. Percy DH, Barthold SW. Rat. In: Pathology of laboratory rodents and rabbits. 3rd edition. Ames: Blackwell Publishing; 2007. p. 146–7.
85. Kohn DF, Clifford CB. Biology and diseases of rats. In: Fox JG, Anderson LC, Loew FM, et al, editors. Laboratory animal medicine. 2nd edition. San Diego: Academic Press; 2002. p. 137–8.
86. Weisbroth SH, Kohn DF, Boot R. Bacterial, mycoplasmal, and mycotic infections. In: Suckow MA, Weisbroth SH, Franklin DL, editors. The laboratory rat. 2nd edition. Orlando: Academic Press; 2002. p. 374–8.
87. Percy DH, Barthold SW. Hamster. In: Pathology of laboratory rodents and rabbits. 3rd edition. Ames: Blackwell Publishing; 2007. p. 192.
88. Hrapkiewicz K, Medina L. Hamsters. In: Clinical laboratory animal medicine. 3rd edition. Ames: Blackwell Publishing; 2007. p. 145.
89. Frisk CS. Bacterial and mycotic infections. In: vanHoosier GL Jr, McPherson CW, editors. Laboratory hamster. Orlando: Academic Press; 1987. p. 129.
90. Goelz MR, Thigpen JE, Mahler J, et al. Efficacy of various therapeutic regimens in eliminating *Pasteurella pneumotropica* from the mouse. Lab Anim Sci 1996; 46:280–5.
91. Schoeb TR. Respiratory diseases of rodents. Vet Clin North Am Exot Anim Pract 2000;3(2):491.
92. Jacoby RO, Fox JG, Davisson M. Biology and diseases of mice. In: Fox JG, Anderson LC, Loew FM, et al, editors. Laboratory animal medicine. 2nd edition. San Diego: Academic Press; 2002. p. 95.
93. Percy DH, Barthold SW. Mouse. In: Pathology of laboratory rodents and rabbits. 3rd edition. Ames: Blackwell Publishing; 2007. p. 69.
94. Weisbroth SH, Kohn DF, Boot R. Bacterial, mycoplasmal, and mycotic infections. In: Suckow MA, Weisbroth SH, Franklin DL, editors. The laboratory rat. 2nd edition. Orlando: Academic Press; 2002. p. 340–4.
95. Percy DH, Barthold SW. Rat. In: Pathology of laboratory rodents and rabbits. 3rd edition. Ames: Blackwell Publishing; 2007. p. 153.
96. Kohn DF, Clifford CB. Biology and diseases of rats. In: Fox JG, Anderson LC, Loew FM, et al, editors. Laboratory animal medicine. 2nd edition. San Diego: Academic Press; 2002. p. 139.
97. Harkness JE, Turner PV, VandeWoude S, et al. Specific diseases and conditions. In: Harkness and Wagner's biology and medicine of rabbits and rodents. 5th edition. Ames: Wiley Blackwell; 2010. p. 380–2.
98. Schoeb TR. Respiratory diseases of rodents. Vet Clin North Am Exot Anim Pract 2000;3(2):489–90.
99. Donnelly T. Small rodents: disease problems. In: Quesenberry KE, Carpenter JW, editors. Ferrets, rabbits, and rodents clinical medicine and surgery. 2nd edition. St Louis: Elsevier Publishing; 2004. p. 304–7.
100. Hrapkiewicz K, Medina L. Rats. In: Clinical laboratory animal medicine. 3rd edition. Ames: Blackwell Publishing; 2007. p. 98.
101. Weisbroth SH, Kohn DF, Boot R. Bacterial, mycoplasmal, and mycotic infections. In: Suckow MA, Weisbroth SH, Franklin DL, editors. The laboratory rat. 2nd edition. Orlando: Academic Press; 2002. p. 346–50.
102. Percy DH, Barthold SW. Rat. In: Pathology of laboratory rodents and rabbits. 3rd edition. Ames: Blackwell Publishing; 2007. p. 149–50.
103. Kohn DF, Clifford CB. Biology and diseases of rats. In: Fox JG, Anderson LC, Loew FM, et al, editors. Laboratory animal medicine. 2nd edition. San Diego: Academic Press; 2002. p. 133–5.

104. Hrapkiewicz K, Medina L. Hamsters. In: Clinical laboratory animal medicine. 3rd edition. Ames: Blackwell Publishing; 2007. p. 145.
105. Percy DH, Barthold SW. Hamster. In: Pathology of laboratory rodents and rabbits. 3rd edition. Ames: Blackwell Publishing; 2007. p. 192.
106. Frisk CS. Bacterial and Mycotic Infections. In: vanHoosier GL Jr, McPherson CW, editors. Laboratory hamster. Orlando: Academic Press; 1987. p. 129.
107. Schoeb TR. Respiratory diseases of rodents. Vet Clin North Am Exot Anim Pract 2000;3(2):492–3.
108. Harkness JE, Turner PV, VandeWoude S, et al. Specific diseases and conditions. In: Harkness and Wagner's biology and medicine of rabbits and rodents. 5th edition. Ames: Wiley Blackwell; 2010. p. 363–4.
109. Percy DH, Barthold SW. Mouse. In: Pathology of laboratory rodents and rabbits. 3rd edition. Ames: Blackwell Publishing; 2007. p. 83–4.
110. Jacoby RO, Fox JG, Davisson M. Biology and diseases of mice. In: Fox JG, Anderson LC, Loew FM, et al, editors. Laboratory animal medicine. 2nd edition. San Diego: Academic Press; 2002. p. 96–8.
111. Percy DH, Barthold SW. Rat. In: Pathology of laboratory rodents and rabbits. 3rd edition. Ames: Blackwell Publishing; 2007. p. 157–8.
112. Kohn DF, Clifford CB. Biology and diseases of rats. In: Fox JG, Anderson LC, Loew FM, et al, editors. Laboratory animal medicine. 2nd edition. San Diego: Academic Press; 2002. p. 152.
113. Weisbroth SH, Kohn DF, Boot R. Bacterial, mycoplasmal, and mycotic infections. In: Suckow MA, Weisbroth SH, Franklin DL, editors. The laboratory rat. 2nd edition. Orlando: Academic Press; 2002. p. 384–9.
114. Percy DH, Barthold SW. Mouse. In: Pathology of laboratory rodents and rabbits. 3rd edition. Ames: Blackwell Publishing; 2007. p. 82.
115. Rehm S, Waalkes MP, Ward JM. Aspergillus rhinitis in Wistar (Crl:(WI)BR) rats. Lab Anim Sci 1998;38:162–6.
116. Hubbs AF, Hahn FF, Lundgren DL. Invasive tracheobronchial aspergillosis in an F-344/N rat. Lab Anim Sci 1991;41:521–3.
117. Royals MA, Getzy DM, Vandewoude S. High fungal spore load in corncob bedding associated with fungal rhinitis in two rats. Contemp Topics 1999;38:64–6.
118. Bornstein S, Iwarsson K. Nasal mites in a colony of Syrian hamsters Lab Anim 1980;14:31–3.
119. Wagner JE. Parasitic diseases. In: vanHoosier GL Jr, McPherson CW, editors. Laboratory hamster. Orlando: Academic Press; 1987. p. 152.
120. Harkness JE, Turner PV, VandeWoude S, et al. Clinical signs and differential diagnoses. In: Harkness and Wagner's biology and medicine of rabbits and rodents. 5th edition. Ames: Wiley Blackwell; 2010. p. 242.
121. Gerardo S, Gerardo C, Mills, et al. Serologic evidence of hantavirus infection in sigmodontine rodents in Mexico. J Wildl Dis 2001;37(2):391–3.
122. Percy DH, Barthold SW. Rat. In: Pathology of laboratory rodents and rabbits. 3rd edition. Ames: Blackwell Publishing; 2007. p. 1132–3.
123. Harkness JE, Turner PV, VandeWoude S, et al. Specific diseases and conditions. In: Harkness and Wagner's biology and medicine of rabbits and rodents. 5th edition. Ames: Wiley Blackwell; 2010. p. 308–9.
124. Lussier G. Murine cytomegalovirus. In: Manual of microbiological monitoring of laboratory animals. 2nd edition. Bethesda: National Institutes of Health Publications; 1994. p. 69–74.
125. Percy DH, Barthold SW. Mouse. In: Pathology of laboratory rabbits and rodents. 3rd edition. Ames: Blackwell Publishing; 2007. p. 19–21.

126. Chen HC, Cover CE. Spontaneous disseminated cytomegalic inclusion disease in an ageing laboratory mouse. J Comp Pathol 1988;98:489–93.
127. Harkness JE, Turner PV, VandeWoude S, et al. Specific diseases and conditions. In: Harkness and Wagner's biology and medicine of rabbits and rodents. 5th edition. Ames: Wiley Blackwell; 2010. p. 278–81.
128. Hrapkiewicz K, Medina L. Mice. In: Clinical laboratory animal medicine. 3rd edition. Ames: Blackwell Publishing; 2007. p. 66.
129. Percy DH, Barthold SW. Mouse. In: Pathology of laboratory rabbits and rodents. 3rd edition. Ames: Blackwell Publishing; 2007. p. 31–6.
130. Harkness JE, Turner PV, VandeWoude S, et al. Specific diseases and conditions. In: Harkness and Wagner's biology and medicine of rabbits and rodents. 5th edition. Ames: Wiley Blackwell; 2010. p. 334–5.
131. Hrapkiewicz K, Medina L. Mice. In: Clinical laboratory animal medicine. 3rd edition. Ames: Blackwell Publishing; 2007. p. 67.
132. Percy DH, Barthold SW. Mouse. In: Pathology of laboratory rabbits and rodents. 3rd edition. Ames: Blackwell Publishing; 2007. p. 44.
133. Karst SM, Wobus CE, Lay M, et al. STAT1-Dependent innate immunity to a Norwalk-like virus. Science 2003;299:1575–8.
134. Percy DH, Barthold SW. Mouse. In: Pathology of laboratory rabbits and rodents. 3rd edition. Ames: Blackwell Publishing; 2007. p. 23–4.
135. Harkness JE, Turner PV, VandeWoude S, et al. Specific diseases and conditions. In: Harkness and Wagner's biology and medicine of rabbits and rodents. 5th edition. Ames: Wiley Blackwell; 2010. p. 334–5.
136. Hrapkiewicz K, Medina L. Mice. In: Clinical laboratory animal medicine. 3rd edition. Ames: Blackwell Publishing; 2007. p. 67.
137. Percy DH, Barthold SW. Mouse. In: Pathology of laboratory rabbits and rodents. 3rd edition. Ames: Blackwell Publishing; 2007. p. 36–7.
138. Jacoby RO, Fox JG, Davisson M. Biology and diseases of mice. In: Fox JG, Anderson LC, Loew FM, et al, editors. Laboratory animal medicine. 2nd edition. San Diego: Academic Press; 2002. p. 71–2.
139. Percy DH, Barthold SW. Rat. In: Pathology of laboratory rabbits and rodents. 3rd edition. Ames: Blackwell Publishing; 2007. p. 134.
140. Kohn DF, Clifford CB. Biology and diseases of rats. In: Fox JG, Anderson LC, Loew FM, et al, editors. Laboratory animal medicine. 2nd edition. San Diego: Academic Press; 2002. p. 146–7.
141. Percy DH, Barthold SW. Hamster. In: Pathology of laboratory rabbits and rodents. 3rd edition. Ames: Blackwell Publishing; 2007. p. 184.
142. Hankensen CF, vanHoosier GL Jr. Biology and diseases of hamsters. In: Fox JG, Anderson LC, Loew FM, et al, editors. Laboratory animal medicine. 2nd edition. San Diego: Academic Press; 2002. p. 184–5.
143. Parker JC, Ganaway JR, Gillett CS. Viral diseases. In: vanHoosier GL Jr, McPherson CW, editors. Laboratory hamster. Orlando: Academic Press; 1987. p. 95–106.
144. Percy DH, Barthold SW. Rat. In: Pathology of laboratory rabbits and rodents. 3rd edition. Ames: Blackwell Publishing; 2007. p. 129–30.
145. Ward JM, Lock A, Collins MJ, et al. Papoviral sialoadenitis in athymic nude rats. Lab Anim 1984;18:84–9.
146. Livingston RS, Besch-Williford I, Myles MH, et al. Pneumocystis carinii infection causes lung lesions indistinguishable from those previously attributed to rat respiratory virus. In: Programs of the 61st AALAS National Meeting (abstract PS101). Atlanta, October 10–14, 2010.

147. Harkness JE, Turner PV, VandeWoude S, et al. Specific diseases and conditions. In: Harkness and Wagner's biology and medicine of rabbits and rodents. 5th edition. Ames: Wiley Blackwell; 2010. p. 373–5.

148. Percy DH, Barthold SW. Mouse. In: Pathology of laboratory rodents and rabbits. 3rd edition. Ames: Blackwell Publishing; 2007. p. 37–9.

149. Jacoby RO, Fox JG, Davisson M. Biology and diseases of mice. In: Fox JG, Anderson LC, Loew FM, et al, editors. Laboratory animal medicine. 2nd edition. San Diego: Academic Press; 2002. p. 59–72.

150. Hrapkiewicz K, Medina L. Mice. In: Clinical laboratory animal medicine. 3rd edition. Ames: Blackwell Publishing; 2007. p. 65–6.

151. Jacoby GA, Gaertner DJ. Viral diseases. In: Suckow MA, Weisbroth SH, Franklin DL, editors. The laboratory rat. 2nd edition. Orlando: Academic Press; 2002. p. 443.

152. Percy DH, Barthold SW. Rat. In: Pathology of laboratory rodents and rabbits. 3rd edition. Ames: Blackwell Publishing; 2007. p. 134–5.

153. Kohn DF, Clifford CB. Biology and diseases of rats. In: Fox JG, Anderson LC, Loew FM, et al, editors. Laboratory animal medicine. 2nd edition. San Diego: Academic Press; 2002. p. 143–4.

154. Percy DH, Barthold SW. Hamster. In: Pathology of laboratory rodents and rabbits. 3rd edition. Ames: Blackwell Publishing; 2007. p. 184–5.

155. Tsukui M, Ito H, Tada M, et al. Protective effect of inactivated virus vaccine on Sendai virus infection in rats. Lab Anim Sci 1982;32:143–6.

156. Iwata H, Tagaya M, Matsumoto K, et al. Aerosol vaccination with a Sendai virus temperature-sensitive mutant (HVJ-pb) derived from persistently infected cells. J Infect Dis 1989;162:402–7.

157. Harkness JE, Turner PV, VandeWoude S, et al. Specific diseases and conditions. In: Harkness and Wagner's biology and medicine of rabbits and rodents. 5th edition. Ames: Wiley Blackwell; 2010. p. 281–3.

158. Fallon MT. Rats and Mice. In: Laber-Laird K, Swindle MM, Flecknall P, editors. Handbook of rodent and rabbit medicine. Tarrytown: Elsevier Science, Inc.; 1996. p. 16–7.

159. Jacoby RO, Fox JG, Davisson M. Biology and diseases of mice. In: Fox JG, Anderson LC, Loew FM, et al, editors. Laboratory animal medicine. 2nd edition. San Diego: Academic Press; 2002. p. 69–71.

160. Percy DH, Barthold SW. Rat. In: Pathology of laboratory rodents and rabbits. 3rd edition. Ames: Blackwell Publishing; 2007. p. 130–2.

161. Jacoby GA, Gaertner DJ. Viral diseaes. In: Suckow MA, Weisbroth SH, Franklin DL, editors. The laboratory rat. 2nd edition. Orlando: Academic Press; 2002. p. 435–42.

162. Hrapkiewicz K, Medina L. Rats. In: Clinical laboratory animal medicine. 3rd edition. Ames: Blackwell Publishing; 2007. p. 100–2.

163. Kohn DF, Clifford CB. Biology and diseases of rats. In: Fox JG, Anderson LC, Loew FM, et al, editors. Laboratory animal medicine. 2nd edition. San Diego: Academic Press; 2002. p. 144–6.

164. Hankensen CF, vanHoosier GL Jr. Biology and diseases of hamsters. In: Fox JG, Anderson LC, Loew FM, et al, editors. Laboratory animal medicine. 2nd edition. San Diego: Academic Press; 2002. p. 184–5.

165. Yoo D, Pei Y, Christie N, et al. Primary structure of the sialodacryoadenitis virus genome: sequence of the structural-protein region and its application for differential diagnosis. Clin Diagn Lab Immunol 2000;7(4):568–73.

166. Schoeb TR. Respiratory diseases of rodents. Vet Clin North Am Exot Anim Prac 2000;3(2):493.

167. Jacoby RO, Fox JG, Davisson M. Biology and diseases of mice. In: Fox JG, Anderson LC, Loew FM, et al, editors. Laboratory animal medicine. 2nd edition. San Diego: Adacemic Press; 2002. p. 113.

168. Percy DH, Barthold SW. Mouse. In: Pathology of laboratory rodents and rabbits. 3rd edition. Ames: Blackwell Publishing; 2007. p. 111–8.

169. Boorman GA, Everitt JI. Neoplastic diseases. In: Suckow MA, Weisbroth SH, Franklin DL, editors. The laboratory rat. 2nd edition. Orlando: Academic Press; 2002. p. 487–8.

170. Stradberg JD. Neoplastic diseases. In: vanHoosier GL Jr, McPherson CW, editors. Laboratory hamster. Orlando (FL): Academic Press; 1987. p. 158–9.

171. Percy DH, Barthold SW. Mouse. In: Pathology of laboratory rodents and rabbits. 3rd edition. Ames: Blackwell Publishing; 2007. p. 93–6, 105–6.

172. Jacoby RO, Fox JG, Davisson M. Biology and Diseases of Mice. In: Fox JG, Anderson LC, Loew FM, et al, editors. Laboratory animal medicine. 2nd edition. San Diego: Academic Press; 2002. p. 105–9.

173. King WW, Russell SP. Metabolic, traumatic, and miscellaneous diseases. In: Suckow MA, Weisbroth SH, Franklin DL, editors. The laboratory rat. 2nd edition. Orlando: Academic Press; 2002. p. 520–2.

174. Percy DH, Barthold SW. Rat. In: Pathology of laboratory rodents and rabbits. 3rd edition. Ames: Blackwell Publishing; 2007. p. 155–6, 164.

175. Kohn DF, Clifford CB. Biology and diseases of rats. In: Fox JG, Anderson LC, Loew FM, et al, editors. Laboratory animal medicine. 2nd edition. San Diego: Academic Press; 2002. p. 153–4.

176. Percy DH, Barthold SW. Hamster. In: Pathology of laboratory rodents and rabbits. 3rd edition. Ames: Blackwell Publishing; 2007. p. 125–6.

177. Hankensen CF, vanHoosier GL Jr. Biology and diseases of hamsters. In: Fox JG, Anderson LC, Loew FM, et al, editors. Laboratory animal medicine. 2nd edition. San Diego: Academic Press; 2002. p. 188–9.

178. Richardson VCG. Hamsters. In: Diseases of small domestic rodents. 2nd edition. Ames: Blackwell Publishing; 2003. p. 161.

179. Hubbard GB, Schmidt RE. Noninfectious diseases. In: vanHoosier GL Jr, McPherson CW, editors. Laboratory hamster. Orlando: Academic Press; 1987. p. 174.

Respiratory System Anatomy, Physiology, and Disease: Guinea Pigs and Chinchillas

Enrique Yarto-Jaramillo, DVM, MSc[a,b],*

KEYWORDS

- Guinea pig • Chinchilla • Respiratory diseases
- Scurvy • Dentition

In the last decade, nontraditional companion mammals have gained increasing interest and popularity both in Mexico and the United States. Rodents are now presented frequently to the exotic animal practitioner for professional medical care.

The order Rodentia comprises the most numerous species of all mammals and includes 2 suborders, one of which, the Hystricognathi, describes guinea pigs and chinchillas. The suborder name derives from the Latin word hystrix (porcupine), in recognition of the porcupinelike nature of these animals. Guinea pigs and chinchillas normally have life expectancies between 5 and 10 years. Improved knowledge of proper diets, husbandry, and veterinary care has led to an improved quality of life and client satisfaction.

Guinea pigs (*Cavia porcellus*), also known as cavies, are classified as members of the family Cavidae and are represented by 14 species. Chinchillas belong to the family Chinchillidae and are represented by 6 species, including long-tailed chinchillas (*Chinchilla laniger*) and short-tailed chinchillas (*Chinchilla brevicaudata*).

Both of these hystricomorph rodents come from South America. Guinea pigs inhabit rocky areas, forest edges, and also swamps in Venezuela, Colombia, Brazil, and Argentina. Chinchillas are rare in the wild and may even be extinct,[1] although other researchers report that *C laniger* may be found in arid areas of the northern Chilean Andes inhabiting rocky crevices at elevations between 3000 and 5000 m; however, the short-tailed species (*C brevicaudata*) has been reported rare or possibly extinct in the wild.[2]

[a] Private Practice, Centro Veterinario México, Cincinnati 22, Colonia Ciudad de los Deportes, 03710 Mexico, DF, México
[b] Department of Ethology, Wildlife and Laboratory Animals, School of Veterinary Medicine, National Autonomus University of Mexico, Ciudad Universitaria 3000, Copilco Universidad, 04360 México, DF, México
* González Calderón 18, Observatorio, CP 11860, México, DF, México.
E-mail address: eyarto@imfac.net

Vet Clin Exot Anim 14 (2011) 339–355
doi:10.1016/j.cvex.2011.03.008
1094-9194/11/$ – see front matter © 2011 Elsevier Inc. All rights reserved.

The word rodent derives from the Latin verb rodere, meaning to gnaw. Although the dental formulas of members of this animal order vary, guinea pigs and chinchillas share the following dental formula:

I 1/1, C 0/0, PM 1/1, M 3/3 = 20

Incisors grow continuously in rodents, a trait classified as elodont. Cheek teeth classification further identifies rodents. The teeth of guinea pigs and chinchillas have long, continuously growing crowns (hypsodont) and no anatomic root (aradicular), whereas rats, mice, and hamsters have short-crowned molars with roots (brachydont) that stop growing once fully erupted.[3–5] Guinea pigs and chinchillas have a diastema, or gap, between the incisors and the cheek teeth, a trait they share with rabbits.[1,4,5]

Dental anatomic adaptations are important in rodent classification, as are features related to feeding habits. The teeth of guinea pigs and chinchillas teeth are adapted to a more abrasive and voluminous diet and have larger chewing surfaces necessary for an herbivorous diet, which also implies pronounced wear in time from prolonged chewing. This cheek teeth wearing is compensated for by constant growth of premolars and molars.[3,5] Guinea pigs exhibit a maxilla wider than the mandible, with a marked occlusal angle of the cheek teeth, in comparison with other rodents.[6]

As with all rodents, the enamel on the incisors of guinea pigs and chinchillas is deposited unevenly (absent on the lingual surface, slight deposition on the mesial and distal surfaces, and full deposition on the labial surface). This feature allows the continuously growing incisor to wear through abrasion, without which the tooth would become too long and prevent feeding. It also helps to sharpen the incisors. The superficial layer of the enamel is pigmented yellow-orange in most rodents, but not in guinea pigs, whose incisors are white.[2–4]

NUTRITION AND HUSBANDRY REQUIREMENTS OF GUINEA PIGS AND CHINCHILLAS
Nutrition

Guinea pigs
In the past, low-quality guinea pig diets with imbalanced mineral concentrations (rich in calcium and phosphorus and deficient in magnesium) were associated with metastatic calcification of soft tissues around elbows and ribs, leading to a wrist stiffness syndrome. Mineralization also involved lungs, aorta, heart, kidneys, sclera, and uterus. The incidence of this condition has been reduced in the last few years because guinea pigs are now generally fed high-quality diets manufactured and balanced according to their specific nutritional requirements.[7]

Guinea pigs, like other mammals (nonhuman primates, humans, and some bat species), require a dietary source of vitamin C (ascorbic acid) because they lack L-gulonolactone oxidase, a hepatic enzyme that converts glucose into ascorbic acid.[2,8]

Vitamin C deficiency may be an underlying factor for any illness in the guinea pig: it produces scurvy, the main clinical signs of which can range from the acute form, with painful joints, generalized immobility, and anorexia, to the chronic form of the disease, characterized by weakness, diarrhea, anorexia, petechia of the mucous membranes, and recurrent chronic diseases including pneumonia and other infections (Fig. 1).[1,7,9,10]

Scurvy in guinea pigs is prevented by the use of proper species-specific commercial diets in which a stable form of vitamin C (as L-ascorbyl 1–2-polyphosphate) is added to the formulation. However, oxidation may deplete the levels of vitamin C in these diets even 90 days after production, and some investigators recommend that supplemental

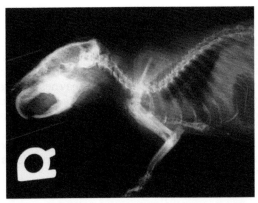

Fig. 1. Cavy radiograph lateral thorax. Pneumonia, dyspnea secondary to vitamin C deficiency. (*Courtesy of* Cathy A. Johnson-Delaney, DVM, Dipl ABVP [Avian], Edmonds, WA.)

ascorbic acid be provided (10 mg/kg daily for nonbreeding animals, 30 mg/kg daily for pregnant sows).[11]

Some investigators recommend supplementing ascorbic acid in the drinking water, but that may add an unpleasant flavor to the water, resulting in refusal to drink and subsequent dehydration. A variety of fresh greens such as cabbage, kale, dandelion, and parsley contain high levels of vitamin C and can be used both for dietary supplementation and environmental enrichment.[2,12]

Another option is the use of specifically manufactured vitamin C supplements in the form of tablets for guinea pigs (Oxbow, Inc, Murdoch, NE, USA).[6,12]

Besides a commercial food and fresh vegetables, high-fiber hay such as grass hay or timothy hay must be offered ad libitum to promote normal gastrointestinal tract function, teeth wearing, and overall health.[11] Because of their high calcium content, clover and alfalfa hays should not be provided because they may cause calcification within the renal system in adults. Guinea pigs consume considerable amounts of food during the day, although maximal intake normally occurs during the late afternoon and evening.[7]

Chinchillas

Chinchillas also require a high-fiber (15%–30% bulk fiber) diet. Pellets manufactured for these rodents should be longer than those for rabbits or guinea pigs to allow easy consumption. The amount of pellets offered daily for a chinchilla must be limited (only 1–2 tablespoons), but high-quality grass hay should be provided in an unlimited fashion.[2,11] Chinchillas must have access to their feed mainly at night because they generally eat most of their daily ration at this time.[7]

Other important nutrients that may affect the overall health of chinchillas include unsaturated fatty acids and vitamin A.[13]

Housing and Bedding

Guinea pigs easily adapt to a variety of climates, although the preferred ambient temperatures for this species range from 18 to 26°C(65–79°F); guinea pigs are more tolerant of heat than chinchillas.[7] Nevertheless, they should not be exposed to high temperatures and humidity.[1]

Chinchillas do best at temperatures ranging from 10 to 20°C (50–60°F) with a humidity less than 40%, so are more tolerant of cold and sensitive to heat.[1,2,7,13,14]

Dust baths should be made available to chinchillas for grooming purposes on a daily basis or at least several times a week; however, excessive use of dust baths could potentially be associated with conjunctivitis and upper respiratory disease.[2,13,14]

Generally, wood shavings are not recommended as a bedding material or substrate for rodents because aromatic hydrocarbons in shavings may cause respiratory problems[7,15]; aromatic oils found in cedar and pine shavings may be important respiratory irritants.[6] More appropriate bedding materials for guinea pigs, chinchillas, and other rodents are newspaper, shredded paper, pelleted recycled paper, aspen shavings, or hay.[1,2,6,16]

Unsanitary conditions including a lack of bedding change and enclosure cleaning can predispose chinchillas and guinea pigs to respiratory problems, pododermatitis, and other health issues.[17]

Behavior

Cavies are not tolerant of abrupt modifications in their environment; even changes in texture, shape, color, or taste of the food or water may lead to refusal to eat or drink.[12]

Knowledge of normal and abnormal behavior in cavies is useful to detect disease signs. Healthy guinea pigs are active, have bright eyes, do not have any nasal or ocular discharge, and have a shiny coat. Lethargy, rough hair coats, and unfocused eyes may indicate disease, including respiratory problems.[12] Clinical signs of pain in guinea pigs such as rapid, shallow breathing and pale mucous membranes may be confused with respiratory signs.[12]

Like most small mammals, chinchillas do not show abnormal behaviors until they exhibit chronic and advanced stages of disease. Being obligate nasal breathers, dyspnea in chinchillas is exhibited only when they undergo severe respiratory compromise.[14]

ANATOMY AND PHYSIOLOGY OF THE RESPIRATORY SYSTEM

In guinea pigs and chinchillas, the oral cavity is small and narrow, and the soft palate extends to the base of the tongue[2,18]; the large and elongated tongue covers most of the floor of the mouth and oropharynx. The soft palate has a small opening called the palatal ostium, which connects the oropharynx with the pharynx (**Fig. 2**).[2,18]

The larynx in these rodents lies dorsally within the oropharynx in close association with the nasopharynx, which makes them obligate nasal breathers. This anatomic feature makes intubation challenging in guinea pigs and chinchillas without the aid of an endoscope.[19–21]

The previously mentioned anatomic features and adaptations to increased airflow make guinea pigs, chinchillas, and other rodents prone to respiratory tract disease such as bacterial invasion.[6,19]

Guinea pigs possess an acute sense of smell, because the caudodorsal nasal cavity is lined by a sensitive olfactory epithelium.[18] Cavies possess a larynx formed by 5 cartilages (epiglottis, thyroid, cricoid, and paired arytenoids), have no laryngeal ventricle, and their vocal folds are small; however, they still command a wide vocal repertoire.[1,2,18,22]

The right lung in cavies is divided into 3 lobes (cranial, caudal, and accessory), whereas the left lung is composed of 4 lobes (cranial, middle, caudal, and accessory) (**Fig. 3**). Chinchillas follow the same pattern.[1,2,23]

The thymus in guinea pigs is located surrounding the trachea instead of lying within the thoracic cavity as in other rodent species.[2]

Lungs are small in guinea pigs because the heart occupies a large portion of the thoracic cavity (**Fig. 4**).[22]

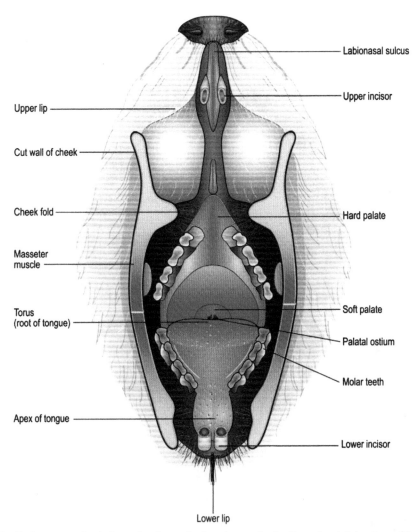

Labionasal sulcus

Upper incisor

Upper lip

Cut wall of cheek

Cheek fold

Masseter
muscle

Torus
(root of tongue)

Apex of tongue

Hard palate

Soft palate

Palatal ostium

Molar teeth

Lower incisor

Lower lip

Fig. 2. Open-mouthed view of guinea pig showing molar teeth and palatal ostium. (*From* Popesko P, Rajtova V, Horak J. A colour atlas of anatomy of small laboratory animals. Vol. 1: rabbit, guinea pig. Elsevier; 1992. p. 189; with permission.)

Unusual Anatomic Characteristics of Guinea Pigs and Chinchillas

Bony spicules composed of dense lamellar bone with different degrees of calcification may appear radiologically in the lungs of guinea pigs and, although there is not reaction in adjacent alveolar septa, these fragments can be misinterpreted as inhaled foreign bodies of bone. These fragments could be diagnosed as osseous metaplasia from a neoplasia, but these are normal radiographic findings.[7]

Reflecting their nocturnal nature, the chinchilla eye has a large cornea, a sensitive retina, a shallow orbit, and a densely pigmented iris.[2,7] Lesions to eye tissues may lead to corneal ulceration and conjunctivitis, which might be confused with, and must be ruled out from, upper respiratory disease.

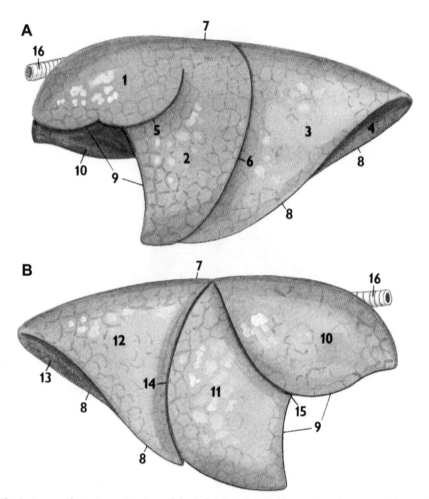

Fig. 3. Lungs of a guinea pig: view of the left (*A*) and right (*B*) costal surfaces. Cranial part of cranial lobe (1), caudal part of cranial lobe (2), caudal lobe (3, 4), cranial lobe (10), medial lobe (11), caudal lobe (12, 13). (*From* Popesko P, Rajtova V, Horak J. A colour atlas of anatomy of small laboratory animals. Vol. 1: rabbit, guinea pig. Elsevier; 1992. p. 189; with permission.)

RESPIRATORY DISEASE IN GUINEA PIGS AND CHINCHILLAS

A handful of factors are involved in the development of respiratory disease in guinea pigs and chinchillas. Among them are overcrowding, improper nutrition, and housing-related issues (poor ventilation, sudden changes in humidity and temperature gradients, cold or hot weather, dusty environments).[15,19]

The exotic pet clinician should use husbandry and nutrition history along with clinical examination to try to identify the factors that could potentially predispose or worsen respiratory disease in each case.[6,19]

Pneumonia is a common disease in guinea pigs and chinchillas when they are housed in damp and drafty conditions, but can occur in any individual (**Fig. 5**).[19,23,24]

Many different pathogens can cause respiratory disease in guinea pigs and chinchillas, including bacterial, viral, and fungal pathogens. Other conditions including

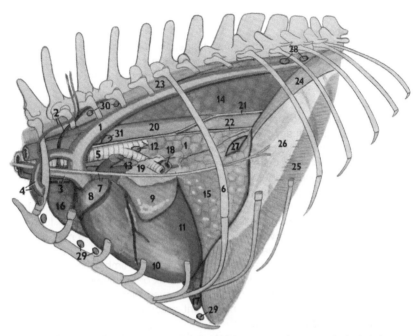

Fig. 4. Lateral view of the thoracic cavity of a guinea pig. Right ventricle (10), left ventricle (11), right accessory lobe of lung (15). (*From* Popesko P, Rajtova V, Horak J. A colour atlas of anatomy of small laboratory animals. Vol. 1: rabbit, guinea pig. Elsevier; 1992. p. 189; with permission.)

cancer, toxins, trauma, foreign-body inhalation, and cardiac disease may affect the respiratory tract and express themselves as respiratory clinical signs.[20,25]

Bacterial

Guinea pigs

There are several bacterial species that can cause pneumonia in guinea pigs, although *Bordetella bronchiseptica* and *Streptococcus pneumoniae* are most frequently

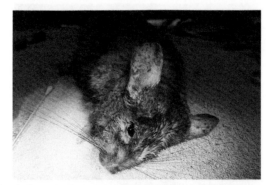

Fig. 5. Sedated chinchilla with chronic ocular discharge and dyspnea related to pneumonia. Husbandry was changed to decrease humidity (removed plastic cover over dustbath frequented by chinchilla). The humidity was high and ventilation poor. (*Courtesy of* Cathy A. Johnson-Delaney, DVM, Dipl ABVP [Avian], Edmonds, WA.)

associated with this condition.[7,25] Both organisms can be found in humans or become a potential zoonotic disease.[11]

Inappropriate husbandry conditions can trigger *B bronchiseptica* infection (**Fig. 6**), because such infections can be expressed when the carrier guinea pig is stressed, or may be acquired from other pets such as dogs or rabbits when all of the species are housed in close proximity.[2,6,20,24]

Infection by *S pneumonia* in guinea pigs can cause pleuropneumonia (presenting similar clinical signs as pneumonia caused by *Bordetella*), pleuritis, and peritonitis. This pathogen is also transmitted by asymptomatic carriers of different species by direct contact, by aerosolization, and on fomites.[6,24,25]

Clinical signs of bacterial pneumonia in guinea pigs are anorexia, ocular and nasal discharge, abnormal respiratory sounds (wheezing, gurgling), lethargy, and sneezing; signs may progress to tachypnea and or dyspnea.[2,6,7,11,25]

Diagnosis of bacterial respiratory disease may be made on evaluation of history, physical examination, and radiographic signs. Consolidation of the lung lobes, bronchioalveolar patterns, as well as exudate-filled tympanic bullae may be present in chronic/advanced cases assessed by radiographic studies.[2,11,23] Care is advised when positioning the patient for radiographs, because the limbs should be extended to avoid rotation and superimposition over the thorax or abdomen.[6]

Confirmation of bacterial diseases can be achieved though microbiology (culture and sensitivity), enzyme-linked immunosorbent assay (ELISA) of the exudates, and indirect immunofluorescence tests.[6,7,11]

Guinea pigs that recover from respiratory disease caused by *Bordetella* species may continue as carriers, so care should be taken not to house them with cagemates and to avoid stressful husbandry situations.[2]

In a group of guinea pigs, *S pneumoniae* infection caused arthritis lesions identified at necropsy as well as pleuritis, pleural effusion, and lung abscesses, which are common postmortem findings in affected individuals.[6]

Treatment options for bacterial pneumonia in guinea pigs include antibiotics (chloramphenicol palmitate, trimethoprim sulfa, and enrofloxacin) for 7 to 21 days depending on the culture/sensitivity results.[2,11] See **Table 1** for antibiotic dosages.

Supportive therapies include analgesics, oxygen and fluid support, vitamin C supplementation, nebulization, and modification of husbandry and nutrition where indicated.[2,7,11]

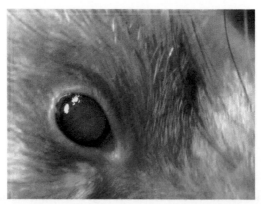

Fig. 6. Cavy with *B bronchiseptica* had corneal lesion, iritis, a possible cataract, and chronic conjunctivitis. The cavy was from a pet store where rabbits and guinea pigs were housed together. (*Courtesy of* Cathy A. Johnson-Delaney, DVM, Dipl ABVP [Avian], Edmonds, WA.)

Table 1
Suggested antibiotics for respiratory disease treatment in guinea pigs and chinchillas

Antibiotic	Dose (mg/kg)	Route	Frequency	Observations
Cefalexin	50	IM	Divided every 12 h	For parenteral use only. May be a cause of dysbiosis
Ceftiofur	1	IM	Once a day	For parenteral use only. May be a cause of dysbiosis
Cephaloridine	10–25	IM	Every 8–12 h	For parenteral use only in guinea pigs
Chloramphenicol	20–50	PO	Every 12 h	
Ciprofloxacin	10	PO	Every 12–24 h	
Enrofloxacin	5–15	PO, SC, IM	Every 12 h	Parenteral injection may cause tissue necrosis if not diluted
Gentamicin	5	SC, IM	Divided every 12 h	Used in synergy with other antibiotics to treat respiratory disease in mammals
Trimethoprim sulfa	15–30	PO, SC	Twice a day	Tissue necrosis may occur when administered SC

Abbreviations: IM, intramuscularly; PO, orally; SC, subcutaneously.
Data from Refs.[2,6,17]

For *B bronchiseptica* infections in guinea pigs, a treatment option making use of an autogenous bacterin is available.[6]

Preventive measures include housing guinea pigs as a single individual or species and far from other potential carriers.[6]

Other bacteria that have been linked to bacterial respiratory disease in guinea pigs are *Haemophilus* species (recovered from the respiratory tract of cavies) and *Streptobacillus moniliformis* (a zoonotic disease from rats that has been implicated in cervical lymphadenitis in guinea pigs).[6,7]

Yersinia pseudotuberculosis can cause septicemic pneumonia in guinea pigs, with death occurring rapidly.[26]

There are reports of cases of pneumonia in guinea pigs involving other bacterial species in addition to those listed earlier. These species include *Staphylococcus aureus* (**Fig. 7**), *Streptococcus pyogenes*, and *Citrobacter freundii* (this is an occasional opportunistic pathogen in guinea pigs and there is a report of fibrinopurulent pleuropneumonia and septic thrombi in the lung, liver, and spleen in one colony of animals).[25]

Cervical lymphadenitis in guinea pigs is caused by *Streptococcus zooepidemicus*, Lancefield group C, and occasionally by *S moniliformis*. The former is part of the normal flora of the nasal cavity and conjunctiva in guinea pigs, and resembles pneumococcal disease. Lesions on the oral mucosa may predispose the animal to bacteria invading the cervical lymph nodes, and sometimes even becoming a systemic disease resulting in necrotizing bronchopneumonia.[24,25]

Treatment is intended to remove the abscess from the lymph nodes (when a sample for culture and sensitivity is taken), along with a broad-spectrum antibiotic. Prevention involves good husbandry management.[24]

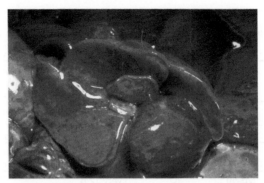

Fig. 7. Cavy pneumonia: gross photograph of the lung. Cultured as *S aureus* coagulase positive, although streptococcal pneumonias are more common and grossly appear the same. (*Courtesy of* Cathy A. Johnson-Delaney, DVM, Dipl ABVP [Avian], Edmonds, WA.)

Chlamydophilosis caused by *Chlamydophila caviae* and also by *C psittaci* (**Fig. 8**) have been reported in guinea pigs, progressing from conjunctivitis and rhinitis to bronchitis and pneumonia. Stress could be a triggering factor. Diagnosis is achieved by cytology, polymerase chain reaction (PCR) of conjunctival scrapings, and at necropsy (submitted samples for histopathology and/or immunohistochemistry). Recently, it has been reported that topical treatment with ointments or drops of tetracyclines or fluoroquinolone might be useful for treating mild cases, or systemic antibiotic therapy such as oral enrofloxacin or parenterally administered doxycycline for more severe cases.[2]

Supportive care for respiratory disease in guinea pigs is the same as for other bacterial diseases.[22]

Chinchillas

Some bacterial species such as *S pneumoniae*, *Pseudomonas*, and *Pasteurella pneumotropica* are part of the normal flora of the respiratory tract of the chinchilla. Nevertheless, pneumonia as a primary disease or as a progression from the upper

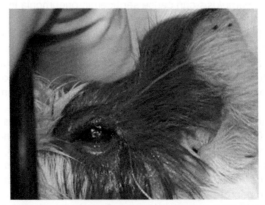

Fig. 8. Guinea pig with confirmed *Chlamydophila psittaci* conjunctivitis, with upper and lower respiratory disease. (*Courtesy of* Cathy A. Johnson-Delaney, DVM, Dipl ABVP [Avian], Edmonds, WA.)

respiratory tract can be caused by *B bronchiseptica* and invasion of the *S pneumoniae* that inhabit the respiratory tract, in stressful conditions.[15,23]

Diagnosis, treatment, supportive care, and prevention are managed as for bacterial respiratory disease in guinea pigs.[23]

An outbreak report of *Klebsiella pneumoniae* infection in chinchillas describes affected animals showing signs of respiratory distress, anorexia, and diarrhea. Postmortem examination findings were suppurative pneumonia and renal tubular necrosis.[27]

Antibiotic Treatment Considerations in Rodents

The ideal antibiotic for rodents and small mammals would be easily administered, bactericidal, and free of antibiotic-induced gastrointestinal disease.[28] Most of the information related to dosing, efficacy, and adverse reactions of antibiotics in rodents is anecdotal, based on clinical experience or extrapolated from other companion animals. Well-known uses for antibiotic therapy in rodents include respiratory disease.[28,29]

Some gram-positive spectrum antibiotics (β-lactams, macrolides, lincosamides) can lead to depletion of normal gut flora and overgrowth of opportunists such as *Clostridium spiroforme*, and *E coli*, especially when these drugs are administer orally.[6,29] The main antibiotic toxicity mechanism in rodents is the disruption of the normal enteric flora (dysbiosis), causing potentially fatal gastrointestinal disease.[29] Overgrowth of opportunistic species contributes to cecal hypotony, with consequent fluid and gas distention.[28,29]

Some of the safer drugs reported for rodent antibiotic treatment include trimethoprim sulfas, chloramphenicol, fluoroquinolones, aminoglycosides, and metronidazole. Nonetheless, some toxic doses of antibiotics that are considered safe (eg, gentamicin) can occur in rodents.[28,29]

Other antibiotics are classified as intermediate in their ability to cause gastrointestinal flora alterations. These antibiotics include parenteral penicillin, oral or injectable cephalosporins, tetracycline, and erythromycin.[11,28]

Ideally, before instituting antibiotics, the clinician should obtain a culture and a minimum database. Not all small mammals die from antibiotic-induced gastrointestinal disease, but the risk of toxicity is reduced when the appropriate treatment is selected.[28]

Viral

Guinea pigs

During the last decade, it was published that bronchopneumonia and death in guinea pigs could be caused by a presumed guinea pig adenovirus.

This respiratory disease has been shown in colonies of cavies during outbreaks of pneumonia. Although the morbidity is considered low, mortality with an acute death is high. A transient subclinical infection caused by the adenovirus is possible in this species of rodent.[2,6,24] However, in at least 1 report, the researchers were not able to experimentally induce the disease in adult guinea pigs, and only in neonatal cavies was the experimental infection possible after exposing the animals to severe stress.[30]

The incubation period of the adenovirus in guinea pigs ranges from 5 to 10 days, and stress may play a role in the development of this infection, which may be suspected when a respiratory disease nonresponsive to antibiotics is present in guinea pigs.[2,6]

Clinical signs of viral pneumonia in guinea pigs include dyspnea, tachypnea, nasal discharge, lethargy, and a hunched posture, or acute death with no clinical signs.[31]

Some reports of infection with adenovirus in guinea pigs do not specify any concurrent clinical signs.[31]

Lesions in diseased lungs are consistent with pulmonary consolidation and emphysema with petechiae; histopathology may reveal necrotizing, exfoliative bronchiolitis with basophilic intranuclear inclusion bodies.[24,31]

Serologic testing is available for the diagnosis of this disease,[2] although it is not a commercial test. Identification of nucleic acids of the DNA adenovirus has been achieved by the use of PCR assay. This PCR test proved that the guinea pig adenovirus was distinct from other adenoviruses.[6,30]

Other factors, such as immune status alteration, poor husbandry, and improper nutritional management, are needed to induce adenoviral respiratory disease in guinea pigs.[31] Because adenoviral infection is self-limiting like other viral infections, supportive care is the only suggested therapy.

Chinchillas

Chinchillas are used as research animals for viral respiratory infections and bacterial associations in human medicine. One report in the late 1990s described the development of otitis media when these rodents were inoculated with pneumococci and influenza A virus in 67% of the chinchilla population, versus 21% when the animals were inoculated with S pneumoniae alone. In the case of chinchillas infected with influenza virus alone, only 4% developed otitis.[32]

These findings do not support that natural infection of chinchillas by the influenza A virus can occur, but they do support the synergy of a viral infection compared with infection with a sole agent in this species of rodents.

Another report on viral disease in a chinchilla with conjunctivitis, uveitis, and neurologic signs has been linked to the infection of the rodent with human herpes simplex virus type 1. Among the pathologic findings in this case, keratouveitis, retinopathy, and unilateral purulent rhinitis were reported,[31] so it is possible that, in the predisposing conditions, this virus could potentially lead to clinical signs that could induce respiratory disease infections in chinchillas.

Fungal Diseases with Respiratory Signs in Rodents

There are only 2 reports of histoplasmosis (Histoplasma capsulatum) affecting chinchillas. In one of the published studies, 17:130 chinchillas died of respiratory disease; confirmation of this fungal agent was achieved exclusively in 1 animal. However, this disease should be considered in companion chinchillas and other rodents because the fungal agent was cultured from food (timothy hay).[33]

Lesions on the lung tissues at necropsy were hemorrhagic foci, alveolar consolidation, and bronchopneumonia.[27]

Adiaspiromycosis caused by Chrysosporium parvum and C crescens can induce respiratory infection in many rodents, leading to macroscopic findings at necropsy such as gray nodules on the lung surface warranting diagnostic studies to identify spherules and conidias in tissues for histopathology and isolation of the fungus.[33]

Systemic antifungal therapy is indicated only for systemic mycoses or resistant cutaneous infections in rodents, because of the danger of adverse effects and overdosing.[33]

Neoplasia

Tumors of the respiratory system

In guinea pigs, bronchogenic papillary adenoma is the most commonly reported tumor, reaching a prevalence of 35% of all neoplasms in this rodent species. It is more common after 3 years of age, and it can be misdiagnosed for pneumonia, a fairly common diagnosis in guinea pigs.[6,34] This tumor is slow growing and does not metastasize, but it does reduce functional lung volume.[23]

Many other tumor types occurring in guinea pigs have been reported, such as bronchogenic and alveologenic adenocarcinoma, and 1 malignant mixed tumor of the mammary gland metastasized to the lungs.[34]

Lymphosarcoma and leukemia in guinea pigs are associated with a type C retrovirus, affecting the mediastinal lymph nodes and leading to dyspnea, so these types of cancer must be taken into account when ruling out respiratory disease in guinea pigs.[19]

Among the most useful diagnostic methods for respiratory disease in rodents are thoracic radiographic studies, which can help the clinician to rule out neoplasia.[6,34]

Reports of neoplasia are rare in chinchillas.[27] There is 1 report of a tumor related to the respiratory system: an adenocarcinoma of the lung. No detailed pathologic descriptions of the organ involved are provided.[34]

Miscellaneous Conditions

Inflammation of the nares in chinchillas
Inflammation of the nares in chinchillas may occur as a precursor to upper respiratory disease, causing the animal to rub its nose frequently. Sometimes a nasal discharge can be seen and, in other more severe cases, infection may damage the nasal sinuses or even cause inflammation that induces meningitis.[13]

Treatment consists of broad-spectrum antibiotics, supportive care including analgesics, and removal of dust baths until the chinchillas' clinical signs have improved.[13]

Heatstroke
Both guinea pigs and chinchillas are susceptible to heat stress because the 2 species are native to cooler regions in South America.

Clinical signs of heatstroke are rapid breathing, thick salivation, lethargy, pale mucous membranes, poor peripheral perfusion, and rectal temperature greater than 39.4°C(103.5°F).[24,27] Diagnosis is made through the history and clinical signs.[2]

Treatment of heatstroke consists of supportive care including cooling the patient in an immersion bath of cool water, parenteral fluids, and, in the case of guinea pigs, corticosteroids may be considered.[6,24,27] Other therapies include antibiotic prevention of clostridial overgrowth, prokinetic drugs, and cholestyramine to prevent endotoxemia.[2] Prognosis is generally guarded.[6,24]

Cardiovascular diseases
Cardiovascular diseases can induce respiratory signs in guinea pigs and chinchillas, and represent another clue for differential diagnosis for the clinician. In guinea pigs, cardiovascular diseases including cardiomyopathy, pericardial effusion, and metastatic or dystrophic mineralization lead to dyspnea, tachypnea, tachycardia, pale mucous membranes, and weakness, among other signs.[6,35] Anecdotal practitioner reports suggest that cardiovascular disease may be common in chinchillas.[27,35]

Diagnosis of cardiac disease in guinea pigs and chinchillas includes observation of cardiac impulse by auscultation or by Doppler probe, careful detection of heart rate and respiratory rate, electrocardiograph, and radiographs. Alveolar edema of cardiac origin and tracheal elevation caused by cardiomegaly can be observed radiographically. Other radiological respiratory signs in rodents with cardiac disease are pleural edema and pleural effusion.[6,35]

Ultrasound showing lung consolidation, and thoracocentesis or pleurocentesis for ruling out infectious and neoplastic causes of effusion, are among other diagnostic techniques for cardiac disease in rodent species.[35]

More research is needed to improve cardiac disease treatment in rodents, although valuable information can be obtained from the laboratory rodent literature and other companion animals.[2,27,35]

Toxicoses

Avocado (Persea americana)

In guinea pigs and other exotic species, leaves, fruit, bark, and seeds of the avocado have been reported to be toxic. The most common clinical signs of avocado toxicosis are respiratory distress, hydropericardium, generalized congestion, anasarca, and death. Avocado toxicosis must be considered when a rodent is presented with respiratory distress and history suggests the possible ingestion of avocado.

Treatment includes toxin removal using activated charcoal, gastric lavage, bulking diets to prevent absorption, oxygen therapy, and diuretics, depending on each case.[36]

Anticoagulant rodenticides

Short-acting (warfarin) and long-acting (pindone, diphacinone, difethialone, chlorophacinone, brodifacoum, and bromadiolone) rodenticides are related to clinical signs such as hemorrhage, pale mucous membranes, dyspnea, coughing, exercise intolerance, and weakness. History is of utmost importance for the clinician to diagnose rodent intoxication with any of these products.[26]

For a rodent or a small mammal exposed to anticoagulants, treatment includes vitamin K therapy (3–5 mg/kg/d orally, divided into 2 or 3 doses) instead of monitoring clotting times. Decontamination is only effective on recently exposed asymptomatic animals.[36] Supportive therapy is advised according to the clinical signs of each patient.

Inhalation Pneumonia

Inhalation pneumonia is a common problem in hand-reared young animals of any species. It often occurs when liquid enters the trachea when a neonate is fed. It may also occur in a clinical setting when administering liquid medications to convalescent, hospitalized patients.

Clinical signs are similar to infectious pneumonia, such as dyspnea, tachypnea, audible respiratory sounds, and pyrexia. Treatment is frequently unrewarding.[13]

RESPIRATORY EMERGENCY MEDICINE

Rodents are commonly presented to the clinician as emergency and critical care patients. Respiratory emergencies may present with pulmonary contusions, pneumonia, electrocution, and foreign-body inhalation/aspiration. The patients may present with variable signs, including dyspnea, pale mucous membranes, nasal discharge, and sometimes a sudden onset of respiratory distress that may be caused by foreign-body inhalation/aspiration.[20]

In guinea pigs and chinchillas, the presence of the palatal ostium (the fusion of the soft palate to the base of the tongue) also complicates orotracheal intubation. In emergency situations in which the clinician wants to provide assisted ventilation, a tracheostomy may be used to access the trachea.[20]

Diagnosis of respiratory emergencies in rodents involves radiographs in which pericardial effusion, pulmonary edema, pulmonary contusions, rib fractures, and/or pneumothorax or hemothorax may be seen, depending on the origin of the disease.[20,37]

Ultrasound is suggested for the evaluation of the thoracic cavity and, if heart disease is suspected, as well as for the diagnosis of some lung lesions like pulmonary consolidation.[20]

Emergency treatment includes oxygen support, proper temperature provision (avoiding hypothermia or hyperthermia), nonsteroidal anti-inflammatory drugs and sedation when required, fluid therapy, broad-spectrum antibiotics, bronchodilators, nebulization, and minimal patient handling.[20,37]

When foreign-body inhalation/aspiration is suspected, saline nebulization is recommended to deliver moisture to the upper respiratory passages and help with the dissolution of food material.[20]

Thoracocentesis using the same technique as for other companion mammals is warranted when fluid is present within the thoracic cavity, as part of the respiratory disease process.[20]

Once the patient is stabilized, or during emergency treatment, samples for cultures obtained from tracheal or bronchoalveolar lavage should be considered and pathogens involved treated accordingly.

SUMMARY

Respiratory diseases are common in guinea pigs and chinchillas. There are multifactorial causes of respiratory involvement in these species of rodents, from infectious (bacterial, viral, and fungal) to neoplastic causes. Toxicoses and diseases affecting other systems may also induce respiratory signs. Knowledge of biology, including husbandry, nutritional requirements, and behavior, are important clues for the clinician to determine the role these issues may play in the development, progression, and prognosis of respiratory clinical cases in rodents. Current approaches in the diagnosis and therapy for respiratory disease in small mammals warrant more research concerning response-to-treatment reports.

REFERENCES

1. Quesenberry KE, Donelly TM, Hillyer EV. Biology, husbandry, and clinical techniques of guinea pigs and chinchillas. In: Quesenberry KE, Carpenter JW, editors. Ferrets, rabbits and rodents, Clinical medicine and surgery. 2nd edition. St Louis (MO): Saunders; 2004. p. 232–44.
2. Johnson-Delaney C. Guinea pigs, chinchillas, degus and duprasi. In: Meredith A, Johnson-Delaney C, editors. BSAVA manual of exotic pets. 5th edition. Gloucester (United Kingdom): British Small Animal Veterinary Association; 2010. p. 28–62.
3. Legendre LF. Oral disorders of exotic rodents. Vet Clin North Am Exot Anim Pract 2003;6(3):601–28.
4. Capello V, Gracis M, Lennox A. Rabbit and rodent dentistry handbook. Hoboken (NJ): Wiley-Blackwell; 2005.
5. Klaphake E. Common rodent procedures. Vet Clin North Am Exot Anim Pract 2006;9:389–413.
6. Riggs SM. Guinea pigs. In: Mitchell MA, Tully TN, editors. Manual of exotic pet practice. St Louis (MO): Saunders Elsevier; 2009. p. 456–73.
7. Donelly TM, Brown CJ. Guinea pig and chinchilla care and husbandry. Vet Clin North Am Exot Anim Pract 2004;7(2):351–73.
8. Dempsey JL. Advances of fruit bat nutrition. In: Fowler ME, Miller RE, editors. Zoo and wild animal medicine, Current therapy. 4th edition. Philadelphia: WB Saunders; 1999. p. 354–9.

9. Clarke GL, Allen AM, Small JD, et al. Subclinical scurvy in the guinea pig. Vet Pathol 1980;17:40–4.
10. Jenkins JR. Diseases of geriatric guinea pigs and chinchillas. Vet Clin North Am Exot Anim Pract 2010;13(1):85–93.
11. Tamura Y. Current approach to rodents as patients. J Exot Pet Med 2010;19(1): 36–55.
12. Bradley T. Guinea pig behavior. In: Bradley Y, Lightfoot T, Mayer J, editors. Exotic pet behavior, birds, reptiles and small mammals. St Louis (MO): Saunders Elsevier; 2006. p. 207–38.
13. Richardson VC. Chinchillas. In: Richardson VCG, editor. Diseases of small domestic rodents. 2nd edition. Oxford (United Kingdom): Blackwell Publishing; 2003. p. 1–53.
14. Johnson DH. Miscellaneous small mammal behavior: chinchillas. In: Bradley Y, Lightfoot T, Mayer J, editors. Exotic pet behavior, birds, reptiles and small mammals. St Louis (MO): Saunders Elsevier; 2006. p. 263–80.
15. Harkness JE, Wagner JE. Specific diseases and conditions. In: Harkness JE, Wagner JE, editors. The biology and medicine of rabbits and rodents. 4th edition. Philadelphia: Williams & Wilkins; 1995. p. 171–322.
16. Brown CJ, Donelly TM. Rodent husbandry and care. Vet Clin North Am Exot Anim Pract 2004;7:201–25.
17. Riggs SM, Mitchell MA. Chinchillas. In: Mitchell MA, Tully TN, editors. Manual of exotic pet practice. St Louis (MO): Saunders Elsevier; 2009. p. 474–91.
18. O'Malley B. Guinea pigs. In: O'Malley MA, editor. Clinical anatomy and physiology of exotic species. Structure and function of mammals, birds and reptiles and amphibians. London: Elsevier Saunders; 2005. p. 197–208.
19. Longley LA. Rodent anesthesia. In: Longley LA, editor. Anaesthesia of exotic pets. London: Saunders Elsevier; 2008. p. 59–84.
20. Hawkins MG, Graham JE. Emergency and critical care of rodents. Vet Clin North Am Exot Anim Pract 2007;10:501–31.
21. Divers SJ. Small mammal anesthesia. In: Proceedings of exotic animal medicine for the clinical practitioner of the American Association of Zoo Veterinarians, Conference. Los Angeles (CA): AAZV; 2008.
22. Johnson-Delaney C, Orosz SE. The respiratory system: exotic companion mammals. In: Proceedings of the 30th Annual Association of Avian Veterinarians Conference and Expo with the AEMV. Milwaukee (WI): AEMV; 2009. p. 41–9.
23. Girling S. Common diseases of small mammals. In: Girling S, editor. Veterinary nursing of exotic pets. Oxford (United Kingdom): Blackwell Publishing; 2003. p. 257–84.
24. O'Rourke DP. Disease problems of guinea pigs. In: Quesenberry KE, Carpenter JW, editors. Ferrets, rabbits and rodents: clinical medicine and surgery. 2nd edition. St Louis (MO): Saunders; 2004. p. 245–54.
25. Schoeb TR. Respiratory diseases of rodents. Vet Clin North Am Exot Anim Pract 2000;3(2):481–96.
26. Rigby C. Natural infections of guinea pigs. Lab Anim 1976;10:119–42.
27. Donnelly T. Disease problems of chinchillas. In: Quesenberry KE, Carpenter JW, editors. Ferrets, rabbits and rodents: clinical medicine and surgery. 2nd edition. St Louis (MO): Saunders; 2004. p. 255–65.
28. Rosenthal KL. Antibiotic treatment protocols for small mammal bacterial diseases. In: Proceedings of the North American Veterinary Conference. Orlando (FL): NAVC; 2007. p. 1676–8.

29. Rosenthal KL. Therapeutic contraindications in exotic pets. Semin Avian Exotic Pet Med 2004;13(1):44–8.
30. Butz N, Ossent P, Homberger FR. Pathogenesis of guinea pigs adenovirus infection. Lab Anim Sci 1999;49(6):600–4.
31. Kashuba C, Hsu C, Krogstad A, et al. Small mammal virology. Vet Clin North Am Exot Anim Pract 2005;8:107–22.
32. Hament JM, Kimpen JL, Fleer A, et al. Respiratory viral infection predisposing for bacterial disease: a concise review. FEMS Immunol Med Microbiol 1999;26: 189–95.
33. Pollock C. Fungal diseases of laboratory rodents. Vet Clin North Am Exot Anim Pract 2003;6:401–13.
34. Greenacre CB. Spontaneous tumors of small mammals. Vet Clin North Am Exot Anim Pract 2004;7:627–51.
35. Heatley JJ. Cardiovascular anatomy, physiology, and diseases of rodents and small exotic mammals. Vet Clin North Am Exot Anim Pract 2009;12:99–113.
36. Lichtenberger M, Richardson JA. Emergency care and managing toxicosis in the exotic animal patient. Vet Clin North Am Exot Anim Pract 2008;11:211–28.
37. Lichtenberger M, Ko J. Critical care monitoring. Vet Clin North Am Exot Anim Pract 2007;10:317–44.

Ferret Respiratory System: Clinical Anatomy, Physiology, and Disease

Cathy A. Johnson-Delaney, DVM, DABVP (Avian), DABVP (Exotic Companion Mammal)[a],*,
Susan E. Orosz, PhD, DVM, DABVP (Avian), DECZM (Avian)[b]

KEYWORDS
- Ferret • Respiratory system • Upper respiratory tract
- Lower respiratory tract • Olfactory system

ANATOMY

The upper and lower respiratory tracts of ferrets have several similarities to humans, and therefore have been used as a research model for respiratory function. The upper respiratory tract of the ferret is complex and starts with the nose and nasal cavity (**Fig. 1**). From here, air moves from the choana into the opening of the larynx, the rima glottis, and then into the trachea. The skin of the nose is unfurred and often pigmented.

The nasal cavity of mammals is considered to have a primary olfactory function, except in primates, including man. This olfactory sense requires a complex nasal cavity that provides optimal temperature and humidity for detecting the chemicals that produce the concept of odor. This part of the respiratory tract also conditions air for normal function of the lower respiratory tract. Ferrets, like most mammals other than primates, are obligatory nose breathers because of the close apposition of the epiglottis to the soft palate. The distance from the nostrils to the nasopharynx is proportional to the size of the head and the length of the snout. This larger olfactory-to-respiratory area ratio is associated with ferrets and other macrosomatic species.[1]

The nasal cavity is divided into right and left nasal passages and has dorsal and ventral nasal conchae that have numerous folds to increase the surface area of the

The authors have nothing to disclose.
[a] Eastside Avian and Exotic Animal Medical Center, 12930 NE 125th Way, Kirkland, WA 98034, USA
[b] Bird and Exotic Pet Wellness Center, 5166 Monroe Avenue, Suite 305, Toledo, OH 43623, USA
* Corresponding author.
E-mail address: cajddvm@hotmail.com

Vet Clin Exot Anim 14 (2011) 357–367
doi:10.1016/j.cvex.2011.03.001
1094-9194/11/$ – see front matter © 2011 Elsevier Inc. All rights reserved.
vetexotic.theclinics.com

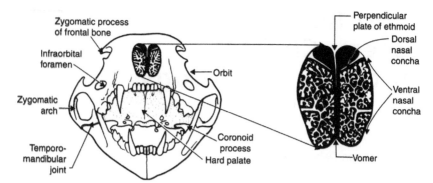

Fig. 1. Ferret skull (rostral view). (*Courtesy of* Howard E. Evans, PhD, Ithaca, NY; with permission.)

epithelium. The maxilloturbinates are composed of a double scroll-like structure that is branched. Histologically, the cranial end of the upper respiratory tract is keratinized squamous epithelium, and then in the area of olfaction it is stratified cuboidal to columnar. Some goblet cells may be present, but this epithelium is characterized as being nonciliated. Goblet cells and ciliated epithelium are characterized more caudally in the nasal cavity.[1]

The nasal cavity is designed to modify the air so that it is appropriate for inhalation into the lung surface. The bends and liner velocities in the airstream and turbulence in air flow are important for the passage of inhaled materials. These quick changes are designed to drop particulate matter out of the airstream to purify the air reaching the lungs. The final fate of particulates is influenced by the mucociliary clearance system and the permeability of secretions, including blood flow.

The hard palate continues as the flexible soft palate that sits over the opening of the larynx (**Fig. 2**). This opening is covered by the epiglottis, which rests above it. This arrangement allows air to move from the nasal cavity directly into the larynx. The larynx of the ferret is similar to that of the human larynx. It closes the airway to raise intra-abdominal pressure along with keeping ingesta from being aspirated into the respiratory tree, and acts as an aid for vocalization. During the normal breathing cycle, the vocal cords remain relaxed. The larynx is innervated by the cranial and caudal laryngeal nerves that are branches of the vagus.

The trachea extends from the larynx to the bifurcation of the primary bronchi, which divides at T5–6. The length of the trachea to this bifurcation is two to three times that of the dog or cat. There is a reduced problem passing an endotracheal tube into just one primary bronchus due to its length. Securing the endotracheal tube can be challenging because ferrets have a small mandible and maxilla. One author often secures the endotracheal tube with ties to the forelegs.

The trachea is composed of C-shaped hyaline cartilages that are connected by smooth muscle. The mucosal surface of the trachea is composed of ciliated and non-ciliated cells with mucus glands. Submucosal glands are present, and are closer in number to a human than a dog. These mucosal and submucosal glands are stimulated by nerves, acetylcholine, and histamine. Secretions can be blocked with atropine, glycopyrolate, and antihistamines.

The thoracic cavity is cone-shaped (**Fig. 3**). The rib cage consists of 14 ribs with 9 sternebrae, with the last several ribs not meeting the distal end of the sternum. The thoracic cage is divided into cranial, middle, and caudal mediastinal cavities.

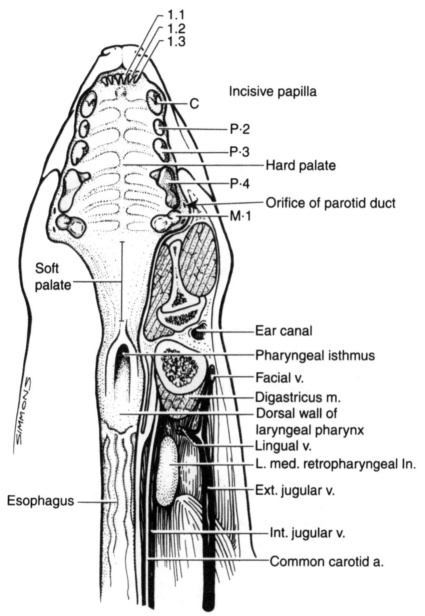

1.1
1.2
1.3

Incisive papilla

C

P·2

P·3

Hard palate

P·4

Orifice of parotid duct

M·1

Soft palate

Ear canal

Pharyngeal isthmus

Facial v.

Digastricus m.

Dorsal wall of laryngeal pharynx

Lingual v.

L. med. retropharyngeal In.

Ext. jugular v.

Esophagus

Int. jugular v.

Common carotid a.

SIMMONS

Fig. 2. Ferret pharynx and structures of interest. (*Courtesy of* Howard E. Evans, PhD, Ithaca, NY; with permission.)

The thoracic cage is compressible and the ferret is sufficiently flexible to turn itself around in the small diameter of the compressed thorax.

Each primary bronchus divides into a lobar or secondary bronchus, with further subdivisions into small lobules of the lung. The lung extends from the first or second up to the tenth or eleventh intercostal spaces (**Fig. 4**). The left lung divides into cranial

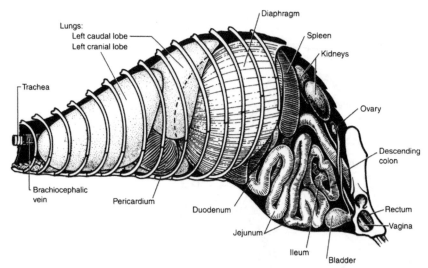

Fig. 3. The thoracic and abdominal viscera by a superficial left lateral view. The dotted line shows the curve of the diaphragm. (*Courtesy of* Howard E. Evans, PhD, Ithaca, NY; with permission.)

and caudal lobes, whereas the right lung has cranial, middle, caudal, and accessory lobes (**Fig. 5**). The accessory lobe of the right lung is irregular and conforms to the shape of the diaphragm, and curves around the caudal vena cava. The number of generations of terminal bronchioles of the ferret (1–2) is intermediate between that of the dog (0–1 generations) and that of humans (3–4 generations).

The pulmonary arteries carry unoxygenated blood from the right ventricle to the parenchyma of the lungs. The pulmonary trunk divides into the right and left pulmonary

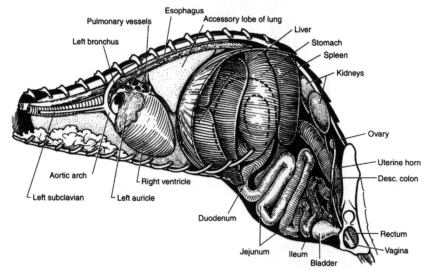

Fig. 4. The ferret thoracic and abdominal viscera on lateral view showing left lung removed. The dotted lines show the stomach passing to the pylorus dorsally and the duodenum. (*Courtesy of* Howard E. Evans, PhD, Ithaca, NY; with permission.)

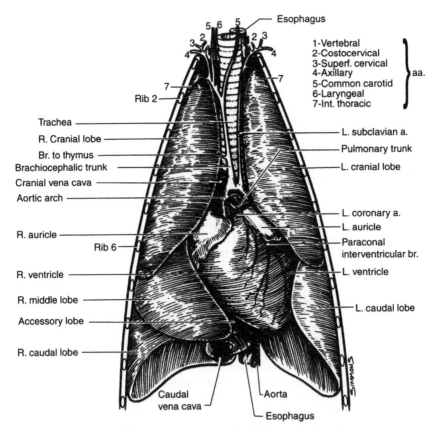

Fig. 5. Ferret heart and lungs (ventral view). (*Courtesy of* Howard E. Evans, PhD, Ithaca, NY; with permission.)

arteries that supply the right and left lung fields. The pulmonary veins carry oxygenated blood from each of the lobes to the left heart. The bronchial arteries supply blood to the parenchyma of the lung. They originate from the first intercostal artery, close to the origin of the aorta.

RESPIRATORY CHARACTERISTICS

The respiratory rate at rest is approximately 33 to 36 breaths per minute. It tends to vary from 27 to 44 breaths per minute when the ferret is under anesthesia. The total lung capacity is very large in ferrets, and this capacity exceeds its predicted value by 297%. The lung capacity measured in 0.6-kg ferrets was similar to that in a 2.5-kg rabbit. The only other mammal with a similar comparative value is the sea otter. In addition to the large lung capacity, the chest wall is very compliant. These two adaptations are believed to be important for successful subterranean hunting.

The ferret lung can adapt to changes in atmospheric pressures. With hypoxia, significant pulmonary vasoconstriction occurs. This effect is similar in humans, who develop pulmonary vasoconstriction in high altitudes. In addition, ozone produces similar epithelial injury in ferrets when compared with nonhuman primates. Ozone-exposed lungs of ferrets had severe, acute infiltration of neutrophils in areas with necrotic epithelial cells. These areas were especially more prominent in the centriacinar region of the lung.[2]

Ferrets exhibit neurogenic inflammation when sensory nerve stimulation causes the release of tachykinins. These substances are found in the nerve terminals of the sensory nerves to the lung parenchyma. Their release causes smooth muscle contraction, submucosal gland secretion, increased vascular permeability, neutrophil adhesion, and cough. Viral diseases, exposure to airborne toxins, including nicotine and other agents, can result in this neurogenic response. Nicotine has been shown to increase the ciliary beat frequency of the epithelial cells. Various air pollutants exacerbate pulmonary disease because they cause smooth muscle contraction and mucosal and submucosal gland secretion.

Studies have shown a difference in the distribution of α1- and β-adrenergic receptors and muscarinic receptors in the pulmonary tree. In small bronchioles, α1-receptors are more numerous but are sparse in the large airways. The β-receptors are relatively high throughout the tree but are highest in the bronchioles. The cholinergic receptors are most dense in the bronchial muscle and decrease in density toward the distal bronchioles.[3,4]

DISEASE, DIAGNOSIS, AND TREATMENT
Influenza

Ferrets are the only domestic animal species naturally susceptible to human influenza viruses, and are often infected by their human owners. Signs are similar to those in humans: photophobia, catarrhal nasal discharge, sneezing, coughing, pyrexia, anorexia, and malaise. They may also act like they have a sore throat or tonsillitis, with marked swallowing efforts. It may progress to pneumonia. During examination, a laryngoscope can be used to better visualize the oral cavity. Clinical course is usually 7 to 14 days. Treatment includes supportive care, antihistamines, cough suppressants without alcohol, and prophylactic antibiotics. Occasionally, for severe tonsillitis or discomfort, a nonsteroidal anti-inflammatory drug (NSAID) such as Metacam (0.2 mg/kg orally every 24 hours) can be provided. To prevent stomach problems, Metacam should not be given with concurrent use of a β_2-histamine blocker such as famotidine (2.5 mg, Pepcid AC, Merck & Co, Inc, Whitehouse Station, NJ, USA).[5] Preventive measures include separation of susceptible ferrets from ferrets or humans affected with influenza. Ferret owners are advised to get influenza vaccinations each year. Although currently vaccinations are not recommended in ferrets, human vaccines are efficacious.

Pneumonia

Bruce Williams, DVM, DACVP, suggests that the most common cause of pneumonia in ferrets is aspiration, either of orally administered medications or of vomitus (personal communication, August 2009). Ferrets often resist liquid oral medication, and may involuntarily inhale part of it. Gross and microscopic pathology are similar to those found in other species with aspiration pneumonia. If aspiration is suspected, prophylaxis with broad-spectrum antibiotics, rest, and supportive care are recommended. Pneumonia and lung consolidation have also been linked to a suspected novel strain of *Mycoplasma* species (Cathy A. Johnson-Delaney, DVM, oral communication, 2011).

Pneumonia from *Bordetella bronchiseptica* and *Pasteurella multocida* has also been reported. *B bronchiseptica* causes upper respiratory signs that respond poorly to antibiotics. Occasionally, as in dogs, ferrets will develop severe pneumonia. Marshall Farms (North Rose, New York) uses a killed *Bordetella* vaccine (Bronchicine, Pfizer, New York, NY, USA) and suggests it is safe and effective. Chloramphenicol and trimethoprim/sulfa may be helpful, along with supportive care. Often, 0.3 to 0.5 mL/kg of a children's formulation of diphenhydramine HCl (6.25 mg/5 mL) will help alleviate nasal congestion. Separating young ferrets from dogs with respiratory disease is recommended, and this is a concern in veterinary hospitals or boarding facilities that take young ferrets and dogs.

Mycoplasma

A novel *Mycoplasma* species was identified in pet ferrets after an outbreak in imported ferrets from a single source.[6] Many ferrets from this source exhibited chronic conjunctivitis, sneezing, wheezing, and coughing. Coughing episodes were chronic, paroxysmal, and harsh.

Radiographs showed mild bronchiolar patterns with mild thickening of bronchi, but these changes were not pathognomic (**Fig. 6**).[7] As some of the ferrets aged, the coughing generally progressed with more frequent bouts. Tonsillitis often accompanied ferrets with severe coughing episodes. Complete blood cell counts and chemistries were within normal ranges.[7,8]

A variety of treatment protocols have been evaluated and administered, including antihistamines, NSAIDs, antibiotics, bronchodilators, and decongestants. Most affected ferrets had no resolution of clinical signs, despite treatment.

One of the authors identified a 2-year-old female that died in 2009 of acute respiratory failure, characterized by a sudden increase in congestion and dyspnea unresponsive to bronchodilators and oxygen (**Fig. 7**). Lung pathology showed lymphoplasmacytic inflammation around the terminal airways, associated with luminal attenuation. Severe, nonsuppurative bronchitis was diagnosed, and lesions resembled those of chronic murine pneumonia caused by *M pulmonis* in rats (**Fig. 8**).[9,10] Immunochemistry of the tissues was positive for *Mycoplasma* spp. Bronchiolar lavage samples and conjunctival swabs were submitted for identification, which led to the identification of a novel *Mycoplasma* spp. Investigations into this disease condition are ongoing.

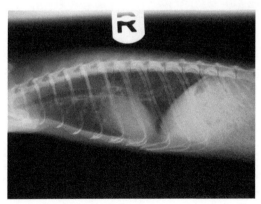

Fig. 6. Lateral radiograph of a ferret with mycoplasma respiratory disease. Note the thickened bronchi. (*Courtesy of* Cathy A. Johnson-Delaney, DVM, Dipl ABVP (Avian), Edmonds, WA; with permission.)

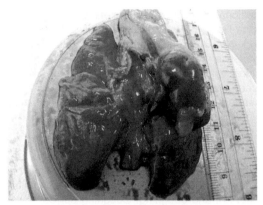

Fig. 7. Gross necropsy of heart and lungs from a ferret with mycoplasma. (*Courtesy of* Cathy A. Johnson-Delaney, DVM, Dipl ABVP (Avian), Edmonds, WA.)

Canine Distemper

Canine distemper is a fatal disease in ferrets. Disease progression ranges from 12 days in ferret-adapted strains to approximately 42 in wild canine strains. Transmission is through direct contact, fomites, or aerosolization of urine, feces, or nasal exudate. The disease has been associated with ferret shows and the intermingling of ferrets that have not been properly vaccinated. The disease is profoundly immunosuppressive, and animals that survive the initial respiratory stages succumb to neurologic dysfunction within several weeks. No treatment exists. Vaccination (Purevax Ferret, Merial, Duluth, Georgia) should begin when the ferret is 6 weeks old, with a second vaccination given at 10 weeks and a third at 14 weeks, with an annual booster. Early clinical signs include anorexia, pyrexia, chin dermatitis, photophobia,

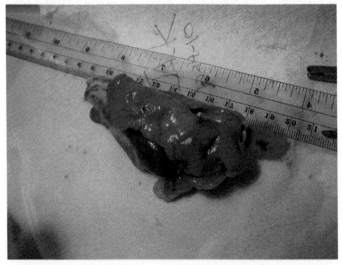

Fig. 8. Gross necropsy of lung abscess from a ferret with mycoplasma respiratory disease. This lesion is one of the gross characteristics seen with mycoplasma infection in ferrets. (*Courtesy of* Cathy A. Johnson-Delaney, DVM, Dipl ABVP (Avian), Edmonds, WA.)

nasal and ocular discharge, and brown crusts around the face. Later clinical signs include bronchopneumonia, hyperkeratosis of the planum nasale and footpads, and central nervous system signs, including tremors, convulsions, coma, and death.

Histologically, eosinophilic viral inclusion bodies are both intracytoplasmic and intranuclear. They may be seen in a wide variety of epithelial cells, neurons, and occasionally in white blood cells and megakaryocytes. The urinary bladder, renal pelvis, and biliary epithelium are the most common sites of inclusions. A nonsuppurative encephalitis with demyelination may be seen in animals showing neurologic disease.

Endogenous Lipid Pneumonia

Endogenous lipid pneumonia is a common incidental finding in mustelids at necropsy and is of no clinical significance. It has been called "foam cell foci" or "subpleural histiocytosis." Practitioners often mistake it at necropsy as a dissemination neoplasm. The cause and origin of the lipid is unknown. Grossly multiple to coalescing white to yellow foci are present within the subpleural pulmonary parenchyma. A transverse cut through one of these foci will reveal its superficial nature. It is an aggregate of lipid-laden macrophages in the alveoli immediately subjacent to the pleura. As the lesions increase in size, they may include moderate numbers of lymphocytes and cholesterol clefts.

Nonspecific Respiratory Conditions

Several ferrets present with chronic sneezing and apparent upper respiratory irritation. Symptoms abate with antihistamines or topical ocular and nasal antibiotics and NSAIDs, but reoccur on cessation of the medications. Some ferrets exhibit seasonal symptoms similar to human allergies or hay fever. Cultures of discharges, nasal flushes, and conjunctival swabs usually contain a variety of bacteria considered normal flora, but nothing specific. Primary or secondary neoplasias affecting the lung may result in respiratory signs, and should be considered as a differential in addition to infectious causes (**Fig. 9**).

H1N1 Influenza

The H1N1 (swine) influenza epidemic that engendered worldwide concern is transmissible to the ferret. Isolation of this virus from pet ferrets has been reported. Affected

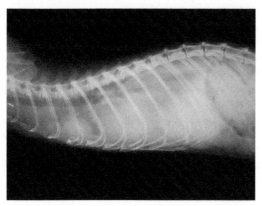

Fig. 9. Lateral radiograph of ferret with metastatic fibrosarcomas that presented in respiratory distress. (*Courtesy of* Cathy A. Johnson-Delaney, DVM, Dipl ABVP (Avian), Edmonds, WA.)

ferrets may present with respiratory disease, tracheitis, anorexia, weight loss, dehydration, and pyrexia. One author has been successful treating ferrets diagnosed with H1N1 with recommended treatment protocols, including bronchodilators, antibiotics for secondary bacterial pneumonias, and meloxicam (0.2 mg/kg, orally, every 24 hours; Metacam, Bohringer-Ingleheim Inc, St Joseph, MO, USA).[6] All treated ferrets recovered. Because of zoonotic potential, practitioners should follow guidelines for the public health reporting system and laboratories in their area when submitting samples for laboratory confirmation. Several clinical laboratories are noted in **Box 1**.

In one outbreak of respiratory disease at a ferret colony, tissues were collected from two juvenile animals for laboratory submission. Bronchointerstitial pneumonia with necrotizing bronchiolitis was revealed microscopically.[1] Immunochemistry and reverse-transcription PCR assay showed the presence of influenza A virus, with a high homology to H1N1 swine influenza viruses. This finding was replicated through additional analysis of the colony premises. Whether an infected ferret can transmit H1N1 influenza to humans is unknown. Prophylactic influenza vaccinations are recommended for individuals who have routine contact with ferrets.[11]

Dental Disease

Dental disease and tooth root abscesses must be investigated whenever a ferret is presented for nasal discharge, whether it is unilateral or bilateral. Intraoral and skull radiographs are useful for examining the tooth roots, because the tooth may seemingly appear healthy. Often these problems arise from a ferret's propensity for trying to break cage doors and chew on hard toys. It is not uncommon to have a fistula through the pulp of the canine extending into the nasal cavity or through the mandible. Ferrets are also notorious for inhaling dusts, hair, spider webs, and other particulates

---

Box 1
Diagnostic laboratories with experience in rabbit polymerase chain reaction, serology, parasitology, histopathology, microbiology, or necropsy

BioReliance Corporation, Laboratory Animal Diagnostic Service; (800) 804–3586; www.bioreliance.com. Available testing: polymerase chain reaction (PCR), serology, parasitology, histopathology, clinical pathology, microbiology.

Charles River Laboratories, Inc, Research Animal Diagnostic Services; (800) 338–9680; www.criver.com. Available testing: PCR, serology, parasitology, histopathology, necropsy, microbiology.

Division of Laboratory Animal Medicine, LSU School of Veterinary Medicine; (225) 578–9643. Available testing: rodent serology.

University of Miami Comparative Pathology Laboratory; (800) 596–7390; http://pathology.med.miami.edu. Available testing: serology, histopathology, necropsy, microbiology, parasitology.

Research Animal Diagnostic Laboratory, University of Missouri; (800) 669–0825; www.radil.missouri.edu. Available testing: PCR, serology, necropsy, histopathology, microbiology, clinical pathology, parasitology.

Zoologix, Inc; (818) 717–8880; www.zoologix.com. Available testing: PCR.

Sound Diagnostics, Woodinville, WA; (206) 363–0787; www.sounddiagnosticsinc.com. Available testing: rabbit serology.

Veterinary Molecular Diagnostics, Milford, OH; (513) 576–1808; www.vmdlabs.com. Available testing: small mammal PCR.

during their environmental investigations. Most of these inhalations result in acute paroxysmal sneezing with clearance of the irritant material. Occasionally the ferret will sneeze so hard that blood will be mixed with the mucus in the discharge. If the sneezing persists, clinicians should consider that a more significant foreign body, rhinitis, or sinusitis may be involved.

REFERENCES

1. Reznik GK. Comparative anatomy, physiology, and function of the upper respiratory tract. Environ Health Perspect 1990;85:171–6.
2. Sterner-Kock A, Kock M, Braun R, et al. Ozone-induced epithelial injury in the ferret is similar to nonhuman primates. Am J Respir Crit Care Med 2000;162(3):1152–6.
3. Whary TM, Andrews PL. Physiology of the ferret. Biology and disease of the ferret. 2nd edition. In: Fox JG, editor. Baltimore (MD): Lippencott Williams & Wilkins; 1998. p. 103–48.
4. Barnes PJ, Basbaum CB, Nadel JA. Autoradiographic localization of autonomic receptors in airway smooth muscles. Am Rev Respir Dis 1983;127:758–62.
5. Johnson-Delaney CA. Ferrets: digestive system and disorders. In: Keeble E, Meredith A, editors. BSAVA manual of rodents and ferrets. Quedgeley, Gloucester (United Kingdom): BSAVA; 2009. p. 275–81.
6. Johnson-Delaney CA. Emerging ferret diseases. J Exotic Pet Med 2010;19(3): 207–15.
7. Schoemaker NJ. Ferrets, skunks and otters. In: Meredith A, Johnson-Delaney C, editors. BSAVA manual of exotic pets. 5th edition. Quedgeley, Gloucester (United Kingdom): BSAVA; 2010. p. 127–38.
8. Orcutt C, Malakoff R. Ferrets: cardiovascular and respiratory system disorders. In: Keeble E, Meredith A, editors. BSAVA manual of rodents and ferrets. Quedgeley, Gloucester (United Kingdom): BSAVA; 2009. p. 282–90.
9. Percy DH, Barthold SW. Rats. Section on mycoplasmal infection: murine respiratory mycoplasmosis. 3rd edition. Ames (IA): Pathology of Laboratory Rodents and Rabbits. Blackwell Publishing Professional; 2007. p. 143–6.
10. Goodman G. Rodents: respiratory and cardiovascular system disorders. In: Keeble E, Meredith A, editors. BSAVA manual of rodents and ferrets. Quedgeley, Gloucester (United Kingdom): BSAVA; 2009. p. 142–9.
11. Patterson AR, Cooper VL, Yoon KJ, et al. Naturally occurring influenza infection in a ferret (*Mustela putorius furo*) colony. J Vet Diagn Invest 2009;21:527–30.

Diagnostic Imaging of the Respiratory System in Exotic Companion Mammals

Vittorio Capello, DVM, DECZM (Small Mammal),
DABVP (Exotic Companion Mammal)[a,b,*],
Angela M. Lennox, DVM, DABVP (Avian)[c]

KEYWORDS

- Respiratory system • Thoracic imaging • Rabbit • Guinea pig
- Chinchilla • Prairie dog • Rat • Ferret • Skunk

The level of care for smaller companion mammals has increased significantly during the past few years. Although not truly exotic, rabbits, rodents, ferrets, and other less common mammal species, including artiodactyls and marsupials, were grouped as undefined, and separate from traditional mammalian pets (dogs and cats). Today, exotic companion mammals represent this group and are acknowledged as a specific area of zoologic medicine. Continuing education is encouraged and supported by specific associations, such as the Association of Exotic Mammal Veterinarians and two dedicated boards of specialties: the American Board of Veterinary Practitioners and the European College of Zoologic Medicine.

Owner demands for a higher level of care is increasing dramatically. Because most of these patients are small (less than 2 kg), this represents a great challenge, in particular for the field of diagnostic imaging.

In addition to routine imaging modalities, such as radiography, oral endoscopy, and to a lesser degree ultrasonography, more diagnostic imaging, including advanced endoscopic techniques, computed tomography (CT), and magnetic resonance (MR), have become available. Many of these techniques are extrapolated from dog and cat medicine, but advances in technology also make them effective for smaller mammals.[1]

This article reviews the 5 main diagnostic imaging modalities currently available for investigation of the respiratory system of exotic companion mammals: radiography, ultrasonography, endoscopy, computed tomography, and magnetic resonance.

The authors have nothing to disclose.

[a] Clinica Veterinaria S. Siro, Via Lampugnano 99, Milano 20151, Italy
[b] Clinica Veterinaria Gran Sasso, Via Donatello 26, Milano, Italy
[c] Avian and Exotic Animal Clinic, 9330 Waldemar Road, Indianapolis, IN 46268, USA
* Corresponding author.
E-mail address: capellov@tin.it

Vet Clin Exot Anim 14 (2011) 369–389
doi:10.1016/j.cvex.2011.03.009   **vetexotic.theclinics.com**
1094-9194/11/$ – see front matter © 2011 Published by Elsevier Inc.

Cardiac disease is part of thoracic imaging and can affect the respiratory system. Nevertheless, cardiology is a specific branch of internal medicine and it is classified separately from thoracic imaging or respiratory disease, and for this reason it will not be discussed in detail in this article.

RADIOGRAPHY

Radiography is the mainstay of diagnostic imaging of the respiratory system, in particular of the thorax and lower respiratory tract, and should be considered the first step in an imaging diagnostic trial. Starting from the information provided by the radiographic examination, further indications for other imaging modalities can be obtained.

Because of the small size of exotic mammal patients, obtaining excellent radiographs must be considered a priority. Most standard radiographic equipment is effective for small exotic mammals. Many factors are involved in the process of taking radiographs, but the two most important are the proper combination of cassette and film, and optimal patient positioning.[2,3]

Mammography film is an ultraslow-speed film used with specific cassettes that include a low-speed intensifying screen. They provide good detail, providing a sharp, nongrainy image, and are therefore especially advantageous in small or very small mammal patients.[2] Despite the fact that low-speed screens and films require more exposure than regular screen/film (including longer exposure time for low-powered radiograph machines), they are rarely affected by patient motion caused by physiologic breathing movements.

Because of small size, behavior, and proper patient positioning, general anesthesia is often required to obtain quality radiographs useful for diagnosis.[3] Critical patients in respiratory distress for which anesthesia represents increased risk may benefit from sedation. Protocols for anesthesia and sedation have been reported elsewhere.[4,5] Manual restraint is rarely an option because of excessive stress during handling.[3] On the other hand, sedation and anesthesia might affect radiographic interpretation because of possible artifacts of pulmonary or cardiac imaging.[3]

The two standard views for radiographic study of the thorax are the latero-lateral and the ventrodorsal (or dorsoventral).[2,3,6] For the latero-lateral projection, patients are placed in right or left lateral recumbency. The thoracic limbs must be extended cranially to prevent superimposition of the brachial muscles over the mediastinal portion cranial to the heart.[2,6] This positioning is important for selected species with short chest lengths, such as prairie dogs, and less critical for other species, such as ferrets. Most common small mammal species do not have a round chest; therefore, lifting of the sternum to prevent oblique artifacts is not a special concern. Even if the radiograph will show superimposition of each hemithorax, the image of the hemithorax leaning directly over the cassette will be more detailed. For this reason, both left-to-right and right-to-left lateral projections should be obtained. This practice is important for several intrapulmonary or extrapulmonary diseases, such as lung or pleural metastasis and pleural effusion. Proper collimation of the radiographic beam is another important factor. The image of the thorax should include all the ribs; therefore, it will include the diaphragm and the cranial portion of the abdomen. More appropriately, the frame for the respiratory system should be enlarged more cranially, to include the cervical portion of the trachea.[2]

The ventrodorsal view is obtained with patients placed in dorsal recumbency.[2,6] The thoracic limbs are extended cranially to prevent superimposition of the scapulae on the lung fields. This position is more stressful for patients in respiratory distress; therefore, the sternal recumbency for the dorsoventral projection may be preferable for selected patients. Optimal symmetry is critical for the sagittal view, and in authors' experience this is easier to obtain from the ventrodorsal projection. Also, the dorso-ventral projection makes cranial extension of forelimbs more difficult.

Radiographs of the nasal cavities are collected with the 5 standard projections of the skull in rabbits and selected rodent species: lateral, ventrodorsal or dorsoventral, right-to-left oblique, left-to-right oblique, and rostrocaudal.[2] They are particularly advantageous when disease of the nasal cavity is secondary to acquired dental disease. In the case of ferrets and other larger carnivore species, open-mouth projections and intraoral films can be used.[2]

Digital systems for radiographic imaging are becoming more and more popular and affordable. Basically, there are 2 digital systems: computed radiography, also named "indirect digital radiography," and direct digital radiography.[2] In the first case, digital detectors are included in the cassette and standard radiographic equipment can be adapted. The cassette is then processed by a dedicated machine and software. Direct digital systems require a specific digital radiographic unit and they send digital information directly to the computer without a reading step.

Digital systems offer several advantages and disadvantages compared with traditional films, and thorough discussion is beyond the purpose of this article. From the visual standpoint, digital radiography allows easier and more flexible adjusting of the gray scale, whereas proper contrast using mammography films depends on the exact setting. Minimal variations can affect the final image of soft-tissue intrathoracic structures, and when suboptimal, the radiograph should be repeated. Minimal variations in the gray scale are critical for visualization of lungs, bronchi, great vessels, and mediastinum, which is why digital radiography might be preferable to mammography films for thoracic imaging, especially for average-sized exotic mammals, such as rabbits, ferrets, skunks, guinea pigs, and prairie dogs. On the other hand, most digital systems do not have a specific high resolution, and the analogic view of a mammography films still remains significantly superior in regard to detail. This superiority is why, in the authors' opinion, mammography films are the best option for thoracic imaging of smaller mammals, such as chinchillas, rats, other small rodent species, hedgehogs, and sugar gliders.

No artifacts or foreign objects should hamper visualization of normal and abnormal anatomic structures; therefore, materials used for optimal positioning of patients (foam positioners, adhesive tape) should be completely radiotransparent, and other monitoring devices (electrocardiogram clips, Doppler) should be properly positioned or temporarily removed. Positioning of the endotracheal tube in patients under general anesthesia is also questionable. Ideally, thoracic radiographs should be taken immediately after induction of anesthesia while oxygen and additional inhalant anesthetic are administered through a facemask, especially in obligate nasal breather species. Endotracheal (ET) intubation should be performed immediately after radiographs are obtained, when general anesthesia must be continued for other reasons. Endotracheal intubation should be evaluated for each patient.

Common indications for collection of diagnostic radiographs of the respiratory system in single species are listed in **Table 1**, and examples of normal and abnormal patterns are shown in **Figs. 1–10, 15–18**.

ULTRASONOGRAPHY

Conduction of ultrasound is enhanced by fluids and hampered by gas. For this reason, ultrasonography of the thorax is difficult because of the presence of air in the lungs, and does not represent the diagnostic imaging of choice. Nevertheless,

Table 1
Common indications for five diagnostic imaging modalities of respiratory system in selected exotic companion mammal species

		Rabbit	Guinea Pigs, Chinchillas, Degus	Prairie Dogs, Squirrels	Rats	Ferrets, Skunks
Radiography	Nasal cavities	Rhinitis or empyema of the nasal cavity/maxillary recess	Rhinitis or empyema of the nasal cavity	—	—	Rhinitis
		—	—	Compressive acquired dental disease (pseudo-odontoma)	—	—
	Esophagus	—	Space-occupying mass (elodontoma)	—	—	Megaesophagus
	Lungs	Bronchopneumonia, intrapulmonary abscesses Metastasis	Bronchopneumonia, intrapulmonary abscesses	—	Bronchopneumonia, intrapulmonary abscesses	Bronchopneumonia
	Mediastinum	Mediastinal mass (thymoma, lymphoma, thymic lymphoma) Pleural effusion Pneumothorax Diaphragmatic hernia (Cardiac disease)	Mediastinal mass Pleural effusion (Cardiac disease)	Pleural effusion (Cardiac disease)	Mediastinal mass (lymphoma) Pleural effusion (Cardiac disease)	Metastasis Mediastinal mass (lymphoma) Pleural effusion Pneumothorax Diaphragmatic hernia (Cardiac disease)
Ultrasonography	Mediastinum	Mediastinal mass (thymoma, lymphoma, thymic lymphoma) Pleural effusion Diaphragmatic hernia (Cardiac disease)	Mediastinal mass (Cardiac disease)	(Cardiac disease)	Mediastinal mass (Cardiac disease)	Mediastinal mass (thymoma, lymphoma, thymic lymphoma) Pleural effusion Diaphragmatic hernia (Cardiac disease)

Endoscopy	Rhinoscopy	Rhinitis; empyema of the nasal cavity/maxillary recess	—	—	—	—
	Laryngoscopy	Laryngeal disease; Aid to endotracheal intubation	Trauma, foreign body; Aid to endotracheal intubation	Aid to endotracheal intubation	Aid to endotracheal intubation	Trauma, foreign body; —
	Tracheoscopy	Tracheitis	—	—	—	Tracheitis
	Bronchoscopy	Bronchopneumonia	—	—	—	Bronchopneumonia
	Thoracoscopy	Inspection and biopsy of mediastinal mass (thymoma, lymphoma, thymic lymphoma)	—	—	—	Inspection and biopsy of mediastinal mass
Computed Tomography	Nasal cavities	Rhinitis; empyema of the nasal cavity/maxillary recess	Rhinitis; empyema of the nasal cavity/maxillary recess	—	—	Rhinitis
			—	Compressive acquired dental disease (pseudo-odontoma)	—	—
			Space-occupying mass (elodontoma)			
	Lungs	Intrapulmonary abscesses	Intrapulmonary abscesses	—	Intrapulmonary abscesses	—
	Mediastinum	Metastasis; Mediastinal mass (thymoma, lymphoma, thymic lymphoma)	Metastasis; Mediastinal mass	—	Mediastinal mass (lymphoma)	Metastasis; Mediastinal mass (lymphoma)
Magnetic Resonance	Nasal cavities	Rhinitis; empyema of the nasal cavity/maxillary recess	—	—	—	—
	Lungs	Metastasis;	Mediastinal mass	—	—	Metastasis;
	Mediastinum	Mediastinal mass (thymoma, lymphoma, thymic lymphoma)				Mediastinal mass (lymphoma)

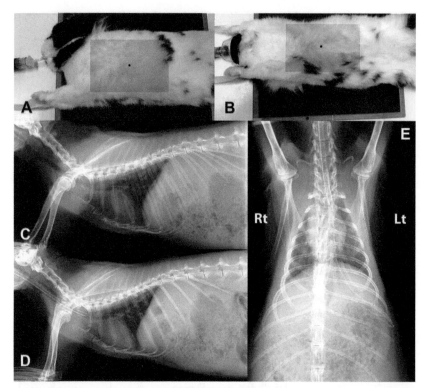

Fig. 1. (*A–E*) Radiography of the thorax in the pet rabbit. (*A*) Lateral projection. The patient is placed in lateral recumbency with the thoracic limbs extended cranially and secured with radiotransparent tape. Both lateral views should be taken. The beam (*dark area*) is collimated over the area of interest. When the cervical tract of the trachea is included in the radiograph, the frame is expanded cranially. The patient is under general anesthesia, and intubated. (*B*) Ventrodorsal projection. The patient is placed in dorsal recumbency with the thoracic limbs extended cranially. Depending on cases, the dorsoventral position can be used, with the patient placed in sternal recumbency. In this example, the patient is under general anesthesia, and oxygen is delivered by face mask. When thoracic limbs are extended, respiration can be impaired especially in dyspneic patients, even if endotracheal intubation is performed. This position should be maintained for only enough time to obtain the radiograph. (*C*) Normal thorax and cervical trachea of a 1.5 kg dwarf rabbit, without intubation. Lateral projection. (*D*) Normal thorax and cervical trachea of a 1.5 kg dwarf rabbit, with intubation. Lateral projection. (*E*) Normal thorax and cervical trachea of a 1.5 kg dwarf rabbit, with intubation. (*From* Vittorio Capello, DVM; with permission.)

ultrasonography may be useful as an adjunct to radiology when fluids or solid densities are present within the thoracic cavity.[3,7]

The use of a high-frequency (7.5–12.0 MHz) probe with a small footprint is critical for optimal results in small exotic companion mammals.[7–9] Other features, such as visualization of both B and M mode, high frame rate, and color Doppler function, are especially useful for echocardiography.

A good ultrasound device should also have a digital recording system.[8]

Fur interferes with ultrasound imaging, so furry patients must be properly shaved before examination. Because small exotic mammals are prone to hypothermia because of their high surface/volume ratio, shaving should be minimized.[7] A small

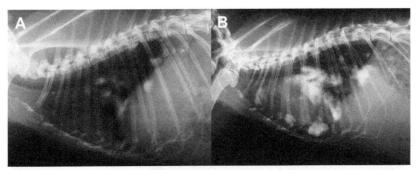

Fig. 2. (*A*, *B*) Pulmonary metastasis from uterine adenocarcinoma in a 7 year old rabbit. (*A*) At the time of diagnosis respiratory symptoms were not detectable. (*B*) Three month later, the patient is showing mild respiratory symptoms. (*From* Vittorio Capello, DVM; with permission.)

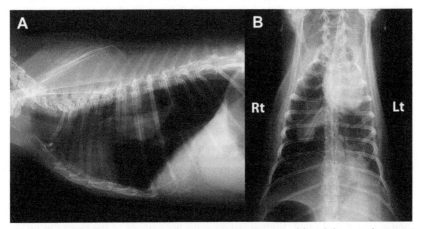

Fig. 3. (*A*, *B*) Pneumothorax in a 8 year old male, 2 kg pet rabbit. (*A*) Lateral projection. A collapsed lobe is visible, surrounded by a large amount of gas in the pleural space. (*B*) ventrodorsal projection. Pneumothorax is lateralized on the right side because radiodensity is present in the left hemithorax. History was unremarkable, and thoracocentesis was unrewarding. The owner declined esplorative thoracotomy. (*From* Vittorio Capello, DVM; with permission.)

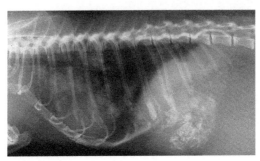

Fig. 4. Pulmonary metastasis from hepatic neoplasia in a 7-year-old female prairie dog. (*From* Angela Lennox, DVM; with permission.)

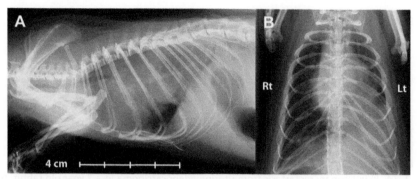

Fig. 5. (*A, B*) Pulmonary abscess in a 1.5-year-old female rat with moderate dyspnea. (*A*) Lateral projection. (*B*) Ventrodorsal projection. Increased radiodensity is present at the caudal portion of the left pulmonary lobe. Both standard projections are needed for a proper diagnosis because a single lateral projection might underestimate or overestimate the extent of lesions (as in this case, where disease is clearly unilateral). The left lung of rats is not divided into lobes (the right lung presents 3 lobes),[26] which explains the uniform pattern of radiodensity on the lateral projection. High-quality radiographs are necessary for proper diagnosis in small patients. (*From* Angela Lennox, DVM; with permission.)

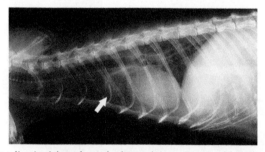

Fig. 6. Enlarged mediastinal lymph node (*arrow*) in a 7-year-old male ferret affected by lymphoma; lateral projection. Normal radiographic appearance of the heart can be evaluated in this radiography. The ferret heart is located more caudally than in the cat or dog, between T5-T8, and between the fifth the seventh intercostal space. The heart shadow is slightly globoid and is normally slightly elevated from the sternum because of the presence of fat in the pericardial ligament.[9] (*From* Vittorio Capello, DVM; with permission.)

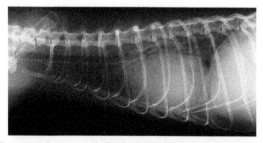

Fig. 7. Dilated cardiomyopathy in a male ferret; lateral projection. Radiographic abnormalities are represented by cardiomegaly, rounding of the cardiac apex, and narrowing of the pericardial space between the heart and the sternum. (*Reprinted from* Capello V, Lennox AM. Radiology of exotic companion mammals. Wiley-Blackwell Publishing, 2008; with permission.)

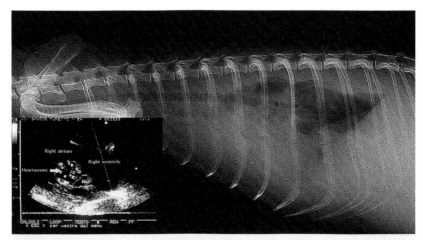

Fig. 8. Pleural effusion in a female ferret, lateral projection. The caudal lung lobes are surrounded by fluid opacity and are partially collapsed. The ventrodorsal projection (not presented here) confirmed bilateralism. Pleural effusion was secondary to heartworm disease, suspected at ultrasonography (*insert*) and confirmed at necropsy. (*Reprinted from* Capello V, Lennox AM. Radiology of exotic companion mammals. Wiley-Blackwell Publishing; 2008; with permission.)

area on both lateral sides of the thorax is usually enough for proper scanning. Water-soluble conduction acoustic gel should be warmed before application to reduce sensitivity and possible hypothermia, and should be dried off after the examination to prevent excessive self-licking.[8] Alcohol should be avoided for conduction or used in minimal amount and carefully washed.

Manual restraint is possible for most rabbits, ferrets, and tame rodents, such as guinea pigs and rats. The technique for restraint differs depending on the species

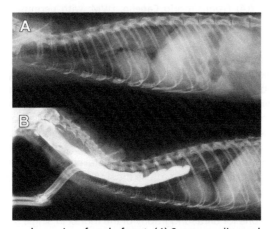

Fig. 9. (*A, B*) Megaesophagus in a female ferret. (*A*) Survery radiograph, lateral projection. Radiotransparency of the craniodorsal mediastinum, severe radiopacity of the lungs and deflection of the trachea are radiographic abnormalities suggestive of megaesophagus. Chronic weight loss and regurgitation were also present. (*B*) Lateral projection, after administration of positive contrast medium (barium sulfate). Megaesophagus is confirmed. (*Reprinted from* Capello V, Lennox AM. Radiology of exotic companion mammals. Wiley-Blackwell Publishing; 2008; with permission.)

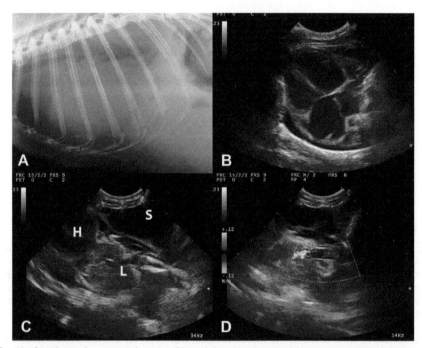

Fig. 10. (A–D) Diaphragmatic hernia of liver lobes in a 9 year old male lop rabbit. (A) Survery radiograph of the thorax, lateral projection. The caudal margin of the cardiac shadow and the diaphragmatic line are not visible. Diffuse pleural effusion covers the lung lobes. (B) Short axis "four chamber" view. Both pericardial and pleural effusion are present. (C) A liver lobe (L) is present just caudal the heart (H). Dorsal to the liver is the fluid filled stomach (S). Ultrasonographic abnormalities were diagnostic for diaphragmatic hernia. (D) Color Doppler ultrasonography demonstrated the presence of large vessels, confirming herniation of part of the liver. ((A) From Vittorio Capello, DVM; with permission; and (B–D) Oriol Domenech, DVM; with permission.)

and should be performed with extreme care by an experienced technician, especially when imaging patients who are dyspneic. Recumbency is preferably dorsal for ferrets and lateral for rabbits, considering that significant respiratory compromise may occur if a rabbit is placed in dorsal recumbency when the stomach or cecum is full.[7] Positioning patients on a slanted table or elevating the thorax while holding patients can significantly reduce the risk of respiratory compromise during imaging.

When manual restraint is not safe, or not feasible for smaller species, ultrasonography can be performed with sedation or with general anesthesia if required. Scanning planes are longitudinal and transverse. The most useful scanning planes for echocardiography are right and left parasternal long-axis 4-chamber view. B mode is used mostly to examine the mediastinum.[8]

Common indications for ultrasonography of the thorax in single species are listed in **Table 1**, and examples of abnormal patterns are shown in **Figs. 8, 10, 17–18**.

ENDOSCOPY

Unlike other diagnostic imaging, endoscopy (meaning *to view inside*) provides direct visualization of internal anatomic structures directly or indirectly related to a real or

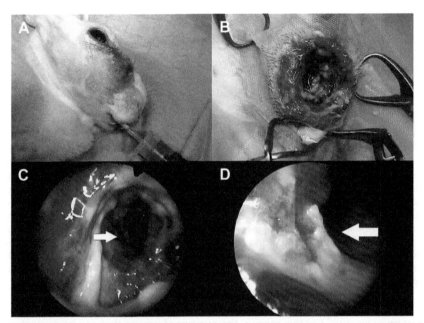

Fig. 11. (*A–D*) Rhinoscopy of the maxillary recess from a lateral approach in a pet rabbit. (*A*) A large facial abscess in a female dwarf rabbit prepared for surgery. The abscess originated from maxillary cheek teeth, and cause empyema of the alveolar bulla and the maxillary recess. (*B*) Intraoperative excision and debridement of the abscess. This surgical aprroach is actually a lateral rhinostomy, entering the maxillary recess through the perforated surface (*facies cribrosa*)[26] of the maxillary bone. (*C*) Rhinoscopy of the maxillary recess. The cavity in the background is the alveolar bulla. An ankylotic fragment of maxillary cheek tooth is till present after intraoral extraction (*arrow*). (*D*) The fragment of reserve crown, at the border-line between alveolar bulla and maxillary recess. This fragment had been missed during stomatoscopy, because inspection of the alveolar bulla is particularly difficult using a rigid endoscope. (*From* Vittorio Capello, DVM; with permission.)

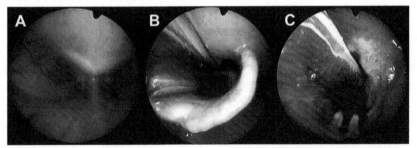

Fig. 12. (*A–C*) Endoscopic-guided orotracheal intubation in a 1.5-kg pet rabbit. (*A*) Normal appearance of the caudal portion of the oropharynx. The physiologic position of the epyglottis in obligate nasal breather species is beneath the caudal margin of the soft palate. The rhinopharynx is separated by the oropharynx. (*B*) Appearance of the epiglottis after the margin has disengaged from the caudal margin of the soft palate. the tip of a transparent, 2 mm uncuffed endotracheal tube is directed to the laryngeal opening. The aritenoid cartilages are visible in the background. (*C*) The endotracheal tube tube has been introduced in between the two arytenoid cartilages, and deeper inside the trachea. The corniculate processes are visible ventrally. (*From* Vittorio Capello, DVM; with permission.)

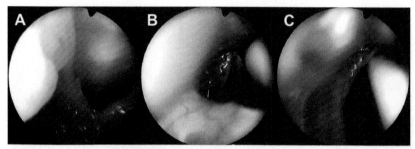

Fig. 13. (*A–C*) Endoscopic-guided orotracheal intubation in a 1-kg prairie dog. (*A*) Orotracheal intubation of intubation of obligate nasal breather rodent species (Guinea pig, Chinchilla, Degus, Prarie dog) is even more challenging than rabbits because of smaller size and because of the presence of the oropharyngeal ostium. The epiglottis is visible in the background behind the ostium. (*B*) The tip of the 2.7 mm, 30° view endoscope passed beyond the oropharingeal ostium, and the disengaged epiglottis. The white tip of a 1.5 mm uncuffed endotracheal tube is visible facing the arytenoids. (*C*) The endotracheal tube has been inserted between the arytenoids and inside the trachea. When feasible, the over-the-endoscope technique is another option for orotracheal intubation, using a larger tracheal tube and a semiflexible endoscope.[13,14] (*From* Vittorio Capello, DVM; with permission.)

virtual body cavity.[10] For this reason, the number of organs that can be evaluated is more limited.

Still, endoscopy carries several diagnostic and therapeutic advantages compared with other methods of diagnostic imaging: the possibility of great magnification of internal structures, the ability to collect biopsies, and the chance for minimally invasive endosurgery in selected cases.[10]

Detailed features of endoscopic instrumentations are reported.[10] The most common used in exotic mammal medicine and surgery are the 2.7-mm system and the 1.9-mm telescope. Both have dedicated sheaths, many with ports and instrument channels. The 1-mm semirigid miniscope is a useful adjunct for smaller exotic mammals.

Indications for the use of endoscopy for the respiratory system of exotic companion mammals are represented by rhinoscopy, tracheoscopy, and bronchoscopy. The endoscope also provides a critical aid for intubation.[11–14] Last, but not least, the use of thoracoscopy has been reported in smaller companion mammals, such as rabbits and ferrets.

Rhinoscopy is mostly performed in rabbits because rhinitis is common in this species. Patients are intubated and placed in sternal recumbency with the head slightly flexed.[11] Position of the head is critical to facilitate reflux of saline used for flushing and to reduce the possibility of inhalation of fluids from around the uncuffed ET tube. Depending on rabbit size, the 2.7-mm rigid endoscope may be used (for rabbits more than 2.0–2.5 kg), otherwise the 1.9-mm is needed for smaller patients. Entering the ventral meatus, the ventral and middle nasal conchae can be scoped. In larger rabbits, it is possible to visualize the rhinopharynx more caudally.[11] Rhinoscopy can also be performed from sites other than the natural nasal openings. Rhinotomy (ie, minimal, temporary rhinostomy) allows inspection, collections of biopsy specimen, and even debridement from a dorsal approach.[11,15] Another possible application is when chronic, septic rhinitis is secondary to advanced dental disease of maxillary cheek teeth. Facial swelling in the zygomatic area can be secondary to empyema of the maxillary recess[16] (in other sources termed the maxillary sinus[17,18]

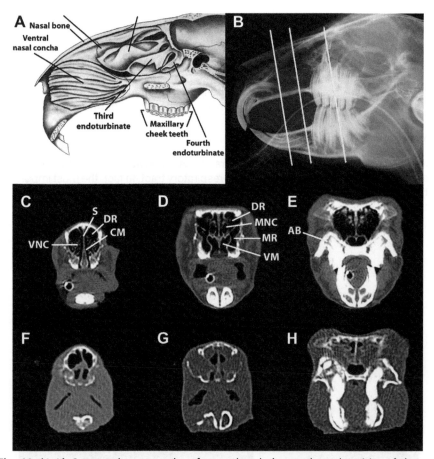

Fig. 14. (A–H) Computed tomography of normal and abnormal nasal cavities of the pet rabbit. (A) Anatomy of the nasal cavities and nasal conchae, sagittal view (*modified from* Popesko). (B) Radiograph of the skull of a normal rabbit, lateral projection, adapted as a scout view for CT axial views. (C–E) Normal nasal cavities. AB, alveolar bulla; CM, common meatus; DR, dorsal recess (otherwise named conchal sinus)[17]; MNC, middle nasal concha; MR, maxillary recess[16]; S, nasal septum; VM, ventral meatus; VNC, ventral nasal concha. (F–H) Empyema of the nasal cavities (including empyema of the maxillary and other recesses) following end-stage acquired dental disease. Nasal cavities are almost completely filled by radiodense, thick pus. The alveolar bullae are deformed. General bone lysis is present because of underlying metabolic bone disease. ([A, B, F–H] From Vittorio Capello, DVM; with permission; and [C–E] Angela Lennox, DVM; with permission.)

or paranasal sinus[11]), which is part of the nasal cavity and lies just cranial to the alveolar bulla. During an extraoral approach to the abscess and the focus of osteomyelitis, the endoscope may provide critical aid in detecting fragments of reserve crowns of cheek teeth and it can be used to enter the maxillary recess.

Inspection of the larynx and the first portion of the trachea can be performed using a rigid 2.7-mm telescope with the intraoral approach while keeping the head of the rabbit extended. Small, flexible endoscopes must be used for examination of the entire trachea and main bronchi.

Few preliminary experiences have been reported regarding thoracoscopy of exotic companion mammals.[11] Indications are related to inspection and biopsy of intrathoracic masses when definitive diagnosis was not achieved with other diagnostic tools. The single-entry approach can be paraxyphoid for most rabbits, and intercostal for rabbits weighing more than 2 kg and for ferrets.[11]

Common indications for endoscopy of the respiratory system in single species are listed in **Table 1**, and examples of normal and abnormal patterns are shown in **Figs. 11–13**.

COMPUTED TOMOGRAPHY

The basic principles of computed tomography as an advanced radiology technique make it ideal for both the upper and lower respiratory tract. In fact, the most important advantage of CT when compared with traditional radiography is the capability to

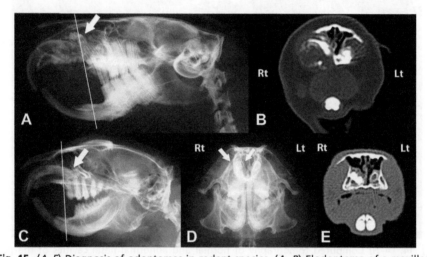

Fig. 15. (A–E) Diagnosis of odontomas in rodent species. (A, B) Elodontoma of a maxillary cheek tooth in a guinea pig. (C–E) Pseudo-odontoma of a maxillary incisor tooth in a prairie dog. (A) Skull radiograph, lateral projection. Abnormal and irregular radiodensity of the infraorbital area is present surrounding the apex and the reserve crown of a maxillary CT1 (arrow). Periosteal soft radiodensity is also visible ventrally to the palatine bone. The lateral radiograph has been used as scout view for the CT axial view (yellow line). (B) Computed tomography of the skull, axial view. Abnormal radiodensity, bone lysis, deformed reserve crown of maxillary CT1, and involvement of the nasal cavity with deviation of the nasal septum are present on the right side. Elodontoma (invasive odontogenic neoplasia) was ultimately diagnosed at necropsy. (C) Skull radiograph, lateral projection. Malocclusion of incisor teeth and apical deformity of one of them are visible (arrow). The other projection demonstrated unilateral pseudo-odontoma (space-occupying odontogenic dysplasia) on the right side. Mild respiratory symptoms were present at this stage. (D) Skull radiograph, rostrocaudal projection. Apical deformity of the right maxillary tooth (arrows). The lateral radiograph has been used as scout view for the CT axial view (yellow line). (E) Computed tomography of the skull, axial view. Space occupying pseudo-odontoma is visible on the right side, and is especially evident when compared with the transverse section of the normal incisive bone and the incisor tooth. Early diagnosis is critical for treatment of pseudo-odontoma, as well as to determine if disease is unilateral or bilateral. The comparison with the rostrocaudal projection of the radiograph of the skull proves that CT is a superior imaging tool for this specific disease. (From Vittorio Capello, DVM; with permission; and (E) Alberto Cauduro, DVM; with permission.)

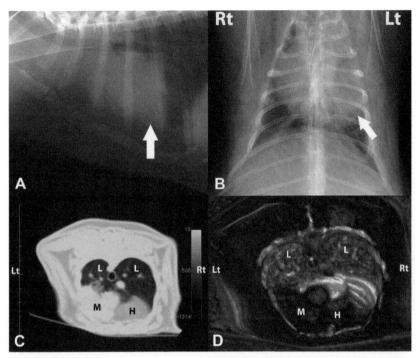

Fig. 16. (A–D) Pulmonary abscess in a rabbit. (A) Radiograph of the thorax, lateral projection. A single large nodule with moderately increased radiodensity is present (arrow). (B) Radiograph of the thorax, ventrodorsal projection. The nodule is located on the left lung (arrow). (C) Computed tomography of the thorax, axial view. It displays the abnormal mass (M), shifting heart (H) on the right side. (D) Computed tomography of the thorax, 3-D volume reconstruction. This special rendering provides even more detailed imaging diagnosis, especially for surgical purposes. Diagnosis was confirmed upon ultrasound-guided fine needle aspirate of the mass. (From Angela Lennox, DVM; with permission.)

provide images without the superimposition of adjacent anatomic structures.[1] The x-ray tube rotating around the patients and computer obtain multiple, parallel, cross-sectional image slices of the tissues of the patients.[19] Modern helical scanners (where patients are continuously moved toward the gantry) allow shorter scanning time, thin slices, and higher resolution. More help is provided by advanced software, software that is even available free of charge. Raw data can be manipulated and rendered in many different ways, including 2-dimensional multiplanar reformation for the 3 standard planes (axial, lateral, and coronal) and 3-dimensional (3-D) virtual volume and surface rendering.[1,19] All these technical features are critical for small patients.

The same axial view can be visualized adjusting different gray scales (windows). The standard windows display hard tissues, soft tissues, and air.[19] Therefore, CT images of the thorax can be examined for the 3 components, with a special emphasis on lungs and possible mediastinal masses. Contrast medium can be injected intravenously to emphasize soft-tissue abnormalities, if they are supported by sufficient blood supply.[20] CT is superior to traditional radiographs for diagnosis of intrapulmonary disease, such as abscesses in rabbits and rats, or lung metastases. They can be visualized in detail, providing higher-quality diagnosis and prognosis.

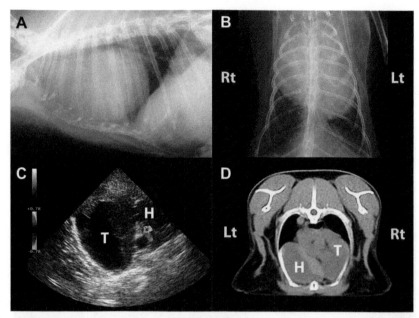

Fig. 17. (*A–D*) Thymoma in an 8-year-old female rabbit. (*A*) Radiograph of the thorax, lateral projection. Abnormal radiodensity is present in the cranial mediastinum, and the cranial margin of the cardiac silhouette is not visible. The trachea is displaced dorsally. (*B*) Radiograph of the thorax, ventrodorsal projection. (*C*) Ultrasonography of the thorax. The mediastinal thymoma (T) was partially cystic, and fluid was drained with thoracocentesis as palliative treatment. H, heart. (*D*) Computed tomography of the thorax, axial view. The thymoma (T) is twice as large as the heart (H). (*From* Vittorio Capello, DVM; with permission; and (*D*) Alberto Cauduro, DVM; with permission.)

Computed tomography of the skull is a critical diagnostic imaging tool also for the nasal cavities, especially in rabbits. Nasal meatuses, nasal septum, turbinates, and maxillary recesses can be visualized in detail; therefore, this diagnostic tool is complementary to rhinoscopy. CT is also critical for diagnosis of space-occupying masses, such as odontomas in rodent species, or for diagnosing masses that compress nasal cavities, such as pseudo-odontomas in prairie dogs.[21]

For CT scanning, patients are usually placed in ventral recumbency, under general anesthesia.[19] The endotracheal tube does not create problems of superimposition as occurs in the case of traditional radiographs.[1] When CT of the nasal cavities is performed, the head is slightly elevated in horizontal position. Proper symmetry is critical for acquisition of images. The scanning plane angle can be adjusted, but it is usually perpendicular to the palatine bone for the head and to the long axis of patients for the thorax.[19]

Common indications for computed tomography of the respiratory system in single species are listed in **Table 1**, and examples of normal and abnormal patterns are shown in **Figs. 14–17**.

MAGNETIC RESONANCE IMAGING

Magnetic resonance imaging (MRI) is a noninvasive imaging modality because it does not use radiation for generating images. Magnetic resonance imaging relies on

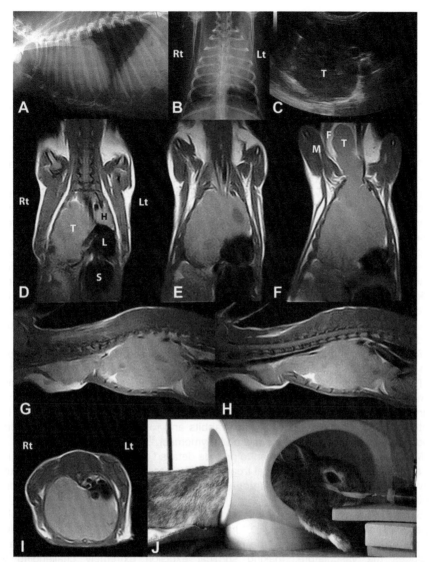

Fig. 18. (*A–J*) Thymoma in a 7-year-old female rabbit. The patient was presented with reduced food intake and mild dyspnea. (*A, B*) Radiograph of the thorax, lateral and ventrodorsal projection. Radiographic findings are similar to those presented in Fig. 17. Ultrasonography of the thorax displayed an enormous mass surrounding the heart (T) that occupied most of the mediastinum. (*D–F*) Magnetic resonance of the thorax, coronal views from dorsal to ventral. The heart (H) is displaced on the left side of the thorax, and a single caudal pulmonary lobe (L) is patent. Caudal to the diaphragm is the gas-filled stomach (S), distended because of aerophagy. In the second frame, the thymoma occupies almost the whole thoracic cavity. In the most ventral frame, the mass spreads outside the thorax in the extravisceral space of the neck. Note the specificity of MRI for soft tissues: neoplastic thymic tissue (T), subcutaneous fat (F), and muscles (M) are clearly distinguished. (*G, H*) Magnetic resonance of the thorax, lateral views from right to left. The cranial portion of the thymoma is visible cranially to the first rib. The second frame scanning the right hemithorax shows the displaced trachea and the small patent lung. (*I*) Magnetic resonance of the thorax, axial view. The section of the trachea and the small lung lobe are visible. MRI proved to be far superior for diagnosis compared with radiography and ultrasonography, which underestimated the size of the thoracic mass. In larger exotic mammal patients and if proper tesla magnet is available, MR might also be considered superior to CT. (*J*) The patient under general anesthesia and intubated is placed in sternal recumbency inside the magnetic field. (*From* Vittorio Capello, DVM; with permission; and (*D–J*) Alberto Cauduro, DVM; with permission.)

computer interpretation of the movements of hydrogen atoms in the body, in reaction to a strong magnetic field placed around patients.[20,22]

MR represents the diagnostic imaging modality of choice for soft tissues. It is most commonly used for the central nervous system, but other soft tissues can be visualized in detail with superior quality than CT.[20] Images are visualized in the 3 standard planes (dorsal, lateral or sagittal, transverse or axial), but complex manipulation and 3-D volume and surface renderings are not possible.

Patients undergoing MR examination are under general anesthesia and are usually positioned in sternal recumbency.

Two potential disadvantages of MR are resolution (especially for small mammals) and prolonged scanning time.[20] Resolution depends on the available magnet. Low-power magnets capable of field strengths of 0.2 to 0.4 T will produce lower-resolution images than magnetic fields of 1.0 T or higher. Acquisition of MR sequences depends on many technical factors that are beyond the scope of this article, but the average time for rabbit patients can range from 20 to 40 minutes, whereas acquisition time for CT scanning can be less than 1 minute. This timing might present potential risks for critical patients. Because of the long acquisition time, images might be affected by patients' respiratory and cardiac rates, which are higher in small-sized mammals.[22] Actually, this does not represent a concern because they respiratory and cardiac rates are significantly reduced under anesthesia.

The dorsal plane is superior for examination of the lungs and mediastinal structure, but the use of all 3 planes is always recommended for complete evaluation of the thorax.[22]

The lungs appear black because of the presence of air inside the parenchyma, and similar to traditional radiographs and CT, it is easy to visualize soft-tissue intrapulmonary abnormalities, but with superior quality. MR is particularly advantageous for detecting intrapulmonary abscesses of rabbits and rodents, metastasis of tumors, and mediastinal masses (lymphomas and thymomas).[18]

MR provides sufficient resolution to provide detailed diagnosis and prognosis, and to access the potential for surgical treatment. The presence of abnormalities should always be confirmed in more than one plane to avoid overinterpretation of various artifacts.[22]

Surgical excision of thymomas can be feasible if they do not envelope the vasculature of the cranial mediastinum.[22–24] In many cases, the vasculature is simply displaced in a lateral position by the mediastinal mass. In other patients, the mass includes the vasculature, making surgical excision extremely challenging to impossible.[22] Because of a specific affinity for soft tissues, MR represents the diagnostic imaging of choice for this disease.

Thick pus, typical of rabbit odontogenic abscesses, results in signal intensities similar to those from soft tissues. For this reason, MR of the skull for purposes other than central nervous system evaluation has interesting applications in pet rabbits.[16] MR provides excellent information when evaluating rabbits with multiple empyema syndrome affecting one or more cavities (nasal cavities, maxillary recess, diseased alveolar bulla, and tympanic bulla)[16] and in cases of retrobulbar and parabulbar abscesses; imaging is superior to even CT, which is less specific for lower radiodensities. CT remains superior for diagnosis of dental disease and related bone infection, and for this reason CT and MRI of the rabbit skull are best used as complementary tests.[16] Because complementary imaging is not feasible in most cases for practical and financial reasons, the clinical examination and survey radiographs are generally used to guide the clinician in selecting the most appropriate diagnostic imaging test.

Common indications for magnetic resonance of the thorax are listed in **Table 1** and examples of abnormal patterns are shown in **Figs. 18, 19**.

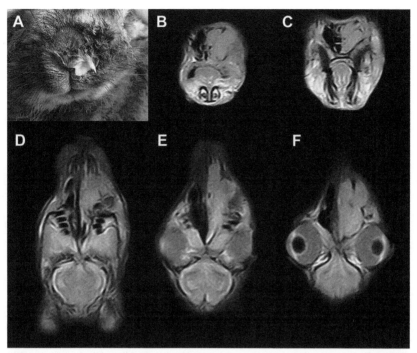

Fig. 19. (*A–F*) Rhinitis and empyema of the nasal cavity in a 2-year-old lop rabbit. (*A*) The rabbit was presented with unilateral thick nasal discharge. (*B, C*) Magnetic resonance of the skull, axial view, from rostral to caudal. The left nasal cavity, including the maxillary recess, is filled with pus with a signal intensity similar to that of soft tissues. (*D–F*) Magnetic resonance of the skull, coronal view, from ventral to dorsal. (*From* Vittorio Capello, DVM; with permission; and Alberto Cauduro, DVM; with permission.)

THE FUTURE OF DIAGNOSTIC IMAGING IN EXOTIC COMPANION MAMMALS

Other advanced imaging modalities, already in use in human medicine, may eventually prove beneficial in exotic mammal medicine.[20]

Fluoroscopy may be useful in selected cases for imaging of the intrathoracic tract of the esophagus, when used in conjunction with contrast medium. Fluoroscopy as an aid for surgical removal of heartworms from the ferret cranial vena cava, like in dogs, may not be an option because of patient size.

Nuclear diagnostic imaging involving injection of radioactive isotope includes scintigraphy and positron emission tomography (PET). This imaging modality provides functional information, rather than morphologic information, and should be used in addition to other standard modalities.[20]

Scintigraphy generates an image by detecting the emission of gamma rays from patients. The use of scintigraphy has been reported in a guinea pig affected by hyperthyroidism, but this technique may provide critical information in cases of neoplasia and aid in the detection of metastases.[25,26]

PET combines CT and MR with the use of radioactive nucleotides.[20]

Disadvantages of nuclear diagnostic imaging include the higher radiation dose administered to patients, the fact that patients remain radioactive after the study, few institutes offer this modality, and cost.[20] Diagnostic value of those modalities has yet to be assessed.

REFERENCES

1. Mackey EB, Hernandez-Divers SJ, Holland M, et al. Clinical technique; application of computed tomography in zoological medicine. J Exotic Pet Med 2008; 17(3):198–209.
2. Capello V, Lennox AM. Clinical radiology of exotic companion mammals. Ames (IA): Blackwell Publishing; 2008.
3. Zwingenberger A, Silverman S. Rodents: diagnostic imaging. In: Keeble E, Meredith A, editors. BSAVA Manual of Rodents and Ferrets. Gloucester (UK): BSAVA; 2009. p. 32–41.
4. Lennox AM. Anesthesia for radiology of exotic companion mammals. In: Advanced imaging of exotic companion mammals. 7th meeting of the Association of Exotic Companion Mammals. Savannah (GA), August 10, 2008. p. 8–9.
5. Lennox AM. It's great to sedate. In: Proceedings of the North American Veterinary Conference. Orlando (Fl): 2009. p. 1863–4.
6. Silverman S, Tell LA, editors. Radiology of rodents, rabbits, and ferrets. An atlas of normal anatomy and positioning. St Louis (MO): Elsevier Saunders; 2005.
7. Antinoff N. Clinically important anatomy of small mammals for diagnostic imaging. In: Advanced imaging of exotic companion mammals. 7th meeting of the Association of Exotic Companion Mammals Savannah (GA), August 10, 2008. p. 1–7.
8. Johnson-Delaney CA. Ultrasonography in ferret practice. In: Lewington JH, editor. Ferret husbandry, medicine and surgery. Philadelphia: BSAVA Manual of Rodents and Ferrets; 2007. p. 417–29.
9. Girling S. Ferrets: diagnostic imaging. In: Keeble E, Meredith A, editors. BSAVA manual of rodents and ferrets. Gloucester (UK): BSAVA; 2009. p. 219–29.
10. Divers SJ. Endoscopy equipment and instrumentation for use in exotic animal medicine. Vet Clin North Am Exot Anim Pract 2010;13(2):171–85.
11. Divers SJ. Exotic mammal diagnostic endoscopy and endosurgery. Vet Clin North Am Exot Anim Pract 2010;13(2):255–72.
12. Lennox AM, Capello V. Tracheal intubation in exotic companion mammals. J Exotic Pet Med 2008;17(3):221–7.
13. Johnson DH. Endoscopic intubation of exotic companion mammals. Vet Clin North Am Exot Anim Pract 2010;13(2):273–89.
14. Johnson DH. Over-the-endoscope endotracheal intubation of small exotic mammals. Exotic DVM 2005;7(2):18–23.
15. Lennox AM. Rhinotomy for treatment of chronic upper respiratory disease in Rabbits. In: Proceedings of the North American Veterinary Conference. Orlando (Fl); 2011.
16. Capello V. Novel diagnostic and surgical techniques for treatment of difficult facial abscesses in pet rabbits. In: Proceedings of the North American Veterinary Conference. Orlando (Fl); 2011. p. 1685–9.
17. Harcourt-Brown FM. Cardiorespiratory disease. In: Harcourt-Brown FM, editor. Textbook of rabbit medicine. Oxford (UK): Butterworth-Heinemann; 2002. p. 324–34.
18. Divers JS. The rabbit respiratory system: anatomy, physiology and pathology. In: Proceedings of the Association of Exotic Mammal Veterinarians Scientific Program. Providence (RI); 2007. p. 61–8.
19. Capello V, Cauduro A, Widmer WR. Introduction to computed tomography in exotic companion mammals. In: Capello V, Lennox AM, editors. Clinical radiology of exotic companion mammals. Ames (IA): Blackwell Publishing; 2008. p. 44–9.

20. Mayer J. Advanced diagnostic imaging in exotic mammals. In: Proc North Am Vet Conf. Orlando (FL); 2008. p. 1856–8.
21. Capello V. Dentistry of other rodent species and ferrets. In: Proceedings of the North American Veterinary Conference. Orlando (Fl); 2011. p. 1681–4.
22. Gavin PR, Holmes SP. Thorax. In: Gavin PR, Bagley RS, editors. Practical small animal MRI. Ames (IA): John Wiley & Sons; 2009. p. 295–308.
23. Bennet RA. Rabbit thoracic surgery. In: Proceedings of the Association of Exotic Mammal Veterinarians Scientific Program. San Diego (CA); 2010. p. 85–91.
24. Morrisey JK, McEntee M. Therapeutic options for thymoma in the rabbit. Sem Avian Exot Pet Med 2005;14(3):175–81.
25. Mayer J, Wagner R, Taeymans O. Advanced diagnostic approaches and current management of thyroid pathologies in guinea pigs. Vet Clin North Am Exot Anim Pract 2010;13(3):509–23.
26. Mayer J. Evidence-based medicine in small mammals. J Exotic Pet Med 2009; 18(3):213–9.

Index

Note: Page numbers of article titles are in **boldface** type.

A

Abscesses, respiratory disorders related to, imaging of, 376, 380, 384, 386–387
    in ferrets, lung, 363–364
        tooth root, 366
    in rabbits, 261–263, 266
    in rodents, 300, 311–312
Acidophilic macrophage pneumonia (AMP), in rodents, 325–326
Adenocarcinoma, of nasal tissue, in rabbits, 265–266
Adenovirus, respiratory disorders related to, in guinea pigs, 349–350
Adiaspiromycosis, respiratory disorders related to, in chinchillas and guinea pigs, 350
Aeromonas hydrophilia, respiratory disorders related to, in pet and ornamental fish, 190
Aerosol therapy, for respiratory disorders, in avians, 249, 254
    in chinchillas and guinea pigs, 353
    in reptiles, 219
    in rodents, 290, 294
Agent-induced pulmonary edema, in rodents, 326
Air sac disease, avian respiratory distress and, 250–254
    anatomy and physiology of, 250–252
    breathing patterns with, 252
    diagnostic tests for, 254
    etiology of, 253–254
    gas exchange dynamics with, 252–253
    history taking for, 252
    physical examination for, 252
    respiratory sounds with, 252
    treatment of, 254
Air-breathing fish, anatomy and physiology of, 181
Airway disease, avian respiratory distress related to. See also *specific anatomy.*
    large airway, 245–247
    lower (parenchymal), 250–254
    small airway, 248–249
    upper airway and infraorbital sinus, 241–245
Airway obstructions. See *Respiratory obstruction.*
Allergic diseases, respiratory disorders related to, in rodents, 326
Alveolar hemorrhage, in rodents, 326
Alveolar histiocytosis, in rodents, 326–327
Alveolar hyperplasia, in rodents, 328
Alveolar lipoproteinosis, in rodents, 326–327
Alveolar proteinosis, in rodents, 326–327
Amyloidosis, respiratory disorders related to, in rodents, 327–328

Vet Clin Exot Anim 14 (2011) 391–420
doi:10.1016/S1094-9194(11)00020-X
1094-9194/11/$ – see front matter © 2011 Elsevier Inc. All rights reserved.

vetexotic.theclinics.com

Anatomy and physiology, of respiratory system, in avians, 241–243, 245–246
    coelomic cavity, 249
    large airway, 245–246
    parenchymal lung or air sac, 250–252
    small airway, 248
    upper airway, 241–243
  in chelonians, 225–226
    lateral view of, 226–227
  in chinchillas, 342–343
  in ferrets, 357–361
    bronchi, 359–360
    heart and lungs, 360–361
    nasal cavity, 357–358
    pharynx, 358–359
    respiratory characteristics, 361–362
    skull view, 357–358
    thorax, 358–360
    trachea, 358
  in guinea pigs, 342–345
  in hedgehogs, 267–269
  in pet and ornamental fish, 179–181
  in rabbits, 257–258
    lung lobes, 258, 260
    paramedian section of, 258
    thymus perspectives, 258–259
  in reptiles, 208–209
  in rodents, 291, 294–296
  in sugar gliders, 269–270
Anesthesia, for imaging, of companion mammals, 370–371, 383, 385
Anticoagulant rodenticides, respiratory disorders related to, in chinchillas and
  guinea pigs, 352
Antifungal agents, for respiratory disorders, in avians, 254
  in chelonians, 233, 235
  in chinchillas and guinea pigs, 350
  in pet and ornamental fish, 199–200
  in reptiles, 217–218
Antimicrobial agents, for respiratory disorders, in avians, 245, 249–250, 254
  in chelonians, 231, 235
  in chinchillas and guinea pigs, 346–349
  in pet and ornamental fish, 198
  in rabbits, 259
  in reptiles, 217–219
  in rodents, 290
Antiparasitic agents, for respiratory disorders, in chelonians, 233, 235
  in pet and ornamental fish, 199–201
  in reptiles, 218–219
Antiviral agents, for respiratory disorders, in chelonians, 232
Arterial blood gas analysis, for respiratory disorders, in reptiles, 220
Ascites, respiratory distress related to, in avians, 250
Aspergillus spp., respiratory disorders related to, in avians, 244, 246–247
  in chelonians, 233

in reptiles, 212
in rodents, 311–312
Aspiration, respiratory obstruction related to, in avians, 253–254
in chinchillas and guinea pigs, 353
Aspiration pneumonia, in rodents, 328
Auscultation, for respiratory disorders, in chinchillas and guinea pigs, 351
in hedgehogs and sugar gliders, 270
Avian respiratory distress, **241–255**
coelomic cavity disease and, 249–250
anatomy and physiology of, 249
ascites and, 250
breathing patterns with, 249
diagnostic tests for, 250
egg binding and, 250
etiology of, 250
history taking for, 249
mass lesions and, 250
organomegaly and, 250
physical examination for, 249
respiratory sounds with, 249
treatment of, 250
large airway disease and, 245–247
anatomy and physiology of, 245–247
breathing patterns with, 246
diagnostic tests for, 246
etiology of, 246–247
history taking for, 246
physical examination for, 246
respiratory sounds with, 246
treatment of, 246
parenchymal disease and, 250–254
anatomy and physiology of, 250–252
breathing patterns with, 252
diagnostic tests for, 254
etiology of, 253–254
gas exchange dynamics with, 252–253
history taking for, 252
physical examination for, 252
respiratory sounds with, 252
treatment of, 254
small airway disease and, 248–249
anatomy and physiology of, 248
breathing patterns with, 248
diagnostic tests for, 249
etiology of, 249
history taking for, 248
physical examination for, 248
respiratory sounds with, 248
treatment of, 249
summary overview of, 241
upper airway and infraorbital sinus disease and, 241–245

Avian respiratory (*continued*)
        anatomy and physiology of, 241–243
        breathing pattern with, 243
        diagnostic tests for, 244–245
        etiology of, 243–244
        history taking for, 242
        physical examination for, 242–243
        respiratory sounds with, 243
        treatment of, 245
Avocado toxicosis, respiratory disorders related to, in chinchillas
    and guinea pigs, 352

B

Bacterial diseases, respiratory disorders related to, in avians, 243–244
        in chelonians, 230–231
        in chinchillas, 342, 348–349
        in guinea pigs, 342, 345–348
            treatment of, 349
        in hedgehogs, 274
        in pet and ornamental fish, 190–191
            treatment of, 198
        in rabbits, 259–265
            bordetellosis, 263
            other pathogens, 264–265
            pasteurellosis, 259–263
            staphylococcosis, 264
        in reptiles, 211–212
            treatment of, 217–219
        in rodents, 297–310
        in sugar gliders, 279
Biopsy, for respiratory disorders, gill, in pet and ornamental fish, 185–186
        in avians, 244, 250, 254
        lung, in chelonians, 229–230
            in reptiles, 217
        ultrasound-guided, in avians, 250
            in rabbits, 266
Bordetella bronchiseptica, respiratory disorders related to, in chinchillas, 349
        in guinea pigs, 345–347
Bordetella spp., respiratory disorders related to, in hedgehogs, 274
        in rabbits, 263
        in rodents, 297
Breathing patterns, of avians, 243, 246, 248–249, 252
    of chelonians, 225–226
    of ferrets, 361–362
    of hedgehogs, 268
    of rabbits, 257–258
    of reptiles, 208–209, 213
    of rodents, 291, 294, 296
    of sugar gliders, 269
Bronchi, of avians, 248, 251–252

of ferrets, 359–360
    sensory nerve stimulation of, 362
of mouse, 291
Bronchial epithelium hyperplasia, in rodents, 328
Bronchioles, of rat, 295–296
Bronchodilators, for respiratory disorders, in avians, 249, 254
    in chinchillas and guinea pigs, 353
    in reptiles, 217, 219
    in rodents, 290, 294
Bronchointerstitial pneumonia, in ferrets, 366
Bronchoscopy, of companion mammals, 373, 379
Brown Norway (BN) rat, eosinophilic granulomatous pneumonia in, 328

C

Candida spp., respiratory disorders related to, in chelonians, 233
    in reptiles, 212
    in rodents, 311
Canine distemper, respiratory disorders related to, in ferrets, 364–365
Capillaria spp., respiratory disorders related to, in avians, 244
    in hedgehogs, 275–276
Capnography, side-stream, for respiratory disorders, in rabbits, 262
Caprinlana sp., respiratory disorders related to, in pet and ornamental fish, 188
Carcinomas, respiratory disorders related to. See *Neoplasia; specific type.*
Cardiomyopathy, respiratory disorders occurring with, imaging of, 376
    in chinchillas and guinea pigs, 351–352
    in hedgehogs, 277–278
Cardiovascular diseases, respiratory disorders occurring with.
    See also *Heart disease.*
    in chinchillas and guinea pigs, 351–352
Cartilage degeneration, in trachea, of rats, 329
Cervical lymphadenitis, respiratory disorders related to, in guinea pigs, 347
Chelonians, respiratory system of, **225–239**. See also *Reptiles.*
    anatomy and physiology of, 208, 225–226
        lateral view of, 226–227
    diagnostics of, 226–230
        biopsy in, 229–230
        culture in, 228, 230, 233, 235
        cytology in, 228
        hematology in, 228
        imaging in, 228–229
        physical exam in, 226–228
    disease signs and symptoms in, 213
    hypovitaminosis A and, 234
    infectious disease in, 230–234
        bacterial, 230–231
        fungal, 233
        iridoviruses, 232–233
        parasitic, 233–234
        viral, 231–232
    noninfectious disease in, 234–235

Chelonians (*continued*)
    summary overview of, 207–208, 221, 225
    therapeutics for, 235
Chilodonella sp., respiratory disorders related to, in pet and ornamental fish, 187
Chinchillas, respiratory system and disorders in, **339–355**
    anatomy and physiology of, 342–343
    behavioral perspectives of, 342
    diagnostic imaging of, 372–373
    emergency management of, 352–353
    housing and bedding factors of, 341–342
    husbandry requirements and, 340–342
    infectious diseases as, 344–345
        bacterial, 342, 348–349
        fungal, 350
        viral, 350
    noninfectious diseases as, 345, 350–352
        heatstroke, 351
        inhalation pneumonia, 352
        miscellaneous conditions, 351–352
        nare inflammation, 351
        neoplasia, 350–351
        toxicosis, 352
        trauma, 352–353
    nutrition perspectives of, 341
    summary overview of, 339–340, 353
Chlamydophila spp., respiratory disorders related to, in avians, 244, 254
    in guinea pigs, 348
    in rabbits, 265
    in rodents, 297–298
Choanal slit, in avians, respiratory disorders and, 244–245
Chronic respiratory disease (CRD), in rats, 304–306
Cilia-associated respiratory bacillus (CARB), in rabbits, 265
    in rodents, 298–300
Clinical signs, of respiratory disorders, in ferrets, 362–366
    in hedgehogs, 270–271, 273–274
    in pet and ornamental fish, 182–183
    in rabbits, 261, 263–266
    in reptiles, 213
    in rodents, 289. See also *specific rodent or disease.*
    in sugar gliders, 270–271, 278–279
Coccidia spp., respiratory disorders related to, in chelonians, 233
Coelomic cavity, respiratory disorders related to, in avians, 249–250
    anatomy and physiology of, 249
    ascites and, 250
    breathing patterns with, 249
    diagnostic tests for, 250
    egg binding and, 250
    etiology of, 250
    history taking for, 249
    mass lesions and, 250
    organomegaly and, 250

physical examination for, 249
respiratory sounds with, 249
treatment of, 250
in reptiles, 221
Coelomocentesis, for avian respiratory distress, 250
Companion mammals, diagnostic imaging of respiratory system in, **369–389**
chinchilla indications, 372–373
computed tomography for, 381–383
examples of, 379–381, 383, 386
specie-specific indications for, 372–373, 383
degus indications, 372–373
endoscopy for, 378–381
examples of, 381, 384–385
specie-specific indications for, 372–373, 381
ferret indications, 372–373, 376–377
future of, 387–388
guinea pig indications, 372–373
magnetic resonance imaging for, 383, 385–387
examples of, 382–383, 387
specie-specific indications for, 372–373, 387
prairie dog indications, 372–373, 375, 379, 383
rabbit indications, 372–374, 380–384, 386–387
radiography for, 370–371
examples of, 371, 374–383
specie-specific indications for, 371–373
rat indications, 372–373, 376
skunk indications, 372–373
squirrel indications, 372–373
summary overview of, 369–370
ultrasonography for, 371, 374, 377–378
examples of, 377–378, 381
specie-specific indications for, 372–373, 378
Companion rodents, respiratory system and disorders in, **339–355**.
See also *Chinchillas; Guinea pigs.*
Computed tomography (CT), of respiratory disorders, in chelonians, 229
in companion mammals, 381–383
examples of, 379–381, 383, 386
specie-specific indications for, 372–373, 383, 387
in hedgehogs and sugar gliders, 273
in reptiles, 214–216
Conjunctivitis, with respiratory disorders, in avians, 244
in chinchillas and guinea pigs, 343, 350
in rabbits, 261–263
Contaminants, respiratory disorders related to. See *Pollutants; Toxins.*
Coronavirus, Parker rat, respiratory disorders related to, in rodents, 322–323
Corynebacterium kutscheri, respiratory disorders related to, in rodents, 300–301
Crenosoma spp., respiratory disorders related to, in hedgehogs, 275–276
Crustacean parasites, respiratory disorders related to, in pet and ornamental fish, 190
Cryptobia spp., respiratory disorders related to, in pet and ornamental fish, 188
Cryptocaryon irritans, respiratory disorders related to, in pet and ornamental fish, 187
Cryptococcus neoformans, respiratory disorders related to, in sugar gliders, 279

Culture(s), for respiratory disorders, in chelonians, 228, 230, 233, 235
    in chinchillas and guinea pigs, 353
    in hedgehogs and sugar gliders, 273
    in rabbits, 264
    in reptiles, 216–217
Cystocentesis, for avian respiratory distress, 250
Cytology. See *Wet mount cytology.*
Cytomegalovirus infections, respiratory disorders related to, in hedgehogs, 275
    in rodents, 313–314

D

Dactylogyrus spp., respiratory disorders related to, in pet and ornamental fish, 189
Decontamination, for respiratory disorders prevention, with rodents, 289–290
Degus, imaging of respiratory system in, 372–373
Dental disease, respiratory disorders related to, in ferrets, 366–367
Dental formula, of chinchillas vs. guinea pigs, 340, 343
Diagnostic evaluation, of respiratory disorders, imaging techniques for.
   See *Imaging.*
    in avians, 244–246, 249–250, 254
    in chelonians, 226–230
    in hedgehogs, 270–273
    in pet and ornamental fish, 182–186
    in rabbits, 264
    in reptiles, 213–217
    in rodents, 287–290. See also *specific rodent or disease.*
    in sugar gliders, 270–273
Diagnostic laboratories, for H1N1 influenza confirmation, in ferrets, 366
   for rodent disease testing, 290, 292–293
Diagnostic samples/sampling, for respiratory disorders. See also *specific test,*
   e.g., Wet mount cytology.
    in avians, 244–245, 250, 254
    in chelonians, 228–230
    in hedgehogs and sugar gliders, 271–273
    in pet and ornamental fish, 185–186
    in rabbits, 264
    in reptiles, 216–217
Diaphragmatic hernia, imaging of, 378
Digital systems, for radiography, in companion mammals, 371
   for ultrasonography, in companion mammals, 374
Dinoflagellates, respiratory disorders related to, in pet and ornamental fish, 189
Disinfection, for respiratory disorders prevention, with rodents, 289–290
Dorsoventral view, in radiography, for companion mammals, 370–371, 383
Drug delivery methods, in pet and ornamental fish, 180
   in reptiles, 219
   in rodents, 290
Drug therapy, for respiratory disorders, in avians, 245, 249–250, 254
    in chelonians, 231–233, 235
    in chinchillas and guinea pigs, 346–349, 353
    in ferrets, 362–363, 366
    in pet and ornamental fish, 197–201

in rabbits, 259, 264
in reptiles, 217–219
in rodents, 290. See also *specific rodent or disease.*

E

Egg binding, avian respiratory distress related to, 250
Electron microscopy, for respiratory disorders, in reptiles, 217
Emergency management, of respiratory disorders,
    in chelonians, 234–235
        in chinchillas and guinea pigs, 352–353
        in pet and ornamental fish, 196–197
        in reptiles, 210, 217, 220–221
Endogenous lipid pneumonia, in ferrets, 365
Endoscopic instrumentations, for exotic mammal medicine, 379
Endoscopic-guided orotracheal intubation, of prairie dog, 385
    of rabbit, 384
Endoscopy, of respiratory disorders, in avians, 244, 246, 254
    in companion mammals, 378–381
        examples of, 381, 384–385
        specie-specific indications for, 372–373, 381
    in hedgehogs and sugar gliders, 273
    in pet and ornamental fish, 186
    in reptiles, 216, 221
Endotracheal intubation, for respiratory disorders, in avians, 246
    in chelonians, 235
    in reptiles, 220
    radiography indications for, in companion mammals, 371
Environmental conditions, respiratory disorders related to, in avians, 249, 253
    in chinchillas and guinea pigs, 342, 352
    in ferrets, 362, 366–367
    in pet and ornamental fish, 194–195
        injury response vs., 181–182
    in reptiles, 210
        treatment considerations of, 217, 219
    in rodents, 288–289
Enzyme-linked immunosorbent assay (ELISA), for respiratory disorders,
    in chelonians, 230–232
    in reptiles, 216–217
Eosinophilic granulomatous pneumonia, in brown Norway rats, 328
Epistylis sp., respiratory disorders related to, in pet and ornamental fish, 188
Epithelial hyalinosis, respiratory disorders related to, in rodents, 325–326
Esophagus, imaging of, in companion mammals, 372, 377

F

Ferrets, respiratory system and disorders of, **357–367**
    anatomy of, 357–361
        bronchi, 359–360
        heart and lungs, 360–361
        nasal cavity, 357–358

Ferrets (*continued*)
      pharynx, 358–359
      skull view, 357–358
      thorax, 358–360
      trachea, 358
   canine distemper as, 364–365
   dental disease and, 366–367
   diagnostic imaging of, 372–373, 376–377
   H1N1 influenza as, 365–366
   influenza as, 362
   Mycoplasma spp. infections as, 363–364
   neoplasia associated with, 365
   nonspecific conditions as, 365
   physiology of, 361–362
   pneumonia as, 362–363
      endogenous lipid, 365
Fish. See *Ornamental fish; Pet fish.*
Flavobacterium spp., respiratory disorders related to, in pet and
   ornamental fish, 190–191
Fluid therapy, for respiratory disorders, in chelonians, 235
   in chinchillas and guinea pigs, 353
   in hedgehogs and sugar gliders, 281
Flukes, respiratory disorders related to, in pet and ornamental fish, 189
Foreign bodies, as respiratory obstruction, in avians, 246, 253
   in chelonians, 234
   in chinchillas and guinea pigs, 353
   in ferrets, 366–367
   in pet and ornamental fish, 196–197
   in reptiles, 210, 221
   in sugar gliders, 281
Freund adjuvant pulmonary granuloma, in rodents, 328
Fungal diseases, respiratory disorders related to, in avians, 246–247, 254
   in chelonians, 233
   in chinchillas and guinea pigs, 350
   in hedgehogs, 275
   in pet and ornamental fish, 193
      treatment of, 199–200
   in reptiles, 212
      treatment of, 217–218
   in rodents, 311–312
   in sugar gliders, 279
Fur removal, for ultrasonography, in companion mammals, 374, 377

G

Gas bubble disease, in pet and ornamental fish, 194–195
Gas exchange physiology. See *Respiration.*
Gas exchange surface, of avian lungs, 252–253
Genetic perspectives, of rodent respiratory disorders, 287–288, 315
Gerbil, respiratory system and disorders in, anatomy and physiology of,
   291–292, 295–296

bordetellosis as, 297
    cilia-associated respiratory bacillus as, 300
    clinical signs of, 289
    diagnostic laboratories for testing of, 290, 292–293
    diagnostic workup of, 287–290
    Mycoplasma pulmonis as, 306
    Pasteurella pneumotropica as, 308
    sanitation and decontamination for, 289–290
    Streptococcus pneumoniae as, 310
Gill anatomy and physiology, in pet and ornamental fish, 179–181
    histologic view of, 180
Gill biopsy, for respiratory disorders, in pet and ornamental
    fish, 185–186
Gill disease, in pet and ornamental fish, 181–182
    anemia presentations with, 184–186
    clinical signs associated with, 182–183
    common diseases, 186–197
Gill injury response, in pet and ornamental fish, 181–182
    focal necrosis as, 184, 192
Glans nictitans infections, in rabbits, 263
Glottis, avian respiratory distress and, 245–247
    anatomy and physiology of, 245–247
    breathing patterns with, 246
    diagnostic tests for, 246
    etiology of, 246–247
    history taking for, 246
    physical examination for, 246
    respiratory sounds with, 246
    treatment of, 246
Glucocorticoids, for respiratory disorders, in reptiles, 217
Guinea pigs, respiratory system and disorders in, **339–355**
    anatomy and physiology of, 342–345
    behavioral perspectives of, 342
    diagnostic imaging of, 372–373
    emergency management of, 352–353
    housing and bedding factors of, 341–342
    husbandry requirements and, 340–342
    infectious diseases as, 344–345
        bacterial, 342, 345–348
            treatment of, 349
        fungal, 350
        viral, 349–350
    noninfectious diseases as, 345, 350–352
        heatstroke, 351
        inhalation pneumonia, 352
        miscellaneous conditions, 351–352
        neoplasia, 350–351
        toxicosis, 352
        trauma, 352–353
    nutrition perspectives of, 340–341
    summary overview of, 339–340, 353

H

H1N1 (swine) influenza, respiratory disorders related to, in ferrets, 365–366

Haemophilus spp., respiratory disorders related to, in guinea pigs, 347
in rodents, 301–302

Hamster, respiratory system and disorders in, alveolar histiocytosis as, 327
amyloidosis as, 328
anatomy and physiology of, 291–292, 295–296
bordetellosis as, 297
cilia-associated respiratory bacillus as, 299
clinical signs of, 289
Corynebacterium kutscheri as, 301
diagnostic laboratories for testing of, 290, 292–293
diagnostic workup of, 287–290
miscellaneous lesions as, 329
mouse cytomegalovirus infection as, 314
Mycoplasma pulmonis as, 306
neoplasia as, 325
Pasteurella pneumotropica as, 308
pneumonia virus as, 317–318
sanitation and decontamination for, 289–290
Sendai virus as, 321
Streptococcus pneumoniae as, 310

Handling, for physical examination, of pet and ornamental fish, 183–184

Hantavirus (HV), respiratory disorders related to, in rodents, 312–313

Harderian gland secretions, of gerbil, respiratory disease associated with, 325–326

Heart anatomy, in ferrets, 360–361

Heart disease, respiratory disorders occurring with, in avians, 250, 254
in chinchillas and guinea pigs, 351–352
in hedgehogs, 277–278
in rodents, 289, 291
in sugar gliders, 280

Heatstroke, respiratory disorders occurring with, in chinchillas and guinea pigs, 351

Hedgehogs, respiratory system and disease of, **267–285**
anatomy and physiology of, 267–269
diagnosis of, 270–273
hibernation and, 268–269, 281
infectious processes in, 268, 273–276
bacterial, 274
fungal, 275
parasitic, 275–276
viral, 274–275
yeast, 275
noninfectious processes in, 277–278
heart disease, 277–278
neoplasia, 277
trauma, 278–279
prevention of, 281
summary overview of, 267, 281–282
torpor and, 268
treatment of, 281

Hematology, in respiratory disorders evaluation, of chelonians, 228
    of pet and ornamental fish, 184–186
Hemorrhage, alveolar, in rodents, 326
Hepatitis virus, respiratory disorders related to, in mouse, 314–315
Herpes virus infections, respiratory disorders related to, in chelonians, 231–232
    in pet and ornamental fish, 191–193
    in reptiles, 210–211
    in rodents, 313–314
Hibernation, by hedgehogs, 268–269, 281
    by sugar gliders, 269–270, 281
High-frequency probe, for ultrasonography, in companion mammals, 374
Histiocytosis, alveolar, in rodents, 326–327
    pulmonary, in rodents, 326–327
Histology, of gill disorders, in pet and ornamental fish, 180
      infectious, 191, 193
      noninfectious, 194
Histoplasmosis, respiratory disorders related to, in chinchillas and guinea pigs, 350
    in hedgehogs, 275
    in sugar gliders, 279
History taking, for respiratory disorders, in avians, 242, 246, 248–249, 252
    in chelonians, 226
    in hedgehogs and sugar gliders, 270
    in pet and ornamental fish, 182–183
    in reptiles, 213
    in rodents, 288
Husbandry, respiratory disorders related to. See also *Environmental conditions.*
    in chinchillas and guinea pigs, 340–342
    in rodents, 288–289
Hyalinosis, epithelial, respiratory disorders related to, in rodents, 325–326
Hyperplasia, alveolar, in rodents, 328
    bronchial epithelium, in rodents, 328
Hypovitaminosis A, respiratory disorders related to, in avians, 243–245
    in chelonians, 234
Hypoxia, in ferrets, 361–362
    in pet and ornamental fish, 182

I

Ichthyobodo sp., respiratory disorders related to, in pet and ornamental fish, 188
Ichthyophthirius multifiliis, respiratory disorders related to, in pet and
    ornamental fish, 187–188
Imaging, of respiratory disorders. See also *specific modality.*
    in avians, 244, 246, 249–250
    in chelonians, 228–229
    in chinchillas, 372–373
    in companion mammals, **369–389**
      computed tomography for, 381–383
        examples of, 379–381, 383, 386
        specie-specific indications for, 372–373, 383
      endoscopy for, 378–381
        examples of, 381, 384–385

Imaging (*continued*)
  specie-specific indications for, 372–373, 381
  future of, 387–388
  magnetic resonance imaging for, 383, 385–387
    examples of, 382–383, 387
    specie-specific indications for, 372–373, 387
  radiography for, 370–371
    examples of, 371, 374–383
    specie-specific indications for, 371–373
  summary overview of, 369–370
  ultrasonography for, 371, 374, 377–378
    examples of, 377–378, 381
    specie-specific indications for, 372–373, 378
  in degus, 372–373
  in ferrets, 372–373, 376–377
  in guinea pigs, 372–373
  in hedgehogs and sugar gliders, 271–273
  in prairie dogs, 372–373, 375, 379, 383
  in rabbits, 372–374, 380–384, 386–387
  in rats, 372–373, 376
  in reptiles, 214–216, 219
  in skunks, 372–373
  in squirrels, 372–373
Immunizations, for canine distemper, in ferrets, 364
  for pasteurellosis, in rabbits, 261
Inclusion body disease (IBD), in snakes, 211
Infectious diseases, respiratory disorders related to, in avians, 243–244,
  246, 249, 253–254
  in chelonians, 230–234
  in chinchillas, 344–345
    bacterial, 342, 348–349
    fungal, 350
    viral, 350
  in ferrets, canine distemper, 364–365
    H1N1 influenza, 365–366
    influenza, 362
    Mycoplasma spp., 363–364
    pneumonia, 362–363
  in guinea pigs, 344–345
    bacterial, 342, 345–348
      treatment of, 349
    fungal, 350
    viral, 349–350
  in hedgehogs, 268, 273–276
    bacterial, 274
    fungal, 275
    parasitic, 275–276
    viral, 274–275
    yeast, 275
  in pet and ornamental fish, 186–193
    bacterial, 190–191

fungal, 193
parasitic, 186–190
viral, 191–193
in rabbits, 258–264
bordetellosis, 263
other bacterial, 264–265
overview of, 258–264
pasteurellosis, 259–263
staphylococcosis, 264
in reptiles, 209–212
bacterial, 211–212
fungal, 212
overview of, 209–210
parasitic, 212
viral, 210–211
in rodents, 290, 297–324
bacterial, 297–310
mycotic, 310–312
parasitic, 312
viral, 312–324
in sugar gliders, 278–280
bacterial, 279
fungal, 279
parasitic, 280
viral, 279
yeast, 279
Inflammation, respiratory disorders related to, neurogenic, in ferrets, 362
of nares, in chinchillas, 351
of nasal mucosa, in rodents, 328
Influenza, respiratory disorders related to, in chinchillas, 350
in ferrets, 362
H1N1 (swine), 365–366
Infraorbital sinus, avian respiratory distress and, 241–245
anatomy and physiology of, 241–243
breathing pattern with, 243
diagnostic tests for, 244–245
etiology of, 243–244
history taking for, 242
physical examination for, 242–243
respiratory sounds with, 243
treatment of, 245
Inhalation pneumonia, in chinchillas and guinea pigs, 352
Injury response, of respiratory system. See *Trauma.*
Iridoviruses, respiratory disorders related to, in chelonians, 232–233

K

Kilham polyomavirus (KPYV), respiratory disorders related to, in rodents, 316
Klebsiella pneumoniae, respiratory disorders related to, in chinchillas, 349
in rodents, 302
Koi herpes virus (KHV), in pet and ornamental fish gills, 191–193

L

Lacrimal duct obstructions, with respiratory disorders, in rabbits, 261–262
    in rodents, 323
Lactic acidosis, therapy for, in chelonians, 235
Large airway disease, avian respiratory distress and, 245–247
        anatomy and physiology of, 245–247
        breathing patterns with, 246
        diagnostic tests for, 246
        etiology of, 246–247
        history taking for, 246
        physical examination for, 246
        respiratory sounds with, 246
        treatment of, 246
Laryngoscopy, of companion mammals, 373, 381
Latero-lateral view, in radiography, for companion mammals, 370
Leeches, on pet and ornamental fish gills, 190
Lipid pneumonia, endogenous, in ferrets, 365
Lipoproteinosis, alveolar, in rodents, 326–327
Lizards, respiratory disease signs and symptoms in, 213
    respiratory medicine for. See *Reptiles.*
    respiratory tract anatomy and physiology of, 209
Lower airway disease, avian respiratory distress and, 250–254.
    See also *Parenchymal disease.*
Lower respiratory tract after Fedde, of avians, 252
Lung biopsy, in chelonians, 229–230
    in reptiles, 217
Lung capacity, of rodents, 294, 296
Lung disease (parenchymal), avian respiratory distress and, 250–254
        anatomy and physiology of, 250–252
        breathing patterns with, 252
        diagnostic tests for, 254
        etiology of, 253–254
        gas exchange dynamics with, 252–253
        history taking for, 252
        physical examination for, 252
        respiratory sounds with, 252
        treatment of, 254
Lung lesions, *Corynebacterium,* in rodents, 300
    in chinchillas and guinea pigs, emergency evaluation of, 353
        primary, 350–351
    lymphohistiocytic, in rodents, 328–329
    Pasteurella, in rabbits, 262–263
Lung lobe aspirate, for respiratory disorders, in hedgehogs and sugar gliders, 272–273
Lung lobes, of avians, 250–252
    of chinchillas, 342
    of ferrets, 360–361
    of guinea pigs, 342–344
    of rabbits, 258, 260
    of rodents, 291, 294
Lung worms, respiratory disorders related to, in hedgehogs, 275–276

Lungs, imaging of, in companion mammals, 372
    primary tumors of, in rodents, 324–325
    septum of, in avians, 248
Lymph disease, respiratory disorders related to, imaging of, 376
        in rabbits, 263, 266
Lymphadenitis, cervical, respiratory disorders related to, in guinea pigs, 347
Lymphohistiocytic lung lesions, in rodents, 328–329
Lymphoid infiltrates, perivascular, in rodents, 329

M

Magnetic resonance imaging (MRI), of respiratory disorders, in companion
    mammals, 383, 385–387
            examples of, 382–383, 387
            specie-specific indications for, 372–373, 387
        in hedgehogs and sugar gliders, 273
        in reptiles, 216
Mammals, companion, diagnostic imaging of respiratory system in, **369–389**.
    See also *Companion mammals.*
Mammography, for companion mammals, 370
Manual restraint, for ultrasonography, of companion mammals, 378
Marsupials. See *Hedgehogs; Sugar gliders.*
Mass lesions. See also *Neoplasia.*
    respiratory disorders related to, in avians, 250
        in chinchillas and guinea pigs, 350–351
        in rodents, 311, 328–329
Mediastinum, imaging of, in companion mammals, 372, 377, 381
Medications, for respiratory disorders. See *Drug entries.*
Megalocytivirus spp., respiratory disorders related to, in pet and ornamental fish, 193
Miscellaneous conditions, respiratory disorders related to, in chinchillas
    and guinea pigs, 351–352
        in ferrets, 365
        in pet and ornamental fish, 196–197
        in rodents, 325–329
Monogeneans, respiratory disorders related to, in pet and ornamental fish, 189
Moraxella catarrhalis, respiratory disorders related to, in rabbits, 264–265
Mouse, respiratory system and disorders in, alveolar vs. bronchial hyperplasia as, 328
            amyloidosis as, 327–328
            anatomy and physiology of, 291, 294
            bordetellosis as, 297
            Chlamydophila spp. as, 297–298
            cilia-associated respiratory bacillus as, 299
            clinical signs of, 289
            Corynebacterium kutscheri as, 301
            cytomegalovirus as, 313–314
            diagnostic laboratories for testing of, 290, 292–293
            diagnostic workup of, 287–290
            Freund adjuvant pulmonary granuloma as, 328
            hepatitis virus as, 314–315
            Kilham polyomavirus as, 316
            macrophagic lesions as, 326–327

Mouse (*continued*)
  murine norovirus as, 315–316
  murine pneumotropic virus as, 316
  Mycobacterium avium-intracellulare as, 302
  Mycoplasma spp. as, 304
  neoplasia as, 324–325
  Parker rat coronavirus as, 322
  Pasteurella pneumotropica as, 307
  perivascular lymphoid infiltrates as, 329
  pneumocystosis as, 310–311
  pneumonia virus as, 316–317
  Proteus mirabilis as, 308
  sanitation and decontamination for, 289–290
  Sendai virus as, 319–321
  sialodacryoadenitis virus as, 322
  Streptococcus pneumoniae as, 309
Mouse cytomegalovirus (MCMV), respiratory disorders related to, in rodents, 313–314
Mouse hepatitis virus (MHV), respiratory disorders related to, in rodents, 314–315
Mucolytic agents, for respiratory disorders, in reptiles, 219
Murine norovirus (MNV-1), respiratory disorders related to, in mouse, 315–316
Murine pneumotropic virus (MPTV), respiratory disorders related to, in rodents, 316
Murine respiratory mycoplasmosis (MRM), in rats, 305–306
Mycobacterium avium-intracellulare, respiratory disorders related to, in rodents, 302
Mycobacterium spp., respiratory disorders related to, in avians, 246
  in hedgehogs, 274
  in pet and ornamental fish, 191
  in rabbits, 265
  in sugar gliders, 279
Mycoplasma spp., respiratory disorders related to, in ferrets, 363–364
  in rodents, 302–306
Mycotic agents, respiratory disorders related to, in reptiles, 212
  in rodents, 310–312

N

Nares, inflammation of, in chinchillas, 351
Nasal cavity, computed tomography of, in companion mammals, 383, 386
  endoscopy of, in companion mammals, 373, 379–381
  imaging of, in companion mammals, 371–373
  magnetic resonance imaging of, in companion mammals, 387
  of ferrets, 357–358
  tumors of, in rodents, 325
Nasal conchae, of avians, 242–243
Nasal glands, respiratory disorders associated with, in gerbil, 325–326
  in hamster, 296
  in rat, 294
Nasal mucosa, inflammation of, in rodents, 328
Nasal swabs/lavage, for respiratory disorders, in avians, 244–245
  in hedgehogs and sugar gliders, 272
  in reptiles, 219
Nasal tissue, of rabbits, 257–258

adenocarcinoma of, 265–266
infections of, 262–263
Nasolacrimal duct, in rabbits, 261–262
Nebulizers. See *Aerosol therapy.*
Necropsy, for respiratory disorders, in chinchillas and guinea pigs, 350
    in ferrets, 363–364
    in hedgehogs and sugar gliders, 273
    in pet and ornamental fish, 186
    in rabbits, 264–265
    in rodents, 290, 300
Needle aspiration, for respiratory disorders, in hedgehogs and
    sugar gliders, 272–273
Neoplasia, respiratory disorders related to, imaging of, 375, 388
    in avians, 246–247, 249–250, 253
    in chinchillas and guinea pigs, 350–351
    in ferrets, 365
    in hedgehogs, 277
    in pet and ornamental fish, 196
    in rabbits, 265–266
    in reptiles, 210, 221
    in rodents, 311, 324–325, 328–329
    in sugar gliders, 280
Neurogenic inflammation, respiratory disorders related to, in ferrets, 362
Noninfectious diseases, respiratory disorders related to, in avians,
    244, 246–247
    in chinchillas and guinea pigs, 345, 350–352
        inhalation pneumonia, 352
        miscellaneous conditions, 351–352
        neoplasia, 350–351
        toxicosis, 352
        trauma, 352–353
    in hedgehogs, 277–278
        heart disease, 277–278
        neoplasia, 277
        trauma, 278–279
    in pet and ornamental fish, 194–197
        environmental, 194–195
        miscellaneous conditions, 196–197
        neoplastic, 196
        nutritional, 195–196
    in reptiles, 209–210
    in rodents, 324–329
    in sugar gliders, 280–281
        heart disease, 280
        neoplasia, 280
        trauma, 280–281
Norovirus, murine, respiratory disorders related to, in mouse, 315–316
Nutritional diseases, respiratory disorders related to, in avians, 243–245
    in chelonians, 226–227
    in chinchillas, 341
    in guinea pigs, 340–341

Nutritional diseases (*continued*)
    in hedgehogs, 278
    in pet and ornamental fish, 195–196
    in rodents, 290
    in sugar gliders, 280

O

Ocular presentations, with respiratory disorders, in chinchillas and
  guinea pigs, 343, 345–346, 350
    in rabbits, 261–263
    in rodents, 324
Olfactory system, of chinchillas and guinea pigs, 342
  of rabbits, 258
Ondontomas, imaging of, 379
Opercular defect, in pet and ornamental fish, 196–197
Ophidian paramyxovirus (OPMV), respiratory disorders related to, in reptiles, 211
Opportunistic infections, respiratory disorders related to, in avians, 254
    in guinea pigs, 346
    in rabbits, 265
Oral cavity, of chinchillas and guinea pigs, 342–343
  of ferrets, 358–359
Organomegaly, avian respiratory distress related to, 250
Ornamental fish, respiratory system disorders in, **179–206**
    anatomy and physiology of, 179–181
    diagnostic evaluation of, 182–186
    gill disease as, 181–182
      clinical signs associated with, 182–183
      common diseases, 186–197
    gill injury response and, 181–182
    infectious diseases as, 186–193
      bacterial, 190–191
        drugs for, 198
      fungal, 193
        drugs for, 199–200
      parasitic, 186–190
        drugs for, 199–201
      viral, 191–193
    noninfectious diseases as, 194–197
      environmental, 194–195
      miscellaneous conditions, 196–197
      neoplastic, 196
      nutritional, 195–196
    summary overview of, 179, 202
    treatment of, 197–201
Orotracheal intubation, endoscopic-guided, of prairie dog, 385
  of rabbit, 384
Oxygen therapy, for respiratory disorders, in avians, 246, 249
    in chelonians, 235
    in chinchillas and guinea pigs, 353
    in reptiles, 220

P

Parabronchi, of avians, 251–252

Paramyxoviridae spp., respiratory disorders related to, in reptiles, 211

Parasitic diseases, respiratory disorders related to, in avians, 244
  in chelonians, 233–234
  in hedgehogs, 275–276
  in pet and ornamental fish, 186–190
    treatment of, 199–201
  in reptiles, 212
    treatment of, 218–219
  in rodents, 312
  in sugar gliders, 280

Parenchymal disease, avian respiratory distress and, 250–254
  anatomy and physiology of, 250–252
  breathing patterns with, 252
  diagnostic tests for, 254
  etiology of, 253–254
  gas exchange dynamics with, 252–253
  history taking for, 252
  physical examination for, 252
  respiratory sounds with, 252
  treatment of, 254

Parker rat coronavirus (PRC), respiratory disorders related to, in rodents, 322–323

Pasteurella pneumotropica, respiratory disorders related to, in chinchillas, 348
  in rodents, 306–308

Pasteurella spp., respiratory disorders related to, in hedgehogs, 274
  in rabbits, 259–263
  in sugar gliders, 279

Pentastomes, respiratory disorders related to, in hedgehogs, 276
  in sugar gliders, 280

Perivascular lymphoid infiltrates, in rodents, 329

Pet fish, respiratory system disorders in, **179–206**
  anatomy and physiology of, 179–181
  diagnostic evaluation of, 182–186
  gill disease as, 181–182
    clinical signs associated with, 182–183
    common diseases, 186–197
  gill injury response and, 181–182
  infectious diseases as, 186–193
    bacterial, 190–191
      drugs for, 198
    fungal, 193
      drugs for, 199–200
    parasitic, 186–190
      drugs for, 199–201
    viral, 191–193
  noninfectious diseases as, 194–197
    environmental, 194–195
    miscellaneous conditions, 196–197
    neoplastic, 196

Pet fish (*continued*)
  nutritional, 195–196
  summary overview of, 179, 202
  treatment of, 197–201
Pharmacologic therapies, for respiratory disorders. See *Drug entries.*
Pharynx, of chinchillas and guinea pigs, 342
  of ferrets, 358–359
Physical examination, for respiratory disorders, in avians,
    242–243, 246, 248–249, 252
    in chelonians, 226–228
    in hedgehogs and sugar gliders, 270–271
    in pet and ornamental fish, 183–184
    in reptiles, 214
    in rodents, 289
Physiology, of respiratory system. See *Anatomy and physiology.*
Pleural effusion, imaging of, 377
    in chinchillas and guinea pigs, 351–352
Pneumocystosis, respiratory disorders related to, in rodents, 310–311
Pneumonia, in avians, 254
    in chelonians, 234
    in chinchillas, 344
      bacterial, 348–350
      inhalation, 352
    in ferrets, 362–363
      bronchointerstitial, 366
      endogenous lipid, 365
    in guinea pigs, 344
      bacterial, 347–348
      inhalation, 352
      Streptococcus, 345–346
      viral, 349–350
    in rabbits, 258, 265
    in reptiles, 217–218, 220–221
      viral, 211
    in rodents, acidophilic macrophage, 325–326
      aspiration, 328
      eosinophilic granulomatous, 328
      Klebsiella, 302
      Streptococcus, 308–310
Pneumonia virus of mice (PVM), respiratory disorders related to, in rodents, 316–318
Pneumothorax, imaging of, 375
Pneumotropic virus, murine, respiratory disorders related to, in rodents, 316
Pollutants, respiratory disorders related to, in chinchillas and guinea pigs, 352
      in ferrets, 362, 366–367
      in pet and ornamental fish, 194–195
        clinical response to, 181–182
      in rodents, 288–289
Polymerase chain reaction (PCR), for respiratory disorders, in avians,
    244, 246, 250, 254
    in chelonians, 230–233
    in guinea pigs, 348, 350

in rabbits, 264
in reptiles, 216–217
Polyoma virus, rat, respiratory disorders related to, in rodents, 318
Positioning, for computed tomography, in companion mammals, 383
for radiography, in companion mammals, 371
Positron emission tomography (PET), of respiratory disorders, in companion
mammals, 387–388
Poxvirus, respiratory disorders related to, in rodents, 318
Prairie dogs, respiratory disorders in, diagnostic imaging of, 372–373, 375, 379, 383
endoscopic-guided orotracheal intubation for, 385
Preventive measures, for respiratory disorders, in hedgehogs, 281
in rabbits, 261
in reptiles, 207–208
in rodents, 289–290, 303
in sugar gliders, 281
Proteinosis, alveolar, in rodents, 326–327
Proteolytic agents, for respiratory disorders, in reptiles, 219
Proteus mirabilis, respiratory disorders related to, in rodents, 308
Pulmonary circulation, in ferrets, 360–361
Pulmonary edema, agent-induced, in rodents, 326
Pulmonary granuloma, Freund adjuvant, in rodents, 328
Pulmonary histiocytosis, in rodents, 326–327
Pulse oximetry, for respiratory disorders, in hedgehogs and sugar
gliders, 270–271
in rabbits, 262

Q

Quarantine programs, for respiratory disorders, in reptiles, 207–208

R

Rabbits, respiratory system and disorders of, **257–266**
anatomy and physiology of, 257–258
lung lobes, 258, 260
paramedian section of, 258
thymus perspectives, 258–259
diagnostic imaging of, 372–374, 380–384, 386–387
endoscopic-guided orotracheal intubation for, 384
infectious diseases as, 258–264
bordetellosis, 263
other bacterial, 264–265
overview of, 258–264
pasteurellosis, 259–263
staphylococcosis, 264
viral, 265
neoplasia as, 265–266
Radiography, of respiratory disorders, in avians, 244, 246, 249
in chelonians, 228–229
in chinchillas and guinea pigs, 351
in companion mammals, 370–371
examples of, 371, 374–383

Radiography (*continued*)
specie-specific indications for, 371–373
in hedgehogs and sugar gliders, 271–272
in rabbits, 262, 265–266
in reptiles, 214–215
Rat, respiratory system and disorders in, anatomy and physiology of, 291, 294–296
mediastinal surfaces of lung, 295
bordetellosis as, 297
cilia-associated respiratory bacillus as, 299
clinical signs of, 289
Corynebacterium kutscheri as, 301
diagnostic imaging of, 372–373, 376
diagnostic laboratories for testing of, 290, 292–293
diagnostic workup of, 287–290
eosinophilic granulomatous pneumonia as, 328
Haemophilus spp. as, 301–302
Kilham polyomavirus as, 316
Klebsiella pneumoniae as, 302
lymphohistiocytic lung lesions as, 328–329
macrophagic lesions as, 327
murine pneumotropic virus as, 316
Mycoplasma pulmonis as, 304–306
Mycoplasma spp. as, 304–306
neoplasia as, 325
Parker rat coronavirus as, 322–323
Pasteurella pneumotropica as, 307–308
pneumocystosis as, 311
pneumonia virus as, 317
polyoma virus as, 318
poxvirus as, 318
respiratory virus as, 318
sanitation and decontamination for, 289–290
Sendai virus as, 321
sialodacryoadenitis virus as, 322–324
Streptobacillus moniliformis as, 308
Streptococcus pneumoniae as, 309–310
tracheal cartilage degeneration as, 329
Rat polyoma virus, respiratory disorders related to, in rodents, 318
Rat respiratory virus, respiratory disorders related to, in rodents, 318
Reptiles, respiratory medicine of, **207–224**
anatomy and physiology of, 208–209
clinical evaluation and diagnostic tests in, 213–217
examination as, 213–214
imaging as, 214–216
samples as, 216–217
disease causes in, 209–212
disease clinical signs in, 213
emergency management in, 210, 220–221
infectious, 209–212
bacterial, 211–212
fungal, 212

overview of, 209–210
    parasitic, 212
    viral, 210–211
noninfectious, 209–210
summary overview of, 207–208, 221
therapy in, 217–221
    for emergencies, 220–221
    medications as, 217–219
    respiratory support and monitoring as, 220
Respiration, in avians, 252–253
    in chelonians, 226
    in ferrets, 361–362
    in hedgehogs, 268
    in pet and ornamental fish, 181
    in reptiles, 209
    in rodents, 291, 294, 296
Respiratory distress, in chelonians, 234–235
    in pet and ornamental fish, 196–197
    in reptiles, 210, 220–221
Respiratory emergencies, management of, in chelonians, 234–235
    in chinchillas and guinea pigs, 352–353
    in pet and ornamental fish, 196–197
    in reptiles, 210, 217, 220–221
Respiratory obstruction, in avians, 246, 253
    in pet and ornamental fish, 196–197
    in reptiles, 210, 217, 221
Respiratory sounds, with respiratory disorders, in avians, 243, 246, 248–249, 252
    in rabbits, 262
Respiratory support and monitoring, for respiratory disorders, in avians, 246
    in chelonians, 235
    in chinchillas and guinea pigs, 352–353
    in hedgehogs and sugar gliders, 281
    in reptiles, 219–220
    in rodents, 290
Respiratory system and disorders. See also *specific species.*
    imaging of. See also *Imaging.*
        in companion mammals, **369–389**
    in pet and ornamental fish, **179–206**
    in rodents, **287–338**
        companion species, **339–355**. See also *Chinchillas; Guinea pigs.*
    of avians, **241–255**
    of chelonians, **225–239**
    of ferrets, **357–367**
    of hedgehogs and sugar gliders, **267–285**
    of rabbits, **257–266**
    of reptiles, **207–224**
Respiratory virus, rat, respiratory disorders related to, in rodents, 318
Rhinitis, allergic, in rodents, 326
Rhinoscopy, of companion mammals, 373, 379–381, 384
Rodenticides, anticoagulant, respiratory disorders related to,
    in chinchillas and guinea pigs, 352

Rodents, dental anatomic adaptations of, 340
    respiratory system and disorders in, **287–338**. See also *specific rodent.*
        anatomy and physiology of, 291, 294–296
        clinical signs of, 289
        companion species, **339–355**. See also *specific specie, e.g., Chinchillas.*
        diagnostic laboratories for testing of, 290, 292–293
        diagnostic workup of, 287–290
        genetic perspectives of, 287–288, 315
        history taking for, 288
        husbandry evaluation for, 288–289
        infectious agents causing, 290, 297–324
            bacterial, 297–310
            mycotic, 310–312
            parasitic, 312
            viral, 312–324
        noninfectious diseases causing, 324–329
            miscellaneous, 325–329
            neoplasia, 324–325
        sanitation and decontamination for, 289–290
        summary overview of, 287
        treatment of, 290

    S

Sagittal view, in radiography, for companion mammals, 371
Saline lavages, for respiratory disorders, in reptiles, 219
Samples/sampling. See *Diagnostic samples/sampling.*
Sanitation, for respiratory disorders prevention, with rodents, 289–290
Scintigraphy, of respiratory disorders, in companion mammals, 388
Scurvy, in guinea pigs, 340–341
Sedation, radiography indications for, in companion mammals, 370
Sendai virus (SeV), respiratory disorders related to, in rodents, 318–321
Serum neutralization (SN) test, for respiratory disorders, in chelonians, 231–233
Shaving, for ultrasonography, in companion mammals, 374, 377
Sialodacryoadenitis virus (SDAV), respiratory disorders related to, in rodents, 322–324
Skull, computed tomography of, 383, 387
    magnetic resonance imaging of, 386–387
Skull view, of ferret upper respiratory tract, 357–358
Skunk, respiratory disorders of, diagnostic imaging of, 372–373
Small airway disease, avian respiratory distress and, 248–249
        anatomy and physiology of, 248
        breathing patterns with, 248
        diagnostic tests for, 249
        etiology of, 249
        history taking for, 248
        physical examination for, 248
        respiratory sounds with, 248
        treatment of, 249
Snakes, respiratory disease signs and symptoms in, 213
    respiratory medicine for. See *Reptiles.*
    respiratory tract anatomy and physiology of, 208

Snuffles, in rabbits, 258
Spleorodens clethrionomys, respiratory disorders related to, in rodents, 312
Squamous cell carcinoma, respiratory disorders occurring with, in hedgehogs, 277
Squirrel, respiratory disorders in, diagnostic imaging of, 372–373
Staphylococcus aureus, respiratory disorders related to, in guinea pigs, 347–348
Staphylococcus spp., respiratory disorders related to, in rabbits, 264
     in sugar gliders, 279
Streptobacillus moniliformis, respiratory disorders related to, in guinea pigs, 347
     in rodents, 308
Streptococcus pneumoniae, respiratory disorders related to, in chinchillas, 348–350
     in guinea pigs, 345–346
     in rodents, 308–310
Streptococcus spp., respiratory disorders related to, in guinea pigs, 345–347
Stress factors, respiratory disorders related to, in guinea pigs, 348
     in pet and ornamental fish, 181–182
     in rodents, 289
Stress response, of gills, in pet and ornamental fish, 181–182
Sugar gliders, respiratory system and disease of, **267–285**
     anatomy and physiology of, 269–270
     diagnosis of, 270–273
     infectious processes in, 278–280
       bacterial, 279
       fungal, 279
       parasitic, 280
       viral, 279
       yeast, 279
     noninfectious processes in, 280–281
       heart disease, 280
       neoplasia, 280
       trauma, 280–281
     prevention of, 281
     summary overview of, 267, 281–282
     torpor and, 269–270
     treatment of, 281
Swine (H1N1) influenza, respiratory disorders related to, in ferrets, 365–366
Syrinx, avian respiratory distress and. See *Trachea to the syrinx.*

T

Thoracocentesis, for respiratory disorders, in chinchillas and guinea pigs, 352–353
     in hedgehogs and sugar gliders, 272
Thoracoscopy, of companion mammals, 373, 380–381
Thorax, computed tomography of, in companion mammals, 382–383
    of ferrets, 358–360
    of guinea pigs, 342, 345
    radiography of, in companion mammals, 371, 374, 378, 380–381, 383
    ultrasonography of, in companion mammals, 371, 374, 377–378
Thymoma, in companion mammals, imaging of, 381–383, 386
     surgical excision of, 385–386
Thymus, of chinchillas and guinea pigs, 342
    of rabbits, 258–259

Thymus (*continued*)
  neoplasia of, 265–266
Torpor, in hedgehogs, 268
  in sugar gliders, 269–270
Tortoise. See *Chelonians.*
Toxins, respiratory disorders related to, in avians, 249, 253
  in chinchillas and guinea pigs, 352
  in ferrets, 362
  in pet and ornamental fish, 194–195
    clinical response to, 181–182
Toxoplasmosis, respiratory disorders related to, in sugar gliders, 280
Trachea, of ferrets, 358
  of hamster, 296
    tumors of, 325
  of rats, 294–295
    cartilage degeneration of, 329
Trachea to the syrinx, avian respiratory distress and, 245–247
  anatomy and physiology of, 245–247
  breathing patterns with, 246
  diagnostic tests for, 246
  etiology of, 246–247
  history taking for, 246
  physical examination for, 246
  respiratory sounds with, 246
  treatment of, 246
Tracheal bifurcation, in avians, 246–247
Tracheal swabs/lavage, for respiratory disorders, in hedgehogs
  and sugar gliders, 272
  in reptiles, 219
Tracheoscopy, of companion mammals, 373, 379
Trauma, to respiratory system, of chelonians, 234–235
  of chinchillas and guinea pigs, 352–353
  of hedgehogs, 278–279
  of pet and ornamental fish, 181–182
  of reptiles, 210
  of sugar gliders, 280–281
Trematodes, respiratory disorders related to, in pet and ornamental
  fish, 189–190
Trichodina sp., respiratory disorders related to, in pet and ornamental
  fish, 187–188
Trichosomoides spp., respiratory disorders related to, in avians, 244
  in rodents, 312
Trichosporon beigelii, respiratory disorders related to, in rodents, 311

  U

Ultrasonography, of respiratory disorders, in avians, 250
  in chinchillas and guinea pigs, 352–353
  in companion mammals, 371, 374, 377–378
    examples of, 377–378, 381, 383
    specie-specific indications for, 372–373, 378

in hedgehogs and sugar gliders, 273
    in reptiles, 214
Ultrasound-guided biopsy, of neoplasia, in avians, 250
    in rabbits, 266
Upper airway disease, avian respiratory distress and, 241–245
    anatomy and physiology of, 241–243
    breathing pattern with, 243
    diagnostic tests for, 244–245
    etiology of, 243–244
    history taking for, 242
    physical examination for, 242–243
    respiratory sounds with, 243
    treatment of, 245
Upper respiratory infection (URI), in avians, 242–243
    differential diagnosis of, 243–244
Upper respiratory tract disease (URTD), in chelonians, 230–232
URD (rhinitis, sinusitis, conjunctivitis, dacryocystitis), in rabbits, 261, 263, 265

V

Vaccines. See *Immunizations.*
Venipuncture trauma, in hedgehogs, 278–279
Ventilation mechanisms, in chelonians, 225–226
    in pet and ornamental fish, 181
    in reptiles, 209
    in rodents, 291, 294, 296
Ventrodorsal view, in radiography, for companion mammals, 370–371, 383
Viral diseases, respiratory disorders related to, in avians, 244, 253
    in chelonians, 231–233
    in chinchillas, 350
    in guinea pigs, 349–350
    in hedgehogs, 274–275
    in pet and ornamental fish, 191–193
    in reptiles, 210–211
    in rodents, 312–324
    in sugar gliders, 279
Vitamin C deficiency, in guinea pigs, 340–341

W

Water quality testing, for respiratory disorders, in pet and ornamental fish,
    184, 194–195, 197
Wet mount cytology, for respiratory disorders, in avians, 244–245, 250
    in chelonians, 228
    in hedgehogs and sugar gliders, 273
    in pet and ornamental fish, examples of, 187–189
        preparation of, 185–186
    in rabbits, 266
    in reptiles, 217

Y

Yeast, respiratory disorders related to, in hedgehogs, 275
    in sugar gliders, 279
Yersinia pseudotuberculosis, respiratory disorders related to, in guinea pigs, 347

Z

Zoonotic potential, of H1N1 influenza, in ferrets, 365–366
    of respiratory disease organisms, in rodents, 290, 312–313
    with necropsy, of rabbits, 265

Moving?

Make sure your subscription moves with you!

To notify us of your new address, find your **Clinics Account Number** (located on your mailing label above your name), and contact customer service at:

Email: journalscustomerservice-usa@elsevier.com

800-654-2452 (subscribers in the U.S. & Canada)
314-447-8871 (subscribers outside of the U.S. & Canada)

Fax number: 314-447-8029

Elsevier Health Sciences Division
Subscription Customer Service
3251 Riverport Lane
Maryland Heights, MO 63043

*To ensure uninterrupted delivery of your subscription,
please notify us at least 4 weeks in advance of move.

Printed and bound by CPI Group (UK) Ltd, Croydon, CR0 4YY

03/10/2024

01040455-0020